Daniels and Worthingham's

MUSCLE TESTING

Techniques of Manual Examination

Helen J. Hislop, Ph.D., Sc.D., FAPTA

Professor Emerita
Department of Biokinesiology and Physical Therapy
University of Southern California
Los Angeles, California

Jacqueline Montgomery, M.A., P.T.

Former Director of Physical Therapy
Rancho Los Amigos National Rehabilitation Center
Downey, California

7th Edition

Daniels and Worthingham's

MUSCLE TESTING

Techniques of Manual Examination

W.B. SAUNDERS COMPANY
An Imprint of Elsevier Science
Philadelphia   London   New York   St. Louis   Sydney   Toronto

W.B. Saunders Company
An Imprint of Elsevier Science

The Curtis Center
Independence Square West
Philadelphia, Pennsylvania 19106

DANIELS & WORTHINGHAM'S MUSCLE TESTING:
Techniques of Manual Examination   ISBN 0-7216-9299-0

Printed in the United States of America

Last digit is the print number: 9   8   7   6   5   4   3   2   1

Dedication

To two of the most illustrious and worthy physical therapists of their day and any other, in grateful appreciation for their majestic contributions to the profession of physical therapy:

CATHERINE A. WORTHINGHAM, P.T., PH.D.
JACQUELIN PERRY, P.T., M.D.

And lest we forget. . .

The 38 physical therapists who participated in muscle testing as part of the Salk vaccine field trials across the United States and whose results proved conclusively that the Salk vaccine was successful as a preventive for paralytic poliomyelitis. The group was organized for this seminal field testing by Lucy Blair, and the instructors for the examiners were Miriam Jacobs and Mary Elizabeth Kolb.

To these physical therapists, we owe a great debt for they sustained and elevated our profession:

Mabel Parker	Helen Blood	Celeste Hayden
Eleanor Malone	Carolyn Bowen	Nina Haugen
Anna Sweeley	Lillie M. Bachanz	Mary Rexroad
Mary A. Gaughan	Alfaretta Wright	Irene Schaper
Myrtle E. Swanson	Mary Elizabeth Kolb	Helen Antman
Jean Bailey	Elizabeth Fellows	Ruth Pratt
Georgianna Harmon	Irene Coons	Sue D. Brooks
Elma Lee Georg	Miriam Jacobs	Edith B. Nichols
Esther D. Hart	Hildegard Kummer	Phyllis Johnson
Winifred L. Rumsey	Carmella Gonella	Paul O'Connor
Deborah Kinsman	Jean McDermott	Margaret S. Arey
Alice Chesrown	Eleanor Westcott	Louise Hayward
Marion Barfknecht	Minna Hildebrandt	

Contributors

Jack E. Turman, Jr., P.T., Ph.D.

Assistant Professor, Department of
Biokinesiology and Physical Therapy,
University of Southern California,
Los Angeles, California

Teresa Van Vranken, D.P.T.

Clinician,
Los Angeles United School District,
Los Angeles, California

Preface

This seventh edition of *Muscle Testing: Techniques of Manual Examination* contains significant new material as well as a reorganization and reworking of existing material. Limb anatomy has been expanded by adding cross-sectional drawings to illustrate the sizes of and relationships among the muscles at a given location on a limb. This addition should help students learn palpation skills and become more familiar with the requirements of wire electrophysiology testing. There is an entirely new chapter on testing the infant and toddler written by Jack Turman, Ph.D., and Teresa Van Vranken, D.P.T. The Ready Reference section, Chapter 9, has been expanded to allow readers, particularly students, to readily refresh their memories about the details of muscle topography, function, and innervation. Also to assist readers, each muscle has been given a reference, or I.D., number to speed cross-referencing and to help them quickly locate the details of any given muscle.

The current authors gratefully acknowledge the basic contributions to this text of the original authors—Lucille Daniels, Marian Williams, and Catherine Worthingham (all now deceased). These pioneers established the format of the book and detailed the muscle testing techniques that have been modified and updated in subsequent editions as new information on muscle performance and structure has become available.

This book is a handbook of manual evaluation of muscular strength and is not intended for use as a comprehensive text for rationale and variations on such testing. Nor does its scope include instrumented methods of evaluation of force, work, and power.

The ultimate message of this book is that here are tried and true methods for assessing and grading skeletal muscle function. The techniques are not such that skill is achieved quickly, despite the considerable detail used to describe them. The only way to acquire mastery of clinical evaluation procedures, including manual muscle testing, is to practice over and over again. As experience with patients matures over time, the nuances that can never be fully described for the wide variety of patients encountered by the clinician will become as much intuition as science. The master clinician will include muscle testing as part and parcel of every patient evaluation, regardless of whether a detailed form is completed, and as a prelude to program planning. It is, indeed, among the most fundamental skills of the physical therapist as well as the occupational therapist and other practitioners. Learn well. Develop a high level of skill, and maintain high standards. The patient will be the beneficiary of how well you achieve high proficiency.

We wish to acknowledge very substantial contributions from a number of persons who assisted with content review and editing and who offered valuable suggestions. These include Jack Turman and Teresa Van Vranken for their new chapter on examining the infant and toddler. Maureen Rodgers reviewed every single test sequence and was a valued consultant in the new edition. Jacquelin Perry's incredible knowledge of functional anatomy was a constant and unerring beacon, which we followed with trust. Arthur Hsu and Edmund S. Crelin also provided anatomical consultation. Judy Burnfield and Ruth McCormick gave generously of their expertise in neurology, which is readily seen in Chapter 7.

Linda Wood, the Developmental Editor for the Sixth Edition, also consulted on this edition, and her insight into design and editing enabled the authors to speak clearly to the reader. Our three illustrators, Larry Ward, Victoria Heim, and Walter Stuart, brought visual reality to the words describing testing procedures and muscle anatomy.

For enlightened computer assistance, we thank Brian Andrews and Kim Pyne.

Manuscript reviewers were Edmund S. Crelin, Ph.D., D.Sc., JoAnne Gronley, D.P.T., and Donna El-Din, Ph.D. Lou Ann Carter and Dorothy Hewitt provided manuscript assistance and moral support.

Finally, we deeply acknowledge the staff at the W.B. Saunders Company for their essential and unfailing support. These include Andrew Allen, Pat Morrison, Karen O'Keefe Owens, Ceil Roberts, Tina Rebane, and Norm Stellander. Special thanks go to Scott Weaver for his wise and patient guidance of the project in its early stages. We are deeply grateful to them all.

HELEN J. HISLOP, PH.D., SC.D., FAPTA
JACQUELINE MONTGOMERY, M.A., P.T.

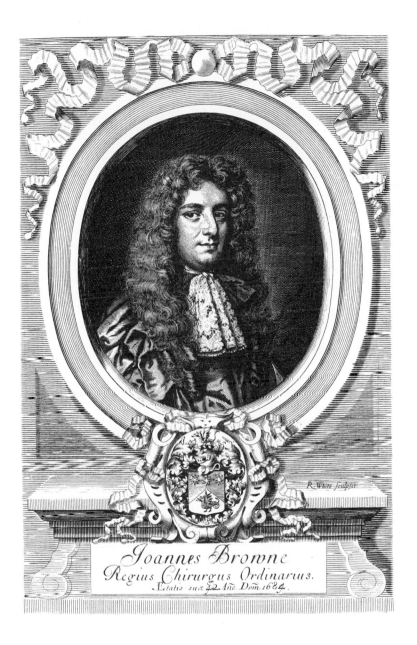

Joannes Browne (1645–1702), a man of another time, became the physician and surgeon to Charles II, King of England in the 17th century. He was appointed by His Majesty as *Regius Chirurgus Ordinarius,* and as a sideline of his royal duties, he prepared an atlas of human muscle anatomy, titled *Myographia Nova Sive Musculorum Omnium (In Corpore Humano hactenus reportorum),* first published in 1684.

This first edition book is presented in calligraphy and written entirely in Latin, as was the custom of scholars of the time. The folio contains text and 40 full-page copperplate engravings drawn by Doctor Browne and possibly influenced by the works of Casserius and Spigelius. The above engraved frontispiece portrait was done by the renowned artist Robert White.

Browne's atlas is considered one of the more important anatomical works of the 17th century. The book was the first to engrave the names of the muscles directly on the plates.

The only known copy in the United States came into the possession of one of the authors (HJH), who is using this opportunity to share some of the beautiful, sometimes whimsical, dissection plates with our readers for their pleasure and appreciation of historic anatomy.

HJH

Contents

Introduction

This book presents an approach to the assessment of muscular strength and function as fundamental components of movement and performance. Classic muscle testing involves manual methods of evaluation and draws on the work and experience of a number of clinical scientists, some of whose work is corroborated by formal research. The majority of manual muscle testing procedures are just coming under scientific scrutiny, but almost a century of clinical use has provided a wealth of clinical corroboration for the empirical validity of such tests.

Use of manual muscle testing is valid in normal persons and those with weakness or paralysis secondary to motor unit disorders (lower motor neuron lesions and muscle disorders). Its use in persons with disturbances of the higher neural centers is flawed because of interference by abnormal sensation, or disturbed tone or motor control. Nevertheless, muscle function must be assessed in such patients, although the procedures used may be quite different. One approach to overall movement analysis that can be used in patients with upper motor neuron disturbances is included in this book. Additional tests for these people remain to be codified, and other procedures, which probably will require the use of extensive technology, may be available for routine clinical use at a future time.

This book, as in its previous editions, directs its focus on manual procedures. Its organization is based on joint motions (e.g., hip flexion) rather than on individual muscles (e.g., iliopsoas). The reason for this approach is that each motion generally is the result of activity by more than one muscle, and although so-called prime movers can be identified, the importance of secondary or accessory movers should never be diminished. Rarely is a prime mover the only active muscle, and rarely is it used under isolated control for a given movement. For example, knee extension is the prerogative of the five muscles of the Quadriceps femoris, yet none of the five extends the knee in isolation from its synergists. Regardless, definitive activity of any muscle in a given movement can be precisely detected only by kinesiologic electromyography, and such studies, although numerous, remain incomplete.

There are examples of manual testing in which an examiner pre-positions a limb with the intent of ruling out a particular muscle from acting in a given movement. Newer work reporting on electromyographic recordings of muscles participating in manual tests, however, will shed light on the actual contributions of participating muscles in specific motions. One example of this is the test used to isolate the Soleus. The Gastrocnemius never turns off in any plantar flexion motion; therefore, it will contaminate any test that purports to isolate the Soleus. The Gastrocnemius does diminish its activity with the knee flexed, most notably when the knee is flexed beyond 45 degrees. The Gastrocnemius still contributes to plantar flexion in that posture, however, so the Soleus is not, in actual fact, totally "isolated." The reader is referred to the tests on plantar flexion for further details.

Range of motion in this book is presented only as information the physical therapist requires to test muscles correctly. A consensus of typical ranges is presented with each test, but the techniques of measurement used are not within the scope of this text.

BRIEF HISTORY OF MUSCLE TESTING

Wilhelmine Wright and Robert W. Lovett, M.D., Professor of Orthopedic Surgery at Harvard University Medical School, were the originators of the muscle testing system that incorporated the effect of gravity.[1,2] Janet Merrill, P.T., Director of Physical Therapeutics at Children's Hospital and the Harvard Infantile Paralysis Commission in Boston, an early colleague of Dr. Lovett, stated that the tests were used first by Wright in Lovett's office gymnasium in 1912.[3] The seminal description of the tests used largely today was written by Wright and published in 1912[1]; this was followed by an article by Lovett and Martin in 1916[4] and by Wright's book in 1928.[5] Miss Wright was a precursor of the physical therapist of today, there being no educational programs in physical therapy in her time, but she headed Lovett's physical therapeutic clinic. Lovett credits her fully in his 1917 book, *Treatment of Infantile Paralysis*,[6] with developing the testing for polio (see Sidebar). In Lovett's 1917 book, muscles were tested using a resistance-gravity system and graded on a scale of 0 to 6. Another early numerical scale in muscle testing was described by Charles L. Lowman, M.D., founder and medical director of Orthopedic Hospital, Los Angeles.[7] Lowman's system (1927) covered the effects of gravity and the full range of movement on all joints and was particularly helpful for assessing extreme weakness. Lowman further described muscle testing procedures in the *Physiotherapy Review* in 1940.[8]

H.S. Stewart, a physician, published a description of muscle testing in 1925 that was very brief and was not anatomically or procedurally consistent with what is done today.[9] His descriptions included a resistance-based grading system not substantially different from that in use today: maximal resistance for a normal muscle; completion of the motion against gravity with no other resistance for a grade of Fair, and so forth. At about the time of Lowman's book, Arthur

Legg, M.D., and Janet Merrill, P.T., wrote a valuable small book on poliomyelitis in 1932. This book, which offered a comprehensive system of muscle testing, was used extensively in physical therapy educational programs during the early 1940s; muscles were graded on a scale of 0 to 5, and a plus or minus designation was added to all grades except 1 and zero.[10]

Among the earliest clinicians to organize muscle testing and support such testing with sound and documented kinesiologic procedures in the way they are used today were Henry and Florence Kendall. Their earliest published documents on comprehensive manual muscle testing became available in 1936 and 1938.[11,12] The 1938 monograph on muscle testing was published and distributed to all Army hospitals in the United States by the U.S. Public Health Service. Another early contribution came from Signe Brunnstrom and Marjorie Dennen in 1931; their syllabus described a system of grading movement rather than individual muscles as a modification of Lovett's work with gravity and resistance.[13]

In this same time period, Elizabeth Kenny came to the United States from Australia, where she had had unique experiences treating polio victims in the Australian back country. Kenny made no contributions to muscle testing, and in her own book and speeches she was clearly against such an evaluative procedure, which she deemed to be harmful.[14] Her one contribution was to heighten the awareness of organized medicine to the dangers of prolonged and injudicious immobilization of the polio patient, something that physical therapists in this country had been saying for some time but were not widely heeded at the time.[12,13,15,16] Kenny also advocated the early use of "hot fomentations" (hot packs) in the acute phase of the disease.[14] In fact, Kenny vociferously maintained that poliomyelitis was not a central nervous system disease resulting in flaccid paresis or paralysis but rather "mental alienation" of muscles from the brain.[15,16] In her system "deformities never occurred,"[14] but neither did she ever present data on muscular strength or imbalance in her patients at any point in the course of their disease.[15,16]

The first comprehensive text on muscle testing still in print (which went through five editions) was written by Lucille Daniels, M.A., P.T., Marian Williams, Ph.D., P.T., and Catherine Worthingham, Ph.D., P.T., and was published in 1946.[17] These three authors prepared a comprehensive handbook on the subject of manual testing procedures that was concise and easy to use. It remains one of the most used texts the world over at the present time and is the predecessor of both the sixth and this seventh edition of *Daniels and Worthingham's Muscle Testing*.

The Kendalls (together and then Florence alone after Henry's death in 1979) developed and published work on muscle testing and related subjects for more than six decades, certainly one of the more remarkable sagas in physical therapy or even medical history.[18-20] Their first edition of *Muscles: Testing and Function* appeared in 1949.[18] Earlier, the Kendalls had developed a percentage system ranging from 0 to 100 to express muscle grades as a reflection of normal; they then reduced the emphasis on this scale, only to return to it in the latest edition (1993), in which Florence again advocated the 0 to 10 scale.[20] The contributions of the Kendalls, however, should not be considered as limited to grading scales. Their integration of muscle function with posture and pain in two separate books[18,19] and then in one book[20] is a unique and extremely valuable contribution to the clinical science of physical therapy.

Muscle testing procedures used in national field trials that examined the use of gamma globulin in the prevention of paralytic poliomyelitis were described by Carmella Gonnella, Georgianna Harmon, and Miriam Jacobs, all physical therapists.[21] The later field trials for the Salk vaccine also used muscle testing procedures.[22] The epidemiology teams at the Centers for Disease Control were charged with assessing the validity and reliability of the vaccine. Because there was no other method of accurately "measuring" the presence or absence of muscular weakness, manual muscle testing techniques were used.

A group from the D.T. Watson School of Physiatrics near Pittsburgh, which included Jesse Wright, M.D., Mary Elizabeth Kolb, P.T., and Miriam Jacobs, P.T., devised a test procedure that eventually was used in the field trials.[23] The test was an abridged version of the complete test procedure but did test key muscles in each functional group and body part. It used numerical values that were assigned grades, and each muscle or muscle group also had an arbitrary assigned factor that corresponded (as closely as possible) to the bulk of the tissue. The bulk factor multiplied by the test grade resulted in an "index of involvement" expressed as a ratio.

Before the trials, Kolb and Jacobs were sent to Atlanta to train physicians to conduct the muscle tests, but it was decided that experienced physical therapists would be preferable to maintain the reliability of the test scores.[23] Lucy Blair, then the Poliomyelitis Consultant in the American Physical Therapy Association, was asked by Catherine Worthingham of the National Foundation for Infantile Paralysis to assemble a team of experienced physical therapists to conduct the muscle tests for the field trials. Kolb and Jacobs trained a group of 67 therapists in the use of the abridged muscle test.[23] A partial list of participants was appended to the Lilienfeld paper in the Physical Therapy Review in 1954 (p. 289).[22] This approach and the evaluations by the physical therapists of the presence or absence of weakness and paralysis in the field trial samples eventually resulted in resounding approval of the Salk vaccine.

Since the polio vaccine field trials, sporadic research in manual muscle testing has occurred as well as continued challenges of its worth as a valid clinical assessment tool. Iddings and colleagues noted that intertester reliability among practitioners varied by about 4 percent, which compares favorably with the 3 percent variation among the carefully trained therapists who participated in the vaccine field trials.[24]

There is growing interest in establishing norms of muscular strength and function. Early efforts in this direction were begun by Willis Beasley[25] (although his earliest work was presented only at scientific meetings) and continued by Marian Williams[26] and Helen J. Hislop,[27,28] which set the stage for objective measures by Bohannon[29] and others. The literature on objective measurement increases yearly, an effort that is long overdue. The data from these studies must be applied to manual testing so that correlations between instrumented muscle assessment and manual assessment can ensue.

In the meantime, until instrumented methods become affordable for every clinic, manual techniques of muscle testing will remain in use. The skill of manual muscle testing is a critical clinical tool that every physical therapist must not only learn but also master. A physical therapist who aspires to recognition as a master clinician will not achieve that status without acquiring exquisite skills in manual muscle testing and precise assessment of muscle performance.

HOW TO USE THIS BOOK

The general principles that govern manual muscle testing are described in Chapter 1. Chapters 2 through 8 present the techniques for testing motions of skeletal muscle groups in the body region covered by that chapter. Each muscle test is described in sequential detail and is accompanied by illustrations that help the user perform the test.

For instant access to anatomical information without carrying a large anatomy text to a muscle testing session, a Ready Reference Anatomy section is given in Chapter 9. This chapter is a synopsis of muscle anatomy, muscles as part of motions, muscle innervation, and myotomes.

To assist readers, each muscle has been assigned an identification number based on a regional sequence, beginning with the head and face and proceeding through the neck, thorax, abdomen, perineum, upper extremity, and lower extremity. This reference number is retained throughout the text for cross-referencing purposes. For example, the Multifidi are referenced as muscle number 94; the Flexor digiti minimi brevis in the hand is number 160; and the muscle of the same name in the foot is number 216. The purpose of these reference numbers is to allow the reader to refer quickly from a muscle listed on the testing page to a more detailed description of its anatomy and innervation in the Ready Reference Anatomy section.

Two lists of muscles with their reference numbers are presented: one alphabetical and one by region to assist readers in finding muscles in the Ready Reference section.

NAMES OF THE MUSCLES

Muscle names have conventions of usage. The most formal usage (and the correct form for many journal manuscripts) is the terminology established by the International Anatomical Nomenclature Committee and approved or revised in 1955, 1960, and 1965.[30] Common usage, however, often neglects these prescribed names in favor of shorter or more readily pronounced names. The authors of this text make no apologies for not keeping strictly to formal usage. The majority of the muscles cited do follow the Nomina Anatomica. Others are listed by the names in most common use. The alphabetical list of muscles (see page 352) gives the name used in this text and the correct Nomina Anatomica term, when it differs, in parentheses.

ANATOMICAL AUTHORITIES

The authors of this book relied on both the American and British versions of *Gray's Anatomy* as principal references for anatomical information; the British edition (Williams et al.) was always the final arbiter because of its finer detail and precision.

THE CONVENTION OF ARROWS IN THE TEXT

Red arrows in the text denote the direction of movement of a body part, either actively by the patient or passively by the examiner. The length and direction of the arrow indicates the relative excursion of the part.

Examples:

Black arrows in the text denote resistance by the examiner. The arrow indicates distance, and the width gives some relative idea of whether resistance is large or small.

Examples:

References

1. Wright WG. Muscle training in the treatment of infantile paralysis. Boston Med Surg J 167:567–574, 1912.
2. Lovett RW. *Treatment of infantile paralysis.* Preliminary report. JAMA 64:2118, 1915.
3. Merrill J. Personal letter to Lucille Daniels dated January 5, 1945.
4. Lovett RW, Martin EG. Certain aspects of infantile paralysis and a description of a method of muscle testing. JAMA 66:729–733, 1916.
5. Wright WG. *Muscle Function.* New York: Paul B. Hoeber, 1928.
6. Lovett RW. *Treatment of Infantile Paralysis,* 2nd ed. Philadelphia: Blakiston's Son & Co., 1917.
7. Lowman CL. A method of recording muscle tests. Am J Surg 3:586–591, 1927.
8. Lowman CL. Muscle strength testing. Physiother Rev 20:69–71, 1940.
9. Stewart HS. *Physiotherapy: Theory and Clinical Application.* New York: Paul B. Hoeber, 1925.
10. Legg AT, Merrill J. Physical therapy in infantile paralysis. *In:* Mock. *Principles and Practice of Physical Therapy,* Vol. 2. Hagerstown, MD: W.F. Prior, 1932.
11. Kendall HO. Some interesting observations about the after care of infantile paralysis patients. J Excep Child 3:107, 1936.
12. Kendall HO, Kendall FP. Care during the recovery period of paralytic poliomyelitis. U.S. Public Health Bulletin No. 242. Washington, D.C.: U.S. Government Printing Office, 1938.
13. Brunnstrom S, Dennen M. Round table on muscle testing. New York: Annual Conference of the American Physical Therapy Association, Federation of Crippled and Disabled, Inc. (mimeographed), 1931.
14. Kenny E. Paper read at Northwestern Pediatric Conference at St. Paul University Club, November 14, 1940.
15. Plastridge AL. Personal report to the National Foundation for Infantile Paralysis after a trip to observe work of Sister Kenny, 1941.
16. Kendall HO, Kendall FP. Report on the Sister Kenny Method of Treatment in Anterior Poliomyelitis made to the National Foundation for Infantile Paralysis. New York, March 10, 1941.
17. Daniels L, Williams M, Worthingham CA. *Muscle Testing: Techniques of Manual Examination.* Philadelphia: W.B. Saunders, 1946.
18. Kendall HO, Kendall FP. *Muscles: Testing and Function.* Baltimore: Williams & Wilkins, 1949.
19. Kendall HO, Kendall FP. *Posture and Pain.* Baltimore: Williams & Wilkins, 1952.
20. Kendall FP, McCreary EK, Provance PG. *Muscles: Testing and Function,* 4th ed. Baltimore: Williams & Wilkins, 1993.

21. Gonella C, Harmon G, Jacobs M. The role of the physical therapist in the gamma globulin poliomyelitis prevention study. Phys Ther Rev 33:337–345, 1953.
22. Lilienfeld AM, Jacobs M, Willis M. Study of the reproducibility of muscle testing and certain other aspects of muscle scoring. Phys Ther Rev 34:279 289, 1954.
23. Kolb ME. Personal communication, October 1993.
24. Iddings DM, Smith LK, Spencer WA. Muscle testing. Part 2: Reliability in clinical use. Phys Ther Rev 41:249–256, 1961.
25. Beasley W. Quantitative muscle testing: Principles and applications to research and clinical services. Arch Phys Med Rehabil 42:398–425, 1961.
26. Williams M, Stutzman L. Strength variation through the range of joint motion. Phys Ther Rev 39:145–152, 1959.
27. Hislop HJ. Quantitative changes in human muscular strength during isometric exercise. Phys Ther 43:21–36, 1963.
28. Hislop HJ, Perrine JJ. Isokinetic concept of exercise. Phys Ther 47:114–117, 1967.
29. Bohannon RW. Manual muscle test scores and dynamometer test scores of knee extension strength. Arch Phys Med Rehabil 67:204, 1986.
30. International Anatomical Nomenclature Committee. *Nomina Anatomica*. Amsterdam: Excerpta Medica Foundation, 1965.

Other Readings

Bailey JC. Manual muscle testing in industry. Phys Ther Rev 41:165–169, 1961.
Bennett RL. Muscle testing: A discussion of the importance of accurate muscle testing. Phys Ther Rev 27:242–243, 1947.
Borden R, Colachis S. Quantitative measurement of the Good and Normal ranges in muscle testing. Phys Ther 48:839–843, 1968.
Brunnstrom S. Muscle group testing. Physiother Rev 21:3–21, 1941.
Currier DP. Maximal isometric tension of the elbow extensors at varied positions. Phys Ther 52:52, 1972.

Downer AH. Strength of the elbow flexor muscles. Phys Ther Rev 33:68–70, 1953.
Fisher FJ, Houtz SJ. Evaluation of the function of the gluteus maximus muscle. Am J Phys Med 47:182–191, 1968.
Frese E, Brown M, Norton BJ. Clinical reliability of manual muscle testing: Middle trapezius and gluteus medius muscles. Phys Ther 67:1072–1076, 1987.
Gonnella C. The manual muscle test in the patient's evaluation and program for treatment. Phys Ther Rev 34:16–18, 1954.
Granger CV. The clinical discernment of muscle weakness. Arch Phys Med 44:430–438, 1963.
Hoppenfeld S. *Physical Examination of the Spine and Extremities.* New York: Appleton-Century-Crofts, 1976.
Janda V. *Muscle Function Testing.* Boston: Butterworths, 1983.
Jarvis DK. Relative strength of hip rotator muscle groups. Phys Ther Rev 32:500–503, 1952.
Kendall FP. Testing the muscles of the abdomen. Phys Ther Rev 21:22–24, 1941.
Lovett RW. Treatment of Infantile Paralysis: Preliminary report. JAMA 64:2118, 1915.
Palmer ML, Epler ME. *Clinical Assessment Procedures in Physical Therapy.* Philadelphia: J.B. Lippincott, 1990.
Salter N, Darcus HD. Effect of the degree of elbow flexion on the maximum torque developed in pronation and supination of the right hand. J Anat 86B:197, 1952.
Smidt GL, Rogers MW. Factors contributing to the regulation and clinical assessment of muscular strength. Phys Ther 62:1283–1289, 1982.
Wadsworth CT, Krishnan R, Sear M, et al. Intrarater reliability of manual muscle testing and hand held dynametric testing. Phys Ther 67:1342–1347, 1987.
Wintz M. Variations in current muscle testing. Phys Ther Rev 39:466 475, 1959.
Zimny N, Kirk C. Comparison of methods of manual muscle testing. Clin Manag 7:6–11, 1987.

Daniels and Worthingham's

MUSCLE
TESTING

Techniques of Manual Examination

CHAPTER 1

Principles of Manual Muscle Testing

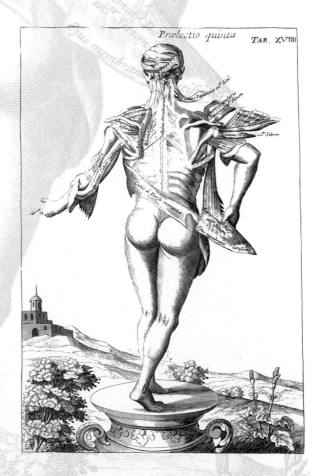

Præelectio quinta   TAB. XVIII

THE GRADING SYSTEM

Grades for a manual muscle test are recorded as numerical scores ranging from zero (0), which represents no activity, to five (5), which represents a "normal" or best-possible response to the test or as great a response as can be evaluated by a manual muscle test. Because this text is based on tests of motions rather than tests of individual muscles, the grade represents the performance of all muscles in that motion. The 5 to 0 system of grading is the most commonly used convention.

Each numerical grade can be paired with a word that describes the test performance in qualitative terms. These qualitative terms, when written, are capitalized to indicate that they too represent a score. This does not mean that the test grades are quantitative in any manner.

Numerical Score	Qualitative Score
5	Normal (N)
4	Good (G)
3	Fair (F)
2	Poor (P)
1	Trace activity (T)
0	Zero (no activity) (0)

These grades are based on several factors of testing and response.

OVERVIEW OF TEST PROCEDURES

The Break Test

Manual resistance is applied to a limb or other body part after it has completed its range of movement or after it has been placed at end range by the examiner. The term "resistance" is always used to denote a force that acts in opposition to a contracting muscle. Manual resistance should always be applied in the direction of the "line of pull" of the participating muscle or muscles. At the end of the available range, or at a point in the range where the muscle is most challenged, the patient is asked to hold the part at that point and not allow the examiner to "break" the hold with manual resistance. For example, a seated subject is asked to flex the elbow to its end range; when that position is reached, the examiner applies resistance at the wrist, trying to force the elbow to "break" its hold and move downward into extension. This is called a break test, and it is the procedure most commonly used in manual muscle testing today.

As a recommended alternative procedure, the examiner may choose to place the muscle group to be tested in the end or test position rather than have the patient actively move it there. In this procedure

the examiner ensures correct positioning and stabilization for the test.

Active Resistance Test

An alternative to the break test is the application of manual resistance against an actively contracting muscle or muscle group (i.e., against the direction of the movement as if to prevent that movement). This may be called an "active resistance" test. During the motion, the examiner gradually increases the amount of manual resistance until it reaches the maximal level the subject can tolerate and motion ceases. This kind of manual muscle test requires considerable skill and experience to perform and is so often equivocal that its use is not recommended.

Application of Resistance

The principles of manual muscle testing presented here and in all published sources since 1921 follow the basic tenets of muscle length-tension relationships as well as those of joint mechanics.[1,2] In the case of the Biceps brachii, for example, when the elbow is straight, the Biceps lever is short; leverage increases as the elbow flexes and becomes maximal (most efficient) at 90°, but as flexion continues beyond that point, the lever arm again decreases in length and efficiency.

In manual muscle testing, the application of external force (resistance) at the end of the range in one-joint muscles allows consistency of procedure rather than an attempt to select the estimated midrange position. In two-joint muscles (e.g., the medial or lateral hamstring muscles), the point of maximum resistance is generally at or near midrange.

The point on an extremity or part where the examiner should apply resistance is near the distal end of the segment to which the muscle attaches. There are two common exceptions to this rule: the hip abductors and the scapular muscles. In testing the hip abductor muscles, resistance would be applied at the distal end of the femur just above the knee. The abductor muscles are so strong, however, that most examiners, in testing a patient with normal knee strength and joint integrity, will choose to apply resistance at the ankle. The longer lever provided by resistance at the ankle is a greater challenge for the abductors and is more indicative of the functional demands required in gait. It follows that when a patient cannot tolerate maximal resistance at the ankle, his muscle cannot be considered Grade 5. In the patient who has an unstable knee, resistance to the abductors of the hip should be applied at the distal femur just above the knee. When using the short lever, hip abductor strength must be graded no better than Grade 4 (Good) even when the muscle takes maximal resistance.

An example of testing with a short lever occurs in the patient with a transfemoral amputation, where the grade awarded, even when the patient can hold against maximal resistance, is Grade 4 (Good). This is done because of the loss of the weight of the leg and is particularly important when the examiner is evaluating the patient for a prosthesis. The muscular force available should not be overestimated in predicting the patient's ability to use the prosthesis.

In testing the vertebroscapular muscles (e.g., Rhomboids), the preferred point of resistance is on the arm rather than on the scapula where these muscles insert. The longer lever more closely reflects the functional demands that incorporate the weight of the arm. Other exceptions to the general rule of applying distal resistance include contraindications such as a painful condition or a healing wound in a place where resistance might otherwise be given.

The application of manual resistance to a part should never be sudden or uneven (jerky). The examiner should apply resistance somewhat slowly and gradually, allowing it to build to the maximum tolerable intensity. Critical to the manual test is the location of the resistance and its consistency over many tests. (The novice examiner should make a note of the point of resistance when a variation is used.) Resistance is applied at a 90° angle to the primary axis of the body part being tested.

The application of resistance permits an assessment of muscular strength when it is applied in the opposite direction to the muscular force or torque. The examiner also should understand that the weight of the limb plus the influence of gravity is part of test responses. When the muscle contracts in a parallel direction to the line of gravity, it is noted as "gravity minimal" (GM). It is suggested that the commonly used term "gravity eliminated" be avoided since, of course, that can never occur except in a zero-gravity environment. Thus, strength is evaluated when weakened muscles are tested in a plane horizontal to the direction of gravity; the body part is supported on a smooth, flat surface in a way that friction force is minimal (Grades 2, 1, and 0). For stronger muscles that can complete a full range of motion in a direction against the pull of gravity (Grade 3), resistance is applied perpendicular to the line of gravity (Grades 4 and 5). Acceptable variations to antigravity and gravity-minimal positions are discussed in individual test sections.

The Examiner and the Value of the Muscle Test

The knowledge and skill of the examiner determine the accuracy and defensibility of a manual muscle test. Specific aspects of these qualities include the following:

- Knowledge of the location and anatomical features of the muscles in a test. In addition to knowing the muscle attachments, the examiner should be able to visualize the location of the tendon and its muscle in relationship to other tendons and muscles and other structures in the same area (e.g., the tendon of the Extensor carpi radialis longus lies on the radial side of the tendon of the Extensor carpi radialis brevis at the wrist).

- Knowledge of the direction of muscle fibers and their "line of pull" in each muscle.

- Knowledge of the function of the participating muscles (e.g., synergists, prime movers, accessories).

- Consistent use of a standardized method for each different test.

- Consistent use of proper positioning and stabilization techniques for each test procedure. Stabilization of the proximal segment of the joint being tested is achieved in several ways. These ways include patient position (via body weight), the use of a firm surface for testing, muscle activity by the patient, and manual fixation by the examiner.

- Ability to identify patterns of substitution in a given test and how they can be detected based on a knowledge of which other muscles can be substituted for the one(s) being tested.

- Ability to detect contractile activity during both contraction and relaxation, especially in minimally active muscle.

- Sensitivity to differences in contour and bulk of the muscles being tested in contrast to the contralateral side or to normal expectations based on such things as body size, occupation, or leisure work.

- Awareness of any deviation from normal values for range of motion and the presence of any joint laxity or deformity.

- Understanding that the muscle belly must not be grasped at any time during a manual muscle test except specifically to assess tenderness or pain and muscle mass.

 Early Kendall

Accuracy in giving examinations depends primarily on the examiner's knowledge of the isolated and combined actions of muscles in individuals with normal, as well as those with weak or paralyzed, muscles.

The fact that muscles act in combination permits substitution of a strong muscle for a weaker one. For accurate muscle examinations, no substitutions should be permitted; that is, the movement described as a test movement should be done without shifting the body or turning the part to allow other muscles to perform the movement for the weak or paralyzed group. The only way to recognize substitution is to know normal function, and realize the ease with which a normal muscle performs the exact test movement.

KENDALL HO, KENDALL FP

From Care During the Recovery Period in Paralytic Poliomyelitis. Public Health Bulletin No. 242. Washington, DC, US Government Printing Office, 1937, 1939, p 26.

- Ability to identify muscles with the same innervation, which will ensure a comprehensive muscle evaluation and accurate interpretation of test results (because weakness of one muscle in a myotome should require examination of all).
- Knowledge of the relationship of the diagnosis to the sequence and extent of the test (e.g., the patient with C7 complete tetraplegia will require definitive muscle testing of the upper extremity but only confirmatory tests in the lower extremities).
- Ability to modify test procedures when necessary while not compromising the test result and understanding the influence of the modification on the result.
- Knowledge of the effect of fatigue on the test results, especially muscles tested late in a long testing session, and a sensitivity to fatigue in certain diagnostic conditions such as myasthenia gravis or Eaton-Lambert syndrome.
- Understanding of the effect of sensory loss on movement.

The examiner also may inadvertently *influence* the test results and should be especially alert when testing in the following situations:

- The patient with open wounds or other conditions requiring gloves, which may blunt palpation skills.
- The patient who must be evaluated under difficult conditions such as the patient in an intensive care unit with multiple tubes and monitors, the patient in traction, the patient in whom turning is contraindicated, the patient on a ventilator, and the patient in restraints.

The novice muscle tester must avoid the temptation to use shortcuts or "tricks of the trade" before mastering the basic procedures lest such shortcuts become an inexact personal standard. One such pitfall for the novice tester is to inaccurately assign a muscle grade from one test position that the patient could not perform successfully to a lower grade without actually testing in the position required for the lower grade.

For example, when testing trunk flexion, a patient partially clears the scapula from the surface with the hands clasped behind the head (the position for the Grade 5 test). The temptation may exist to assign a grade of 4 to this test, but this may "overrate" the true strength of trunk flexion unless the patient is actually tested with the arms across the chest to confirm Grade 4.

The good clinician never ignores a patient's comments and must be a good listener, not just to questions but also to the words the patient uses and their meaning. This quality is the first essential of good communication and the means of encouraging understanding and respect between therapist and patient. The patient is the best guide to a successful muscle test.

Population Variation

Most of the papers that report muscle testing results are studies done on normal adults, and on specific subpopulations such as athletes, sedentary persons, and the elderly. Children remain in their own category. With this wide variation, it is necessary to modify grading procedures but not testing technique. Some also believe that the assigned grade should be consistent with those used with the normal adult population standards, but this requires innate understanding that an 80-year-old woman will be further down the grade scale than a 30-year-old woman; that a husky football player may be "off the scale" in contrast to the nonathletic white-collar worker. A grade of 4 will be very different in a child of 10 years versus a teen of 18 years. Chapter 6 provides a different testing procedure for children before they reach school age.

Some muscles, such as the muscles of the face and head, cannot be evaluated by these standard methods; these are included with a different scale and criteria in Chapter 7.

Validity and Reliability from the Literature

Manual muscle testing is well embedded as a testing device in physical therapy, having come onto the scene during the poliomyelitis epidemic in New England prior to World War I. (See Brief History of Muscle Testing in Introduction.) Credit for development of the early procedures belongs primarily to Wilhelmine Wright[3] (as what today we would call a physical therapist), who worked with orthopedic surgeon Robert Lovett.[4,5] The techniques she used to evaluate muscles are not radically different now, though refined and extended.

The first statistical measures systematically applied to manual muscle testing did not occur until after World War II when they were used to evaluate the presence and severity of paralytic poliomyelitis.[6,7] The seminal gamma globulin field trials were conducted in 1952, followed by more elaborate field trials in 1955 and 1956 when controlled trials were used before and after Salk vaccine administration.[8,9] These evaluations of the subjective manual muscle test results were quite positive and showed that they did, indeed, test muscular strength and torque (validity). The muscles that showed "weakness" were compared with functional tests (such as walking) of those muscles, though the correlation was much lower. These tests were done prior to the availability of instrumented dynamometers, but the validity was good enough to continue manual testing for almost 90 years after such testing began.

The analysis of the effectiveness of gamma globulin was planned and conducted in 1952.[8] The test was modified for the 1953 gamma globulin trials in which muscles were grouped slightly differently. The muscles innervated by the cranial nerves were not overlooked because Gonnella described their involvement, albeit with somewhat different techniques.[10]

The results of these preliminary tests were impressive but did show the importance of using examiners who were experienced, as well as the importance of training examiners for the procedure to be used (standardization). The results revealed minor differences between experienced examiners, and wide variance between the new and experienced therapists. Many studies have followed the polio era ones and in general, validity is high while reliability shows greater differences.[11-16]

Since manual muscle testing is subjective, the conventional acceptability for reliability is that among examiners and in successive tests with the same examiner, the results should be within one-half of a grade (or within a plus or minus of the base grade).[16] Others maintain that within the same grade is acceptable, pluses and minuses notwithstanding.[17]

Reliability is increased by adhering to the same procedure for each test (for one or several examiners), by providing clear instructions to the subject, and by having a quiet and comfortable environment for the test.

Some studies after the poliomyelitis years reported muscular strength grades as congruent 50 percent of the time; grades were within a plus or minus of the base grade 66 percent of the time; and 90 percent of the time they were identical within a full testing grade.[12,13,15,19] These results were obtained with grouped data; between examiners the agreement of grade assigned dropped off sharply.[22-24]

In muscles with grades below 3 (Fair) reliability declines.[12,15,22,23] Other studies pointed up that differences in technique could account for their low reliability.[22,23] The Grade 4 (Good) muscle presents considerable variance because Grade 4 can be so broad and can be interpreted differently by different examiners: in small muscle groups the relative strength of the examiner may not be capable of accurate discrimination between Lumbricals and wrist flexors or extensors; and similarly by the small woman examiner testing the arm flexors of a large injured football lineman.

As stated earlier, reliability is affected by the experience of the examiners as was shown in the 1950s trials. In both the gamma globulin and the polio trials the examiners all were experienced and also trained by the same instructors for the specific tests to be used in the trials.[8,9] Since 38 physical therapists and a small number of physicians and nurses performed the muscle examinations across the country, reproducibility among examiners was a critical factor. This was indeed a definitive factor in the tests that proved the efficacy of the Salk vaccine.

When the instructors and trainees were compared in a variety of combinations, they agreed within a plus or minus grade 95 percent of the time and agreed completely 70 percent of the time. Blair reported similar results in 1957 after the Salk vaccine trials.[9] In the same chronological period, Williams reported that two examiners agreed on the manual muscle testing grade 60 to 75 percent of the time.[13] Iddings et al., in the early 1960s, reported intertester and intratester scores to be in agreement in 48 percent of tests and within a plus or minus in 91 percent of the tests.[11] Surprisingly, in the Iddings study the test procedures used by the examiners were not homogeneous.

In later years (1980s and 1990s) investigators used statistical analyses to interpret data in studies that looked at examiner experience; comparison between test procedures and their standardization; influence of muscle weakness (e.g., Good tests and those below Fair) on the grade assigned; and the reliability of intertester versus intratester performance. In most testing, reliability was acceptable for these subjective tests.[20-24]

The issue of reliability of manual muscle testing has not gone away, but neither has manual testing been replaced by instrumented dynamometers, which have their own issues that await resolution. More work is needed to assess the problems found in testing at the Grade 4 (Good) level and in solving the conundrums in grades below 3 (Fair). Examiners, especially novices, must be cautious about their test procedures and make vigorous attempts to standardize their methods.

Despite the multiple issues and problems with manual muscle testing, both reliability and validity are satisfactory for clinical use and can never be "perfect" because of the subjectivity of the measures.

Influence of the Patient on the Test

The intrusion of a living, breathing, feeling person into the neat test package may distort scoring for the unwary examiner. The following circumstances should be recognized:

- There may be variation in the assessment of the true effort expended by a patient in a given test (reflecting the patient's desire to do well or to seem more impaired than is actually the case).
- The patient's willingness to endure discomfort or pain may vary (e.g., in the stoic, the whiner, the high competitor).
- The patient's ability to understand the test requirements may be limited in some cases because of comprehension and language barriers.
- The motor skills for the test may be beyond some patients (e.g., the clumsy or inept patient who just cannot perform as requested).

Principles of Testing (1925)

The following points are applicable to nearly every case requiring muscle [testing] and are of the utmost importance for successful work:

1. Determine just what muscles are involved by careful testing and chart the degree of power in each muscle or group to be treated.
2. Insist on such privacy and discipline as will gain the patient's cooperation and undivided attention. . . .
3. Use some method of preliminary warming up of the muscles . . . doubly essential in the cold, cyanotic and weakened muscles. . . .
4. Have the entire part free from covering and so supported as not to bring strain . . . from gravity . . . or antagonists.

HARRY EATON STEWART, M.D.

From *Physiotherapy: Theory and Clinical Application.* New York: Hoeber, 1925.

- Lassitude and depression may cause the patient to be indifferent to the test and the examiner.
- Cultural, social, and gender issues may be associated with palpation and exposure of a body part for testing.
- Though not an individual variation but causing considerable differences in grading are the size and noncomparability between big versus small muscles (e.g., the gluteus medius versus a finger extensor). There is a huge variability in maximum torque between such muscles and the examiner must use care not to assign a grade that is not consistent with muscle size and architecture.

CRITERIA FOR ASSIGNING A MUSCLE TEST GRADE

The grade given on a manual muscle test comprises both subjective and objective factors. Subjective factors include the examiner's impression of the amount of resistance to give before the actual test and then the amount of resistance the patient actually tolerates during the test. Objective factors include the ability of the patient to complete a full range of motion or to hold the position once placed there, and to move the part against gravity or an inability to move it at all. All these factors require clinical judgment, which makes manual muscle testing an exquisite skill that requires considerable experience to master. An accurate test grade is important not only to establish a functional diagnosis but also to assess the patient's longitudinal progress during the period of recovery and treatment.

The Grade 5 (Normal) Muscle

The wide range of "normal" muscle performance leads to a considerable underestimation of a muscle's capability. If the examiner has no experience in examining persons who are free of disease or injury, it is unlikely that there will be any realistic judgment of what is Normal and how much normality can vary. Generally, a physical therapy student learns manual muscle testing by practicing on classmates, but this provides only minimal experience compared to what is needed to master the skill. It should be recognized, for example, that the average physical therapist cannot "break" knee extension in a reasonably fit young man, even by doing a handstand on his leg! This and similar observations were derived by objective comparisons of movement performance acquired by assessing the amount of resistance given and then testing the muscle group's maximal capacity on an electronic dynamometer.[15,28–30]

The examiner should test normal muscles at every opportunity, especially when testing the contralateral limb in a patient with a unilateral problem. In almost every instance when the examiner cannot break the patient's hold position, a grade of 5 (Normal) is assigned. This value must be accompanied by the ability to complete a full range of motion or maintain end-point range against maximal resistance.

The Grade 4 (Good) Muscle

The grade of 4 (Good) represents the true weakness in manual muscle testing procedures (pun intended). Sharrard counted alpha motor neurons in the spinal cords of poliomyelitis victims at the time of autopsy.[27] He correlated the manual muscle test grades in the patient's chart with the number of motor neurons remaining in the anterior horns. His data revealed that more than 50 percent of the pool of motor neurons to a muscle group were gone when the muscle test result had been recorded as Grade 4 (Good). Thus, when the muscle can withstand considerable but less than "normal" resistance, it has already been deprived of at least half of its innervation.

Grade 4 is used to designate a muscle group that is able to complete a full range of motion against gravity and can tolerate strong resistance without breaking the test position. The Grade 4 muscle "gives" or "yields" to some extent at the end of its range with maximal resistance. When maximal resistance clearly results in a break, the muscle is assigned a grade of 4 (Good).

The Grade 3 (Fair) Muscle

The Grade 3 muscle test is based on an objective measure. The muscle or muscle group can complete a full range of motion against only the resistance of gravity. If a tested muscle can move through the full range against gravity but additional resistance, however mild, causes the motion to break, the muscle is assigned a grade of 3 (Fair).

Sharrard cited a residual autopsy motor neuron count of 15 percent in polio-paretic muscles that had been assessed as Grade 3, meaning that 85 percent of the innervating neurons had been destroyed.[27]

Direct force measurements have demonstrated that the force level of the Grade 3 muscle usually is low, so that a much greater span of functional loss exists between Grades 3 and 5 than between Grades 3 and 1. Beasley, in a study of children aged 10 to 12 years, reported the Grade 3 (Fair) in 36 muscle tests as no greater than 40 percent of normal (one motion), the rest being 30 percent or below a normal "strength" and the majority falling between 5 and 20 percent of a rated normal.[26] A grade of 3 (Fair) may be said to represent a definite *functional threshold* for each movement tested, indicating that the muscle or muscles can achieve the minimal task of moving the part upward against gravity through its range of motion. Although this ability is significant for the upper extremity, it falls far short of the functional requirements of many lower extremity muscles used in walking, particularly such groups as the hip abductors and the plantar flexors. The examiner must be sure that muscles given a grade of 3 are not in the joint "locked" position during the test (e.g., locked elbow when testing elbow extension).

The Grade 2 (Poor) Muscle

The Grade 2 (Poor) muscle is one that can complete the full range of motion in a position that minimizes the force of gravity. This position often is described as the horizontal plane of motion.

The Grade 1 (Trace) Muscle

The Grade 1 (Trace) muscle means that the examiner can detect visually or by palpation some contractile activity in one or more of the muscles that participate in the movement being tested (provided that the muscle is superficial enough to be palpated). The examiner also may be able to see or feel a tendon pop up or tense as the patient tries to perform the movement. There is, however, no movement of the part as a result of this minimal contractile activity.

A Grade 1 muscle can be detected with the patient in almost any position. When a Grade 1 muscle is suspected, the examiner should passively move the part into the test position and ask the patient to hold the position and then relax; this will enable the examiner to palpate the muscle or tendon, or both, during the patient's attempts to contract the muscle and also during relaxation.

The Grade 0 (Zero) Muscle

The Grade 0 (Zero) muscle is completely quiescent on palpation or visual inspection.

Plus (+) and Minus (−) Grades

Use of a plus (+) or minus (−) addition to a manual muscle test grade is discouraged except in three instances—Fair+, Poor+, and Poor−. Scalable gradations in other instances can be described in documentation as improved or deteriorated within a given test grade (such as Grade 4) without resorting to the use of plus or minus labels. The purpose of avoiding the use of plus or minus signs is to restrict the variety of manual muscle test grades to those that are meaningful and defendable.

The Grade 3+ (Fair+) Muscle

The Grade 3+ muscle can complete a full range of motion against gravity, and the patient can hold the end position against mild resistance. There are functional implications associated with this grade.

For example, the patient with weak wrist extensors at Grade 3 cannot use a wrist-hand orthosis (WHO) effectively, but a patient with a Grade 3+ muscle can use such a device. Likewise, the patient with only Grade 3 ankle dorsiflexion cannot use a shoe-insert type of ankle-foot orthosis functionally. The patient with Grade 3+ dorsiflexors can tolerate the added weight of the brace, which is comparable to the mild resistance used in the test.

The plus addition to Grade 3 is considered by many clinicians to represent not just strength but the additional endurance that is lacking in a simple Grade 3 muscle.

The Grade 2+ (Poor+) Muscle

The Grade 2+ is given when assessing the strength of the plantar flexors when either of the following two conditions exist. The first is when the patient, while weight bearing, can complete a partial heel rise using correct form (see test for plantar flexion). The second condition is when the test is performed non−weight bearing and the patient takes maximum resistance and completes full available range. The 2+ Grade clearly distinguishes it from Grade 2 which indicates that full range is completed and takes no resistance. A grade of 3 or better can be given to the plantar flexors only when the patient is weight bearing.

The Grade 2− (Poor−) Muscle

The Grade 2− (Poor−) muscle can complete partial range of motion in the horizontal plane, the gravity-minimized position. The difference between Grade 2 and Grade 1 muscles represents such a broad functional difference that a minus sign is important in assessing even minor improvements in return of function. For example, the patient with infectious neuronitis (Landry-Guillain-Barré syndrome) who moves from muscle Grade 1 to Grade 2− demonstrates a quantum leap forward in terms of recovery and prognosis.

Available Range of Motion

When any condition limits joint range of motion, the patient can perform only within the range available. In this circumstance, the *available range* is the full range of motion for that patient at that time, even though it is not "normal." This is the range used to assign a muscle testing grade.

For example, the normal knee extension range is 135° to 0°. A patient with a 20° knee flexion contracture is tested for knee extension strength. This patient's maximal range into extension is −20°. If this range (in sitting) can be completed with maximal resistance, the grade assigned would be a 5 (Normal). If the patient cannot complete that range, the grade assigned MUST be less than 3 (Fair). The patient then should be repositioned in the side-lying position to ascertain the correct grade.

SCREENING TESTS

In the interests of time and cost-efficient care, it is rarely necessary to perform a muscle test for the entire body. Two exceptions among several are patients with Landry-Guillain-Barré syndrome and those with incomplete spinal cord injuries. To screen for areas that need definitive testing, the examiner can use a number of maneuvers to rule out parts that do not need testing. Observation of the patient before the examination will provide valuable clues to muscular weakness and performance deficits. For example, the examiner can

- Watch the patient as he or she enters the treatment area to detect gross abnormalities of gait.
- Watch the patient sit and rise from a chair, fill out admission or history forms, or remove street clothing.
- Ask the seemingly normal patient to walk on the toes and then on the heels.
- Ask the patient to grip the examiner's hand.
- Perform gross checks of bilateral muscle groups.

PREPARING FOR THE MUSCLE TEST

The examiner and the patient must work in harmony if the test session is to be successful. This means that some basic principles and inviolable procedures should be second nature to the examiner.

1. The patient should be as free as possible from discomfort or pain for the duration of each test. It may be necessary to allow some patients to move or be positioned differently between tests.
2. The environment for testing should be quiet and nondistracting. The temperature should be comfortable for the partially disrobed subject.
3. The plinth or mat table for testing must be firm to help stabilize the part being tested. The ideal is a hard surface, minimally padded or not padded at all. The hard surface will not allow the trunk or limbs to "sink in." Friction of the surface material should be kept to a minimum. When the patient is reasonably mobile a plinth is fine, but its width should not be so narrow that the patient is terrified of falling or sliding off. When the patient is severely paretic, a mat table is the more practical choice. The height of the table should be adjustable to allow the examiner to use proper leverage and body mechanics.
4. Patient position should be carefully organized so that position changes in a test sequence are minimized. The patient's position must permit adequate stabilization of the part or parts being tested by virtue of body weight or with help provided by the examiner.
5. All materials needed for the test must be at hand. This is particularly important when the patient is anxious for any reason or is too weak to be safely left untended.

Materials needed include the following:

- Muscle test documentation forms (Fig. 1–1)
- Pen, pencil, or computer terminal
- Pillows, towels, pads, and wedges for positioning
- Sheets or other draping linen
- Goniometer
- Interpreter (if needed)
- Assistance for turning, moving, or stabilizing the patient
- Emergency call system (if no assistant is available)
- Reference material

SUMMARY

From the foregoing, it should be clear that manual muscle testing is an exacting clinical skill. Experience, experience, and more experience are essential to bring such a skill to an acceptable level of clinical proficiency, to say nothing of clinical mastery.

DOCUMENTATION OF MUSCLE EXAMINATION

LEFT				RIGHT		
3	2	1	Date of Examination Examiner's Name	1	2	3
			NECK			
			Capital extension			
			Cervical extension			
			Combined extension (capital plus cervical)			
			Capital flexion			
			Cervical flexion			
			Combined flexion (capital plus cervical)			
			Combined flexion and rotation (Sternocleidomastoid)			
			Cervical rotation			
			TRUNK			
			Extension—Lumbar			
			Extension—Thoracic			
			Pelvic elevation			
			Flexion			
			Rotation			
			Diaphragm strength			
			Maximal inspiration less full expiration (indirect intercostal test)(inches)			
			Cough (indirect forced expiration) (F, WF, NF, O)			
			UPPER EXTREMITY			
			Scapular abduction and upward rotation			
			Scapular elevation			
			Scapular adduction			
			Scapular adduction and downward rotation			
			Shoulder flexion			
			Shoulder extension			
			Shoulder scaption			
			Shoulder abduction			
			Shoulder horizontal abduction			
			Shoulder horizontal adduction			
			Shoulder external rotation			
			Shoulder internal rotation			
			Elbow flexion			
			Elbow extension			
			Forearm supination			
			Forearm pronation			
			Wrist flexion			
			Wrist extension			
			Finger metacarpophalangeal flexion			
			Finger proximal interphalangeal flexion			
			Finger distal interphalangeal flexion			
			Finger metacarpophalangeal extension			
			Finger abduction			
			Finger adduction			
			Thumb metacarpophalangeal flexion			
			Thumb interphalangeal flexion			

FIGURE 1–1
Documentation of muscle examination.
Illustration continued on following page

MUSCLE EXAMINATION - Page 2

LEFT				RIGHT		
3	2	1		1	2	3
			Thumb metacarpophalangeal extension (motion superior to plane of metacarpals)			
			Thumb interphalangeal extension			
			Thumb carpometacarpal abduction (motion perpendicular to plane of palm)			
			Thumb carpometacarpal abduction and extension (motion parallel to plane of palm)			
			Thumb adduction			
			Thumb opposition			
			Little finger opposition			
			LOWER EXTREMITY			
			Hip flexion			
			Hip flexion, abduction, and external rotation with knee flexion (Sartorius)			
			Hip extension			
			Hip extension (Gluteus maximus)			
			Hip abduction			
			Hip abduction and flexion			
			Hip adduction			
			Hip external rotation			
			Hip internal rotation			
			Knee flexion			
			Knee flexion with leg external rotation			
			Knee flexion with leg internal rotation			
			Knee extension			
			Ankle plantar flexion			
			Ankle plantar flexion (soleus)			
			Foot dorsiflexion and inversion			
			Foot inversion			
			Foot eversion with plantar flexion			
			Foot eversion with dorsiflexion			
			Great toe metatarsophalangeal flexion			
			Toe metatarsophalangeal flexion			
			Great toe interphalangeal flexion			
			Toe interphalangeal flexion			
			Great toe metatarsophalangeal extension			
			Toe metatarsophalangeal extension			
			Great toe interphalangeal extension			
			Toe interphalangeal extension			

Comments: _____

_____

_____

_____

_____

Diagnosis _____ Onset _____ Age _____ Birth date _____

Patient Name _____
            last   first   middle   ID number

FIGURE 1-1
Continued

References

Cited References

1. LeVeau B. *Williams and Lissner's Biomechanics of Human Motion,* 3rd ed. Philadelphia: WB Saunders, 1992.
2. Soderberg GL. *Kinesiology: Application to Pathological Motion.* Baltimore: Williams & Wilkins, 1997.
3. Wright WG. Muscle training in the treatment of infantile paralysis. Boston Med Surg J 167:567–574, 1912.
4. Wright WG. *Muscle Function.* New York: Hoeber, 1928.
5. Lovett RW. *Treatment of Infantile Paralysis,* 2nd ed. Philadelphia; Blakiston's, 1917.
6. Lovett RW, Martin EG. Certain aspects of infantile paralysis and a description of a method of muscle testing. JAMA 66:729–733, 1916.
7. Martin EG, Lovett RW. A method of testing muscular strength in infantile paralysis. JAMA 65:1512–1513, 1915.
8. Lilienfeld AM, Jacobs M, Willis M. Study of the reproducibility of muscle testing and certain other aspects of muscle scoring. Phys Ther Rev 34:279–289, 1954.
9. Blair L. Role of the physical therapist in the evaluation studies of the poliomyelitis vaccine field trials. Phys Ther Rev 37:437–447, 1957.
10. Gonnella C, Harmon G, Jacobs M. The role of the physical therapist in the gamma globulin poliomyelitis prevention study. Phys Ther Rev 33:337–345, 1953.
11. Iddings DM, Smith LK, Spencer WA. Muscle testing. Part 2. Reliability in clinical use. Phys Ther Rev 41:249–256, 1961.
12. Wintz M. Variations in current manual muscle testing. Phys Ther Rev 39:466–475, 1959.
13. Williams M. Manual muscle testing: Development and current use. Phys Ther Rev 36:797–805, 1956.
14. Beasley WC. Influence of method on estimates of normal knee extensor force among normal and post-polio children. Phys Ther Rev 36:21–41, 1956.
15. Beasley WC. Quantitative muscle testing: Principles and application to research and clinical services. Arch Phys Med Rehabil 42:398–425, 1961.
16. Lamb R. Manual muscle testing. *In* Rothstein JM (ed). *Measurement in Physical Therapy.* New York: Churchill-Livingstone, 1985.
17. Palmer ML, Epler ME. *Fundamentals of Musculoskeletal Assessment Techniques,* 2nd ed. Philadelphia: Lippincott Williams & Wilkins, 1998.
18. Kolb, ME. Personal communication, 2001.
19. Daniels L, Williams M, Worthingham CA. *Muscle Testing: Techniques of Manual Examination,* 5th ed. Philadelphia: WB Saunders, 1986.
20. Zimny N, Kirk C. A comparison of methods of manual muscle testing. Clin Manage Phys Ther 7:6–11, 1987.
21. Brandsma JW, Schreuders TAR, Birke JA, et al. Manual muscle strength testing: Intraobserver and interobserver reliabilities for the intrinsic muscles of the hand. J Hand Ther 8:185–190, 1995.
22. Florence JM, Pandya S, King WM, et al. Intrarater reliability of manual muscle test (Medical Research Council Scale) grades in Duchenne's muscular dystrophy. Phys Ther 72:115–126, 1992.
23. Frese F, Brown M, Norton BJ. Clinical reliability of manual muscle testing: Middle trapezius and gluteus medius muscles. Phys Ther 67:1072–1076, 1987.
24. Keyweg RP, Van Der Meche FGA, Schmitz PIM. Interobserver agreement in the assessment of muscle strength and functional abilities in Guillain-Barré syndrome. Muscle Nerve 14:1103–1109, 1991.
25. Ikai M, Steinhaus AH. Some factors modifying the expression of human strength. J Appl Physiol 26:157–163, 1961.
26. Beasley WC. Normal and fair muscle systems: Quantitative standards for children 10 to 12 years of age. Presented at 39th Scientific Session of the American Congress of Rehabilitative Medicine, Cleveland, August 1961.
27. Sharrard WJW. Muscle recovery in poliomyelitis. J Bone Joint Surg Br 37:63–69, 1955.
28. Williams M, Stutzman L. Strength variation through the range of motion. Phys Ther Rev 39:145–152, 1959.
29. Bohannon RW. Test retest reliability of hand held dynamometry during single session of strength assessment. Phys Ther 66:206–209, 1986.
30. Bohannon RW. Manual muscle test scores and dynamometer test scores of knee extension strength. Arch Phys Med Rehabil 67:390–392, 1986.

Other Readings

Dvir, Z. Grade 4 in manual muscle testing: The problem with submaximal strength assessment. Clin Rehabil 11:36–41. 1997.
Herbison GJ, Issac Z, Cohen ME, et al. Strength post–spinal cord injury: Myometer vs manual muscle test. Spinal Cord 34:543–548, 1996.
Schwartz S, Cohen ME, Herbison GJ, et al. Relationship between two measures of upper extremity strength: Manual muscle test compared to hand-held myometry. Arch Phys Med Rehabil 73:1063–1068, 1992.

CHAPTER 2

Testing the Muscles of the Neck

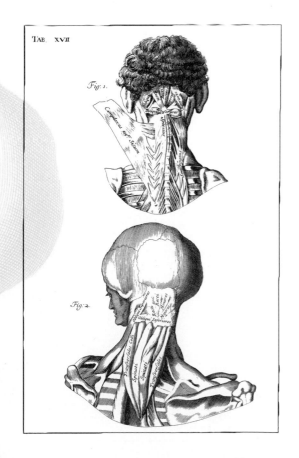

Note: This section of the book on testing the neck muscles
is divided into tests for capital and cervical extension and
flexion and their combination. This distinction was first described by Perry and Nickel as a necessary and effective
way of managing nuchal weakness or paralysis.[1] All muscles
acting on the head are inserted on the skull. Those muscles
that lie behind the coronal midline are termed capital extensors. Motion is centered at the atlanto-occipital and atlantoaxial joints.[2,3]

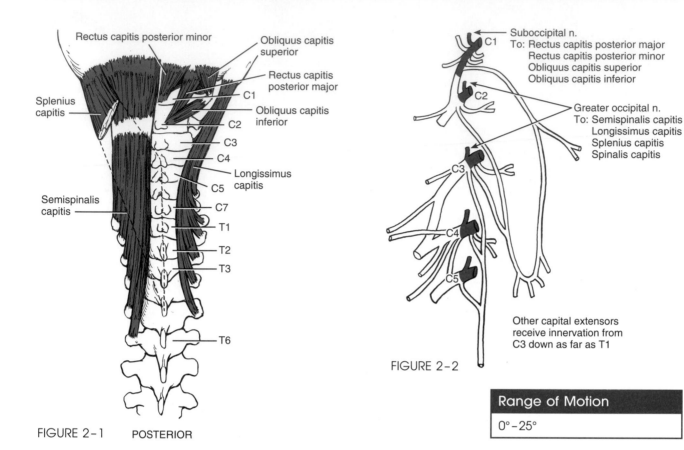

FIGURE 2–1   POSTERIOR

FIGURE 2–2

Range of Motion

0°–25°

Table 2-1   CAPITAL EXTENSION

I.D.	Muscle	Origin	Insertion
56	Rectus capitis posterior major	Axis (spinous process)	Occiput (inferior nuchal line laterally)
57	Rectus capitis posterior minor	Atlas (tubercle of posterior arch)	Occiput (inferior nuchal line medially)
60	Longissimus capitis	T1–T5 vertebrae (transverse processes) C4–C7 vertebrae (articular processes)	Temporal bone (mastoid process, posterior surface)
58	Obliquus capitis superior	Atlas (transverse process)	Occiput (between superior and inferior nuchal lines)
59	Obliquus capitis inferior	Axis (lamina and spinous process)	Atlas (transverse process, inferior-posterior surface)
61	Splenius capitis	Ligamentum nuchae C7–T4 vertebrae (spinous processes)	Temporal bone (mastoid process) Occiput (below superior nuchal line)
62	Semispinalis capitis (distinct medial part often named Spinalis capitis)	C7–T6 vertebrae (transverse processes) C4–C6 vertebrae (articular processes)	Occiput (between superior and inferior nuchal lines)
124	Trapezius (upper)	Occiput (external protuberance and superior nuchal line, middle 1/3) C7 (spinous process) Ligamentum nuchae	Clavicle (posterior border of lateral 1/3)
63	Spinalis capitis	Medial part of Semispinalis capitis, usually blended inseparably	Occiput (between superior and inferior nuchal lines)

Other

83	Sternocleidomastoid (posterior)		

Grade 5 (Normal) and Grade 4 (Good)

Position of Patient: Prone with head off end of table. Arms at sides.

Position of Therapist: Standing at side of patient next to the head. One hand provides resistance over the occiput (Fig. 2–3). The other hand is placed beneath the overhanging head, prepared to support the head should it give way with resistance which is applied directly opposite to the movement of the head.

Test: Patient extends head by tilting chin upward in a nodding motion. (Cervical spine is not extended.)

Instructions to Patient: "Look at the wall. Hold it. Don't let me tilt your head down."

Grading

Grade 5 (Normal): Patient completes available range of motion without substituting cervical extension. Tolerates maximal resistance. (This is a strong muscle group.)

Grade 4 (Good): Patient completes available range of motion without substituting cervical extension. Tolerates strong to moderate resistance.

Grade 3 (Fair)

Position of Patient: Prone with head off end of table and supported by therapist. Arms at sides.

Position of Therapist: Standing at side of patient's head. One hand should remain under the head to catch it should the muscles fail to hold position (Fig. 2–4).

Instructions to Patient: "Look at the wall."

Test: Patient completes available range of motion with no resistance.

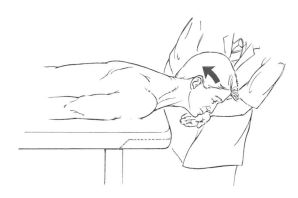

FIGURE 2–4

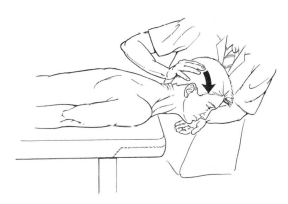

FIGURE 2–3

Grade 2 (Poor), Grade 1 (Trace), and Grade 0 (Zero)

Position of Patient: Supine with head on table. Arms at sides. Note: The gravity minimized position (sidelying) is not recommended for any of the tests of the neck for grades 2 (Poor) and below because test artifacts are created by the examiner in attempting to support the head without providing assistance to the motion.

Position of Therapist: Standing at end of table facing patient. Head is supported with two hands under the occiput. Fingers should be placed just at the base of the occiput lateral to the vertebral column to attempt to palpate the capital extensors (Fig. 2–5). Head may be slightly lifted off table to reduce friction.

Test: Patient attempts to look back toward examiner without lifting the head from the table.

Instructions to Patient: "Tilt your chin up," OR "Look back at me. Don't lift your head."

Grading

Grade 2 (Poor): Patient completes limited range of motion.

Grade 1 (Trace) and Grade 0 (Zero): Palpation of the capital extensors at the base of the occiput just lateral to the spine may be difficult; the Splenius capitis lies most lateral and the Recti lie just next to the spinous process.

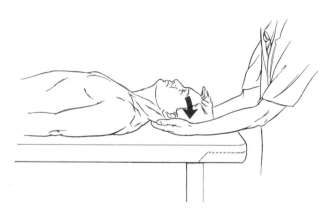

FIGURE 2–5

Helpful Hints

- Clinicians are reminded that the head is a very heavy object suspended on thin support. Whenever testing with the patient's head off the table, extreme caution should be used for the patient's safety, especially in the presence of suspected or known neck or trunk weakness. Always place a hand under the head to catch it should the muscles give way.

- Significant weakness of the capital extensor muscles combined with laryngeal and pharyngeal weakness can result in a nonpatent airway. There also may be inability to swallow. Both of these problems occur because the loss of capital extensors leaves the capital flexors unopposed, and the resultant head position favors the chin tucked on the chest, especially in the supine position.[1] This problem is not limited to patients with severe polio paralysis; it is also evident in patients with severe rheumatoid arthritis. Patients with chronic forward head posture also commonly have weak cervical extensors.

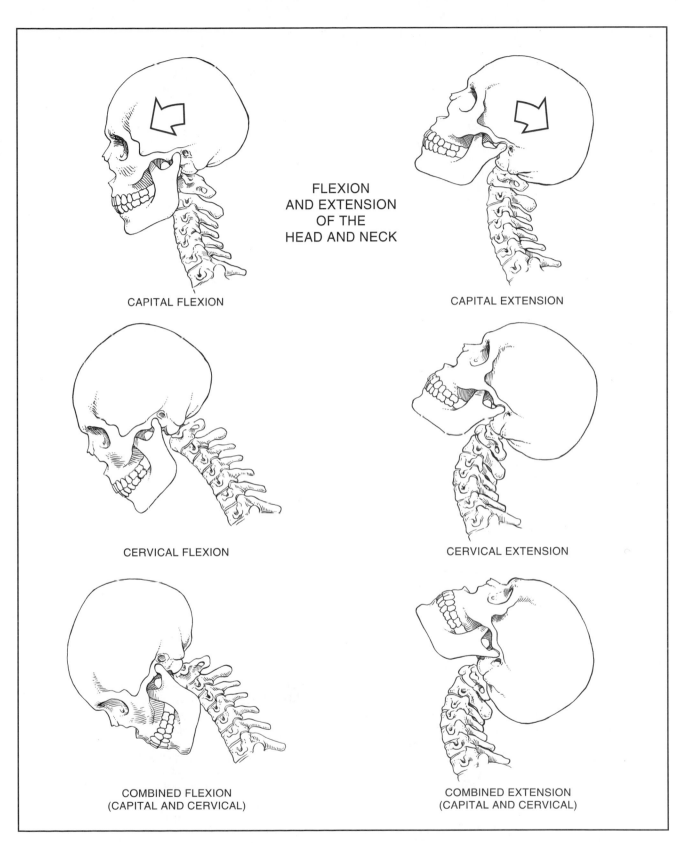

FLEXION
AND EXTENSION
OF THE
HEAD AND NECK

CAPITAL FLEXION

CAPITAL EXTENSION

CERVICAL FLEXION

CERVICAL EXTENSION

COMBINED FLEXION
(CAPITAL AND CERVICAL)

COMBINED EXTENSION
(CAPITAL AND CERVICAL)

PLATE 1

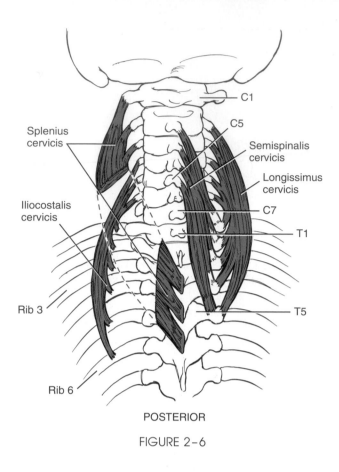

Splenius cervicis

Iliocostalis cervicis

Rib 3

Rib 6

C1

C5

Semispinalis cervicis

Longissimus cervicis

C7

T1

T5

POSTERIOR

FIGURE 2–6

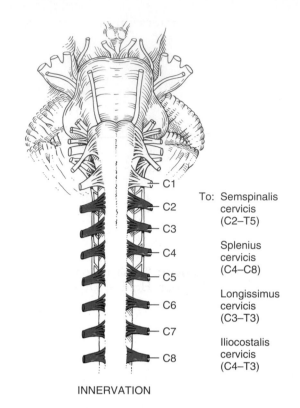

C1

C2

C3

C4

C5

C6

C7

C8

To: Semspinalis cervicis (C2–T5)

Splenius cervicis (C4–C8)

Longissimus cervicis (C3–T3)

Iliocostalis cervicis (C4–T3)

INNERVATION

FIGURE 2–7

Range of Motion

0° to less than 30°

Table 2-2 CERVICAL EXTENSION

I.D.	Muscle	Origin	Insertion
64	Longissimus cervicis	T1–T5 vertebrae (transverse processes) variable	C2–C6 vertebrae (transverse processes)
65	Semispinalis cervicis	T1–T5 vertebrae (transverse processes)	Axis (C2)–C5 vertebrae (spinous processes)
66	Iliocostalis cervicis	Ribs 3–6 (angles)	C4–C6 vertebrae (transverse processes, posterior tubercles)
67	Splenius cervicis (may be absent or variable)	T3–T6 vertebrae (spinous processes)	C1–C3 vertebrae (transverse processes)
124	Trapezius (upper)	Occiput (protuberance and superior nuchal line, middle 1/3) C7 (spinous process) Ligamentum nuchae T1–T12 vertebrae occasionally	Clavicle (posterior border of lateral 1/3)
68	Spinalis cervicis (often absent)	C7 and often C6 vertebrae (spinous processes) Ligamentum nuchae T1–T2 vertebrae occasionally	Axis (spinous process) C2–C3 vertebrae (spinous process)

Others

69	Interspinales cervicis		
70	Intertransversarii cervicis		
71	Rotatores cervicis		
94	Multifidi		
127	Levator scapulae		

The cervical extensor muscles are limited to those that act only on the cervical spine with motion centered in the lower cervical spine.[2,3]

Grade 5 (Normal) and Grade 4 (Good)

Position of Patient: Prone with head off end of table. Arms at sides.

Position of Therapist: Standing next to patient's head. One hand is placed over the parieto-occipital area for resistance (Fig. 2–8). The other hand is placed below the chin, ready to catch the head if it gives way suddenly during resistance.

Test: Patient extends neck without tilting chin.

Instructions to Patient: "Push up on my hand but keep looking at the floor. Hold it. Don't let me push it down."

Grading

Grade 5 (Normal): Patient completes full range of motion and holds against maximal resistance. Examiner must use clinical caution because these muscles are not strong, and their maximal effort will not tolerate much resistance.

Grade 4 (Good): Patient completes full range of motion against moderate resistance.

Grade 3 (Fair)

Position of Patient: Prone with head off end of table. Arms at sides.

Position of Therapist: Standing next to patient's head with one hand supporting (or ready to support) the forehead (Fig. 2–9).

Test: Patient extends neck without looking up or tilting chin.

Instructions to Patient: "Lift your forehead from my hand and keep looking at the floor."

Grading

Grade 3 (Fair): Patient completes range of motion but takes no resistance.

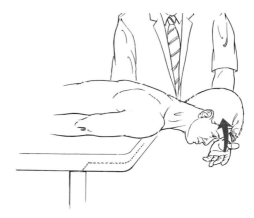

FIGURE 2-9

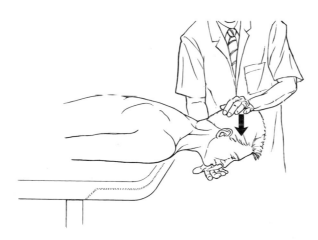

FIGURE 2-8

Alternate Test for Grade 3. This test should be used if there is known or suspected trunk extensor weakness. The examiner should always have an assistant participate to provide protective guarding under the patient's forehead. This test is identical to the preceding Grade 3 test except that stabilization is provided by the therapist if needed to accommodate trunk weakness. Stabilization is provided to the upper back by the forearm placed over the upper back with the hand cupped over the shoulder (Fig. 2–10).

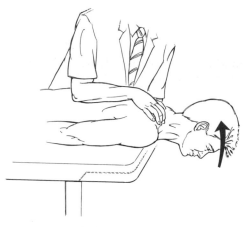

FIGURE 2–10

Grade 2 (Poor), Grade 1 (Trace), and Grade 0 (Zero)

Position of Patient: Supine with head fully supported by table. Arms at sides.

Position of Therapist: Standing at head end of table facing the patient. Both hands are placed under the head. Fingers are distal to the occiput at the level of the cervical vertebrae for palpation (Fig. 2–11).

Test: Patient attempts to extend neck into table.

Instructions to Patient: "Try to push your head down into my hands."

Grading

Grade 2 (Poor): Patient moves through small range of neck extension by pushing into therapist's hands.

Grade 1 (Trace): Contractile activity palpated in cervical extensors.

Grade 0 (Zero): No palpable muscle activity.

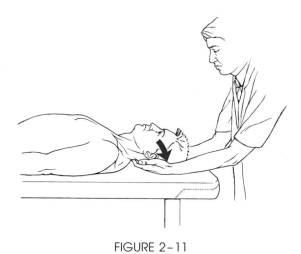

FIGURE 2–11

Range of Motion
0°–45°

Grade 5 (Normal) and Grade 4 (Good)

Position of Patient: Prone with head off end of table. Arms at sides.

Position of Therapist: Standing next to patient's head. One hand is placed over the parieto-occipital area to give resistance, which is directed both down and forward (Fig. 2–12). The other hand is below the chin ready to catch the head if muscles give way during resistance.

Test: Patient extends head and neck through available range of motion by lifting head and looking up.

Instructions to Patient: "Lift your head and look at the ceiling. Hold it. Don't let me push your head down."

Grading

Grade 5 (Normal): Patient completes available range of motion against maximal resistance.

Grade 4 (Good): Patient completes available range of motion against moderate resistance.

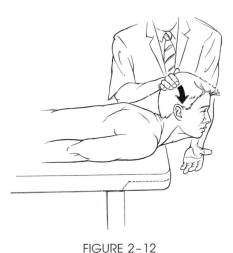

FIGURE 2–12

Grade 3 (Fair)

Position of Patient: Patient prone with head off end of table. Arms at sides.

Position of Therapist: Standing next to patient's head.

Test: Patient extends head and neck by raising head and looking up (Fig. 2–13).

Instructions to Patient: "Raise your head from my hand and look up to the ceiling."

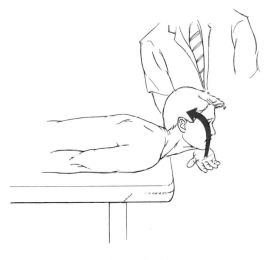

FIGURE 2–13

Grading

Grade 3 (Fair): Patient completes available range of motion without resistance except that of gravity.

Alternate Test for Grade 3: This test is used when the patient has trunk or hip extensor weakness. The test is identical to the previous test except that stabilization of the upper back is provided by the therapist (Fig. 2–14).

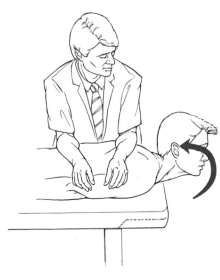

FIGURE 2–14

Grade 2 (Poor), Grade 1 (Trace), and Grade 0 (Zero)

Position of Patient: Patient prone with head fully supported on table. Arms at sides.

Position of Therapist: Standing next to patient's upper trunk. Both hands on cervical region and base of occiput for palpation.

Test: Patient attempts to raise head and look up.

Instructions to Patient: "Try to raise your head off the table and look at the ceiling."

Grading

Grade 2 (Poor): Patient moves through partial range of motion.

Grade 1 (Trace): Palpable contractile activity in both capital and cervical extensor muscles, but no movement.

Grade 0 (Zero): No palpable activity in muscles.

Helpful Hints

Extensor muscles on the right (or left) may be tested by having the patient rotate the head to the right (or left) and extend the head and neck.

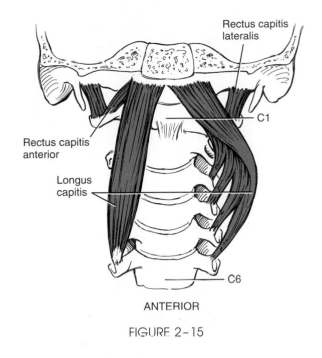

ANTERIOR

FIGURE 2-15

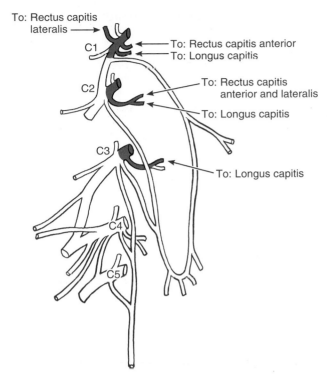

FIGURE 2-16

Range of Motion
0° to 10°–15°

Table 2-3 CAPITAL FLEXION

I.D.	Muscle	Origin	Insertion
72	Rectus capitis anterior	Atlas (C1) transverse process and lateral mass	Occiput (basilar part, inferior surface)
73	Rectus capitis lateralis	Atlas (transverse process)	Occiput (jugular process)
74	Longus capitis	C3–C6 vertebrae Transverse processes, anterior tubercles)	Occiput (basilar part, inferior surface)
Others			
	Suprahyoids:		
75	Mylohyoid		
76	Stylohyoid		
77	Geniohyoid		
78	Digastric		

All muscles that act on the head are inserted on the skull. Those that are anterior to the coronal midline are termed capital flexors. Their center of motion is in the atlanto-occipital or atlantoaxial joints.[2,3]

Starting Position of Patient: In all capital, cervical, and combined flexion tests, patient is supine with head supported on table and arms at sides (Fig. 2–17). See note, page 16, Position of Patient.

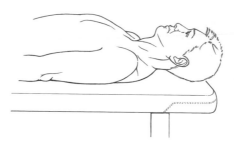

FIGURE 2–17

Grade 5 (Normal) and Grade 4 (Good)

Position of Patient: Supine with head on table. Arms at sides.

Position of Therapist: Standing at head of table facing patient. Both hands are cupped under the mandible to give resistance in an upward and backward direction (Fig. 2–18).

Test: Patient tucks chin into neck without raising head from table. No motion should occur at the cervical spine. This is the downward motion of nodding.

Instructions to Patient: "Tuck your chin. Don't lift your head from the table. Hold it. Don't let me lift up your chin."

Grading

Grade 5 (Normal): Patient completes available range of motion against maximal resistance. These are very strong muscles.

Grade 4 (Good): Patient completes available range of motion against moderate resistance.

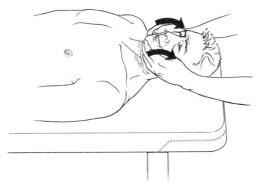

FIGURE 2–18

Grade 3 (Fair)

Position of Patient: Supine with head supported on table. Arms at sides.

Position of Therapist: Standing at head of table facing patient.

Test: Patient tucks chin without lifting head from table (Fig. 2–19).

Instructions to Patient: "Tuck your chin into your neck. Do not raise your head from the table."

Grading

Grade 3 (Fair): Patient completes available range of motion with no resistance.

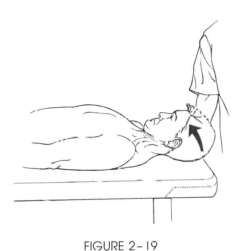

FIGURE 2–19

Grade 2 (Poor), Grade 1 (Trace), and Grade 0 (Zero)

Position of Patient: Supine with head supported on table. Arms at sides.

Position of Therapist: Standing at head of table facing patient.

Test: Patient attempts to tuck chin (Fig. 2–20).

Instructions to Patient: "Try to tuck your chin into your neck."

Grading

Grade 2 (Poor): Patient completes partial range of motion.

Grade 1 (Trace): Contractile activity may be palpated in capital flexor muscles but it is difficult and only minimal pressure should be used.

Grade 0 (Zero): No contractile activity.

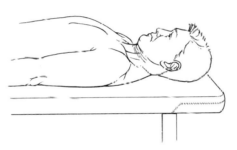

FIGURE 2–20

Helpful Hints

- Palpation of the small and deep muscles of capital flexion may be a difficult task unless the patient has severe atrophy. *It is NOT recommended that much pressure be put on the neck in such attempts.* Remember that the ascending arterial supply (carotids) to the brain runs quite superficially in this region.

- In patients with lower motor neuron lesions (including poliomyelitis) that do not affect the cranial nerves, capital flexion is seldom lost. This can possibly be attributed to the suprahyoid muscles, which are innervated by cranial nerves. Activity of the suprahyoid muscles can be identified by control of the floor of the mouth and the tongue as well as by the absence of impairment of swallowing or speech.[1]

- When capital flexion is impaired or absent, there usually is serious impairment of the cranial nerves, and other CNS signs are present which may require further evaluation by the physical therapist.

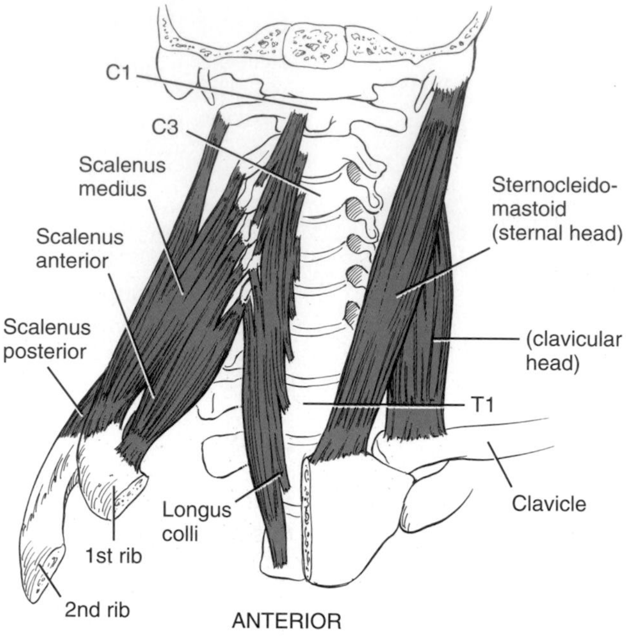
C1
C3
Scalenus medius
Scalenus anterior
Scalenus posterior
Sternocleido-mastoid (sternal head)
(clavicular head)
T1
Clavicle
Longus colli
1st rib
2nd rib
ANTERIOR

FIGURE 2–21

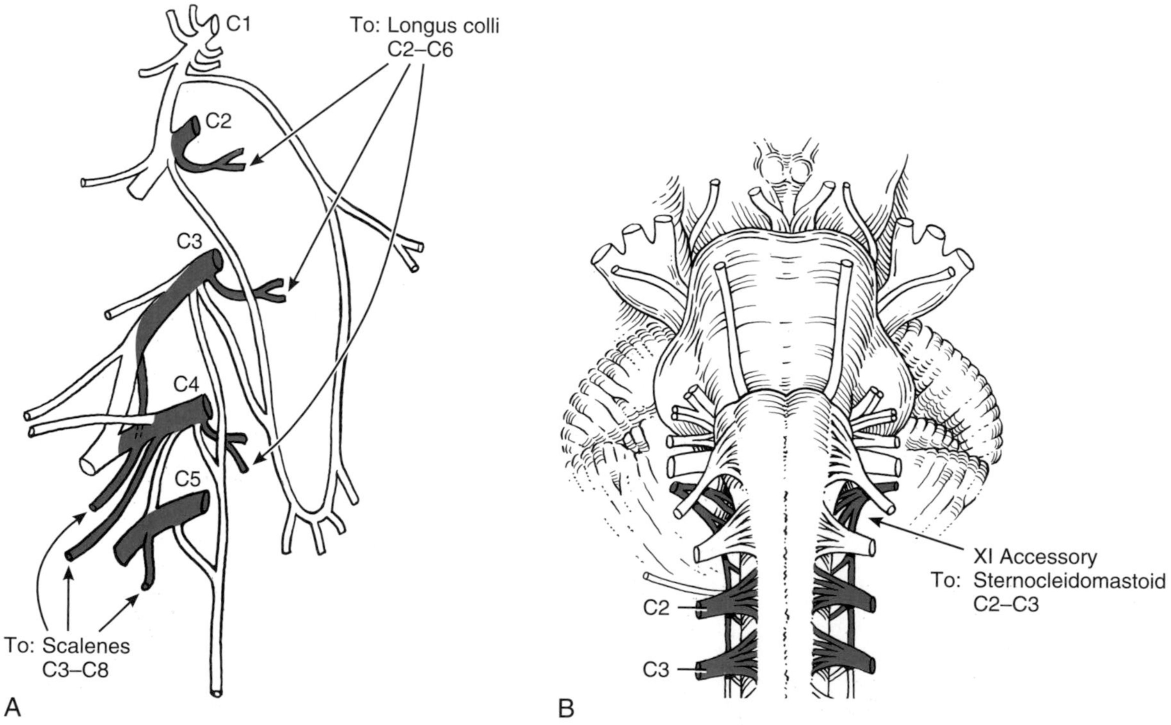
C1
To: Longus colli C2–C6
C2
C3
C4
C5
To: Scalenes C3–C8
A
XI Accessory
To: Sternocleidomastoid C2–C3
C2
C3
B

FIGURE 2–22 A, B

Range of Motion
0° to 35°–45°
Note: Women have greater cervical lordosis than men, so it is likely that they will have a greater arc of motion.

Table 2-4 CERVICAL FLEXION

I.D.	Muscle	Origin	Insertion
83	Sternocleidomastoid		
	Sternal head	Sternum (Manubrium, upper anterior aspect)	Two heads blend in middle of neck; occiput (lateral half of superior nuchal line)
	Clavicular head	Clavicle (medial 1/3 superior and anterior surfaces)	Temporal bone (mastoid process)
79	Longus colli		
	Superior oblique head	C3–C5 vertebrae (transverse processes)	Atlas (anterior arch, tubercle)
	Vertical intermediate head	T1–T3 and C5–C7 vertebrae (anterolateral bodies)	C2–C4 vertebrae (anterior bodies)
	Inferior oblique head	T1–T3 vertebrae (anterior bodies)	C5–C6 vertebrae (transverse processes, anterior tubercles)
80	Scalenus anterior	C3–C6 vertebrae (transverse processes, anterior tubercles)	1st rib (scalene tubercle)
Others			
81	Scalenus medius		
82	Scalenus posterior		
	Infrahyoids:		
84	Sternothyroid		
85	Thyrohyoid		
86	Sternohyoid		
87	Omohyoid		

The muscles of cervical flexion act only on the cervical spine with the center of motion in the lower cervical spine.[2,3]

Grade 5 (Normal) and Grade 4 (Good)

Position of Patient: Refer to starting position for all flexion tests. Supine with arms at side. Head supported on table.

Position of Therapist: Standing next to patient's head. Hand for resistance is placed on patient's forehead. Use two fingers only (Fig. 2–23). Other hand may be placed on chest, but stabilization is needed only when the trunk is weak.

Test: Patient flexes neck by lifting head straight up from the table without tucking the chin. This is a weak muscle group.

Instructions to Patient: "Lift your head from the table; keep looking at the ceiling. Do not lift your shoulders off the table. Hold it. Don't let me push your head down."

Grading

Grade 5 (Normal): Patient completes available range of motion against moderate two-finger resistance.

Grade 4 (Good): Patient completes available range of motion against mild two-finger resistance.

Grade 3 (Fair)

Positions of Patient and Therapist: Same as for Normal test. No resistance is used on the forehead.

Test: Patient flexes neck, keeping eyes on the ceiling (Fig. 2–24).

Instructions to Patient: "Bring your head off the table, keeping your eyes on the ceiling. Keep your shoulders completely on the table."

Grading

Grade 3 (Fair): Patient completes available range of motion.

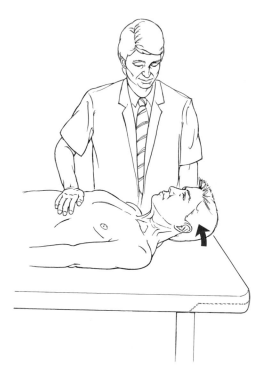

FIGURE 2–24

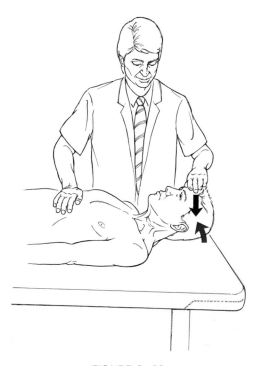

FIGURE 2–23

Grade 2 (Poor), Grade 1 (Trace), and Grade 0 (Zero)

Position of Patient: Supine with head supported on table. Arms at sides.

Position of Therapist: Standing at head of table facing patient. Fingers of both hands (or just the index finger) are placed over the Sternocleidomastoid muscles to palpate them during test (Fig. 2–25).

Test: Patient rolls head from side to side, keeping head supported on table.

Instructions to Patient: "Roll your head to the left and then to the right."

Grading

Grade 2 (Poor): Patient completes partial range of motion. The right Sternocleidomastoid produces the roll to the left side and vice versa.

Grade 1 (Trace): No motion occurs, but contractile activity in one or both muscles can be detected.

Grade 0 (Zero): No motion and no contractile activity detected.

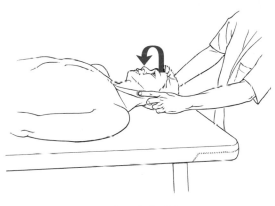

FIGURE 2–25

Substitution

The Platysma may attempt to substitute for weak or absent Sternocleidomastoid muscles during cervical or combined flexion. When this occurs, the corners of the mouth pull down; a grimacing expression or "What do I do now?" expression is seen. Superficial muscle activity will be apparent over the anterior surface of the neck, with skin wrinkling.

(Capital plus Cervical)

Grade 5 (Normal) and Grade 4 (Good)

Position of Patient: Supine with head supported on table. Arms at sides.

Position of Therapist: Standing at side of table at level of shoulder. Hand placed on forehead of patient to give resistance (Fig. 2–26). One arm may be used to provide stabilization of the thorax if there is trunk weakness. In such cases, the forearm is placed across the chest at the distal margin of the ribs. Although this arm does not offer resistance, considerable force may be required to maintain the trunk in a stable position. In a large patient, both arms may be required to provide such stabilization, the lower arm anchoring the pelvis. Examiner must use caution and not place too much weight or force over vulnerable nonbony areas like the abdomen.

Test: Patient flexes head and neck, bringing chin to chest.

Instructions to Patient: "Bring your head up until your chin is on your chest, and don't raise your shoulders. Hold it. Don't let me push it down."

Grading

Grade 5 (Normal): Patient completes available range of motion and tolerates strong resistance. (This combined flexion test is stronger than the capital or cervical component alone.)

Grade 4 (Good): Patient completes available range of motion and tolerates moderate resistance.

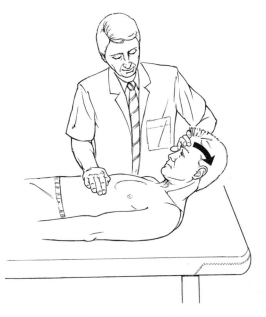

FIGURE 2–26

Grade 3 (Fair)

Position of Patient: Supine with head supported on table. Arms at sides.

Position of Therapist: Standing at side of table at about chest level. No resistance is given to the head motion. In the presence of trunk weakness, the thorax is stabilized.

Test: Patient flexes neck with chin tucked until the available range is completed (Fig. 2–27).

Instructions to Patient: "Bring your chin up on your chest. Don't raise your shoulders."

Grading

Grade 3 (Fair): Patient completes available range of motion without resistance.

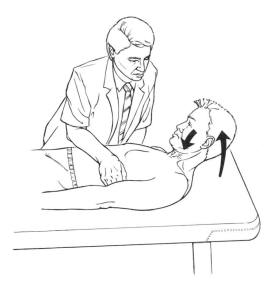

FIGURE 2–27

Grade 2 (Poor), Grade 1 (Trace), and Grade 0 (Zero)

Position of Patient: Supine with head fully supported on table. Arms at sides.

Position of Therapist: Standing at head of table facing the patient. Fingers of both hands, or preferably just the index finger, should be used to palpate the Sternocleidomastoid muscles bilaterally.

Test: Patient attempts to roll the head from side to side. The Sternocleidomastoid on one side rotates the head to the opposite side. Most of the capital flexors rotate the head to the same side.

Instructions to Patient: "Try to roll your head to the right and then back and all the way to the left."

Grading

Grade 2 (Poor): Patient completes partial range of motion.

Grade 1 (Trace): Muscle contractile activity palpated, but no motion occurs. Use considerable caution when palpating anterior neck.

Grade 0 (Zero): No palpable contractile activity.

Helpful Hints

If the capital flexor muscles are weak and the Sternocleidomastoid is relatively strong, the latter muscle action will increase the extension of the cervical spine because its posterior insertion on the mastoid process makes it a weak extensor. This is true only if the capital flexors are not active enough to pre-fix the head in flexion. When the capital flexors are normal, they fix the spine in flexion, and the Sternocleidomastoid functions in its flexor mode. If the capital flexors are weak, the head can be raised off the table, but it will be in a position of capital extension with the chin leading.

COMBINED FLEXION TO ISOLATE A SINGLE STERNOCLEIDOMASTOID

Range of Motion
0° to 45°–55°

This test should be performed when there is suspected or known asymmetry of strength in these neck flexor muscles.

Grade 5 (Normal), Grade 4 (Good), and Grade 3 (Fair)

Position of Patient: Supine with head supported on table and turned to the left (to test right Sternocleidomastoid).

Position of Therapist: Standing at head of table facing patient. One hand is placed on the temporal area above the ear for resistance (Fig. 2–28).

Test: Patient raises head from table.

Instructions to Patient: "Lift up your head, keeping your head turned."

Grading

Grade 5 (Normal): Patient completes available range of motion and takes strong resistance. This is usually a very strong muscle group.

Grade 4 (Good): Patient completes available range of motion and takes moderate resistance.

Grade 3 (Fair): Patient completes available range of motion with no resistance (Fig. 2–29).

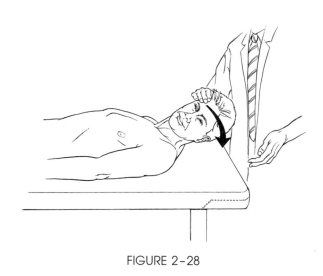

FIGURE 2–28

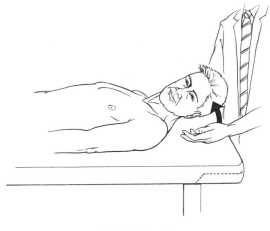

FIGURE 2–29

Grade 2 (Poor), Grade 1 (Trace), and Grade 0 (Zero)

Position of Patient: Supine with head supported on table.

Position of Therapist: Standing at head of table facing patient. Fingers are placed along the side of the head and neck so that they (or just the index finger) can palpate the Sternocleidomastoid (see Fig. 2–25).

Test: Patient attempts to roll head from side to side.

Instructions to Patient: "Roll your head to the right and then to the left."

Grading

Grade 2 (Poor): Patient completes partial range of motion.

Grade 1 (Trace): Palpable contractile activity in the Sternocleidomastoid, but no movement.

Grade 0 (Zero): No palpable contractile activity.

Grade 5 (Normal), Grade 4 (Good), and Grade 3 (Fair)

Position of Patient: Supine with cervical spine in neutral (flexion and extension). Head supported on table with face turned as far to one side as possible. Sitting is an alternative position for all tests.

Position of Therapist: Standing at head of table facing patient. Hand for resistance is placed over the side of head above ear. (Grades 5 and 4 only.)

Test: Patient rotates head to neutral against maximal resistance. This is a strong muscle group. Repeat for rotators on the opposite side. Alternatively, have patient rotate from left side of face on table to right side of face on table.

Instructions to Patient: "Turn your head and face the ceiling. Hold it. Do not let me turn your head back."

Grading

Grade 5 (Normal): Patient rotates head through full available range of motion to both right and left against maximal resistance.

Grade 4 (Good): Patient rotates head through full available range of motion to both right and left against moderate resistance.

Grade 3 (Fair): Patient rotates head through full available range to both right and left without resistance.

Grade 2 (Poor), Grade 1 (Trace), and Grade 0 (Zero)

Position of Patient: Sitting. Trunk and head may be supported against a high-back chair. Head posture neutral.

Position of Therapist: Standing directly in front of patient.

Test: Patient tries to rotate head from side to side, keeping the neck in neutral (chin neither down nor up).

Instructions to Patient: "Turn your head as far to the left as you can. Keep your chin level." Repeat for turn to right.

Grading

Grade 2 (Poor): Patient completes partial range of motion.

Grade 1 (Trace): Contractile activity in Sternocleidomastoid or posterior muscles visible or evident by palpation. No movement.

Grade 0 (Zero): No palpable contractile activity.

Participating Muscles in Cervical Rotation (with reference numbers)

56. Rectus capitis posterior major
59. Obliquus capitis inferior
60. Longissimus capitis
61. Splenius capitis
62. Semispinalis capitis
65. Semispinalis cervicis
67. Splenius cervicis
71. Rotatores cervicis
74. Longus capitis
79. Longus colli (Inferior oblique)
80. Scalenus anterior
81. Scalenus medius
82. Scalenus posterior
83. Sternocleidomastoid
124. Trapezius
127. Levator scapulae

References

Cited References

1. Perry J, Nickel VL. Total cervical spine fusion for neck paralysis. J Bone Joint Surg Am 41:37–60, 1959.
2. Fielding JW. Cineroentgenography of the normal cervical spine. J Bone Joint Surg Am 39:1280–1288, 1957.
3. Ferlic D. The range of motion of the "normal" cervical spine. Johns Hopkins Hosp Bull 110:59, 1962.

Other Readings

Eriksson PO, Zafar H, Nordh E. Concomitant mandibular and head-neck movements during jaw opening-closing in man. J Oral Rehabil 25:859–870, 1998.

Takebe K, Vitti M, Basmajian JV. The functions of semispinalis capitis and splenius capitis muscles: An electromyographic study. Anat Rec 179:477–480, 1974.

Zafar H, Nordh E, Eriksson PO. Temporal coordination between mandibular and head-neck movements during jaw opening-closing tasks in man. Arch Oral Biol 45:675–682, 2000.

CHAPTER 3

Testing
the Muscles
of the Trunk

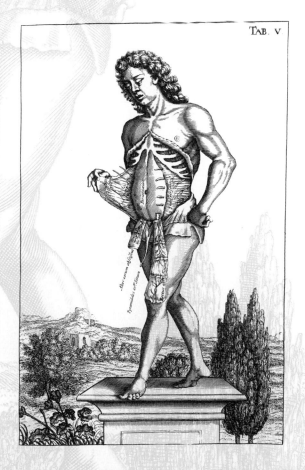

TAB. V

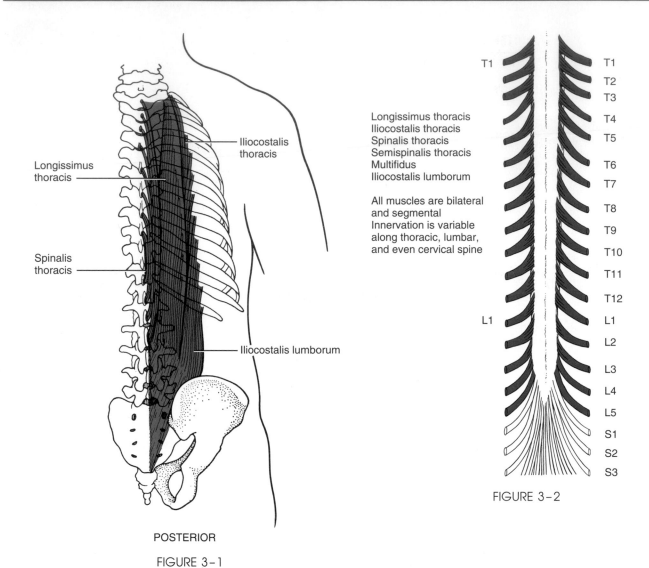

Iliocostalis
thoracis

Longissimus
thoracis

Spinalis
thoracis

Iliocostalis lumborum

Longissimus thoracis
Iliocostalis thoracis
Spinalis thoracis
Semispinalis thoracis
Multifidus
Iliocostalis lumborum

All muscles are bilateral
and segmental
Innervation is variable
along thoracic, lumbar,
and even cervical spine

T1 T1
T2
T3
T4
T5
T6
T7
T8
T9
T10
T11
T12
L1 L1
L2
L3
L4
L5
S1
S2
S3

FIGURE 3-2

POSTERIOR

FIGURE 3-1

Table 3-1 TRUNK EXTENSION

I.D.	Muscle	Origin	Insertion
89	Iliocostalis thoracis	Ribs 12 up to 7 (angles)	Ribs 6 up to 1 (angles) C7 vertebra (transverse processes)
90	Iliocostalis lumborum	Tendon of Erector spinae (anterior surface) Thoracolumbar fascia Iliac crest (external lip) Sacrum (posterior surface)	Ribs 6–12 (angles)
91	Longissimus thoracis	Tendon of Erector spinae Thoracolumbar fascia L1–L5 vertebrae (transverse processes)	T1–T12 vertebrae (transverse processes) Ribs 2–12 (between angles and tubercles)
92	Spinalis thoracis (often indistinct)	Common tendon of Erector spinae T11–L2 vertebrae (spinous processes)	T1–T4 vertebrae (or to T8, spinous processes) Blends with Semispinalis thoracis
93	Semispinalis thoracis	T6–T10 vertebrae (transverse processes)	C6–T4 vertebrae (spinous processes)
94	Multifidi	Sacrum (posterior) Erector spinae (aponeurosis) Ilium (PSIS) and crest Sacroiliac ligaments L1–L5 vertebrae (mamillary processes) T1–T12 vertebrae (transverse processes) C4–C7 vertebrae (articular processes)	Spinous processes of higher vertebra (may span 2–4 vertebrae before inserting)
95, 96	Rotatores thoracis and lumborum (11 pairs)	Thoracic and lumbar vertebrae (transverse processes; variable in lumbar area)	Next highest vertebra (lower border of lamina)
97, 98	Interspinales thoracis and lumborum	Thoracis: (3 pairs) between spinous processes of contiguous vertebrae (T1–T2; T2–T3; T11–T12) Lumborum: (4 pairs) lie between the 5 lumbar vertebrae; run between spinous processes	See origin
99	Intertransversarii thoracis and lumborum	Thoracis: (3 pairs) between transverse processes of contiguous vertebrae T10–T12 and L1 Lumborum: medial muscles; accessory process of superior vertebra to mamillary process of vertebra below Lateral muscles: fill space between transverse processes of adjacent vertebrae	See origin
100	Quadratus lumborum	Ilium (crest and inner lip) Iliolumbar ligament	12th rib (lower border) L1–L4 vertebrae (transverse processes) T12 vertebra (body)

Other

182	Gluteus maximus (provides stable base for trunk extension by stabilizing pelvis)		

LUMBAR SPINE

Grade 5 (Normal) and Grade 4 (Good)

Note: The Grade 5 and Grade 4 tests for spine extension are different for the lumbar and thoracic spines. Beginning at Grade 3, the tests for both levels are combined.

Position of Patient: Prone with hands clasped behind head.

Position of Therapist: Standing so as to stabilize the lower extremities just above the ankles if the patient has Normal hip strength (Fig. 3–3).

Alternate Position: Therapist stabilizes the lower extremities using body weight and both arms placed across the pelvis if the patient has hip extension weakness. It is very difficult to stabilize the pelvis adequately in the presence of significant hip weakness (Fig. 3–4).

Test: Patient extends the lumbar spine until the entire thorax is raised from the table (clears umbilicus).

Instructions to Patient: "Raise your head, shoulders, and chest off the table. Come up as high as you can."

Grading

Grade 5 (Normal) and Grade 4 (Good): The examiner distinguishes between Grade 5 and Grade 4 muscles by the nature of the response (see Figs. 3–3 and 3–4). The Grade 5 muscle holds like a lock; the Grade 4 muscle yields slightly because of an elastic quality at the end point. The patient with Normal back extensor muscles can quickly come to the end position and hold that position without evidence of significant effort. The patient with Grade 4 back extensors can come to the end position but may waver or display some signs of effort.

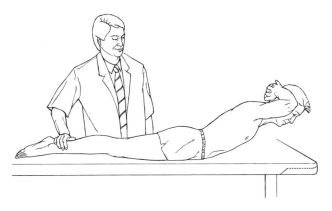

FIGURE 3–3

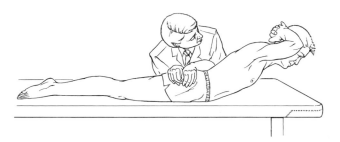

FIGURE 3–4

THORACIC SPINE

Grade 5 (Normal) and Grade 4 (Good)

Position of Patient: Prone with head and upper trunk extending off the table from about the nipple line (Fig. 3–5).

Position of Therapist: Standing so as to stabilize the lower limbs at the ankle.

Test: Patient extends thoracic spine to the horizontal.

Instructions to Patient: "Raise your head, shoulders, and chest to table level."

Grading

Grade 5 (Normal): Patient is able to raise the upper trunk quickly from its forward flexed position to the horizontal (or beyond) with ease and no sign of exertion (Fig. 3–6).

Grade 4 (Good): Patient is able to raise the trunk to the horizontal level but does it somewhat laboriously.

LUMBAR AND THORACIC SPINE

Grade 3 (Fair)

Position of Patient: Prone with arms at sides.

Position of Therapist: Standing at side of table. Lower extremities are stabilized just above the ankles.

Test: Patient extends spine, raising body from the table so that the umbilicus clears the table (Fig. 3–7).

Instructions to Patient: "Raise your head, arms, and chest from the table as high as you can."

Grading

Grade 3 (Fair): Patient completes the range of motion.

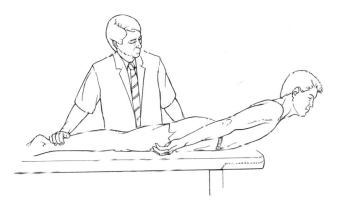

FIGURE 3–7

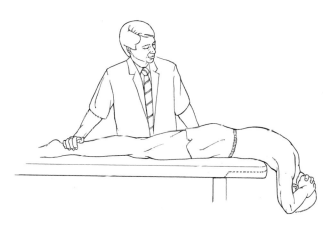

FIGURE 3–5

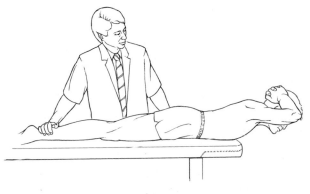

FIGURE 3–6

Grade 2 (Poor), Grade 1 (Trace), and Grade 0 (Zero)

These tests are identical to the Grade 3 test except that the examiner must palpate the lumbar and thoracic (Fig. 3–8 and 3–9) spine extensor muscle masses adjacent to both sides of the spine. The individual muscles cannot be isolated.

Grading

Grade 2 (Poor): Patient completes partial range of motion.

Grade 1 (Trace): Contractile activity is detectable but no movement.

Grade 0 (Zero): No contractile activity.

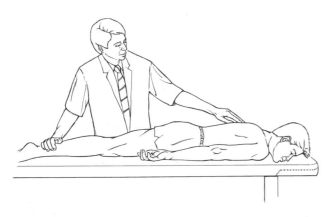

FIGURE 3–8

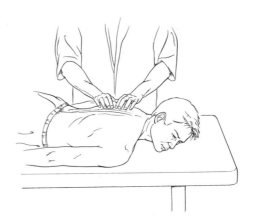

FIGURE 3–9

Helpful Hints

- Tests for hip extension and neck extension should precede tests for trunk extension.

  When the spine extensors are weak and the hip extensors are strong, the patient will be unable to raise the upper trunk from the table. Instead, the pelvis will tilt posteriorly while the lumbar spine moves into flexion (low back flattens).

  When the back extensors are strong and the hip extensors are weak, the patient can hyperextend the low back (increased lordosis) but will be unable to raise the trunk without very strong stabilization of the pelvis by the examiner.

- If the neck extensors are weak, the examiner may need to support the head as the patient raises the trunk.

- The position of the arms (clasped behind the head) provides added resistance for Grades 5 and 4; the weight of the head and arms essentially substitutes for manual resistance by the examiner.

- If the patient is a complete paraplegic, the test should be done on a mat table. Position the subject with both legs and pelvis off the mat. This allows the pelvis and limbs to contribute to stabilization, and the examiner holding the lower trunk has a chance to provide the necessary support. (If a mat table is not available, an assistant will be required, and the lower body may rest on a chair.)

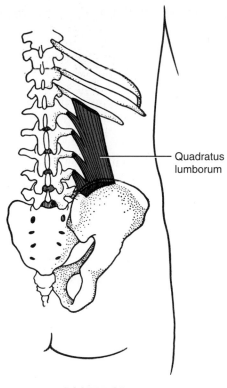

POSTERIOR

FIGURE 3-10

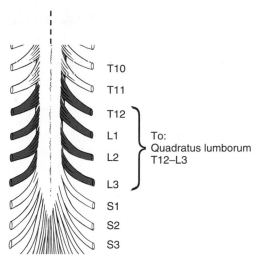

To:
Quadratus lumborum
T12–L3

FIGURE 3-11

Range of Motion
Approximates pelvis to lower ribs; range not precise

Table 3-2 ELEVATION OF THE PELVIS

I.D.	Muscle	Origin	Insertion
100	Quadratus lumborum	Ilium (crest and inner lip) Iliolumbar ligament	Rib 12 (lower border) L1–L4 vertebrae (transverse processes, apex) T12 vertebra (body; occasionally)
110	Obliquus externus abdominis	Ribs 5–12 (interdigitating on external and inferior surfaces)	Iliac crest (outer border) Linea alba Aponeurosis from 9th costal cartilage to ASIS; both sides meet at midline to form linea alba Pubic symphysis (upper border)
111	Obliquus internus abdominis	Iliac crest (anterior 2/3 of intermediate line) Thoracolumbar fascia Inguinal ligament (lateral 2/3 of upper aspect)	Ribs 9–12 (inferior border and cartilages by digitations that appear continuous with internal intercostals) Ribs 7–9 (cartilages) Aponeurosis to linea alba

Others

130	Latissimus dorsi (arms fixed)		
90	Iliocostalis lumborum		

Grade 5 (Normal) and Grade 4 (Good)

Position of Patient: Supine or prone with hip and lumbar spine in extension. The patient grasps edges of the table to provide stabilization during resistance (not illustrated).

Position of Therapist: Standing at foot of table facing patient. Therapist grasps test limb with both hands just above the ankle and pulls caudally with a smooth, even pull (Fig. 3–12). Resistance is given as in traction.

Test: Patient hikes the pelvis on one side, thereby approximating the pelvic rim to the inferior margin of the rib cage.

Instructions to Patient: "Hike your pelvis to bring it up to your ribs. Hold it. Don't let me pull your leg down."

Grading

Grade 5 (Normal): This motion, certainly not attributable solely to the Quadratus lumborum, is one that tolerates a huge amount of resistance that is not readily broken when the muscles involved are Normal.

Grade 4 (Good): Patient tolerates very strong resistance. Testing this movement requires more than a bit of clinical judgment.

Grade 3 (Fair) and Grade 2 (Poor)

Position of Patient: Supine or prone. Hip in extension; lumbar spine neutral or extended.

Position of Therapist: Standing at foot of table facing patient. One hand supports the leg just above the ankle; the other is under the knee so the limb is slightly off the table to decrease friction (Fig. 3–13).

Test: Patient hikes the pelvis unilaterally to bring the rim of the pelvis closer to the inferior ribs.

Instructions to Patient: "Bring your pelvis up to your ribs."

Grading

Grade 3 (Fair): Patient completes available range of motion.

Grade 2 (Poor): Patient completes partial range of motion.

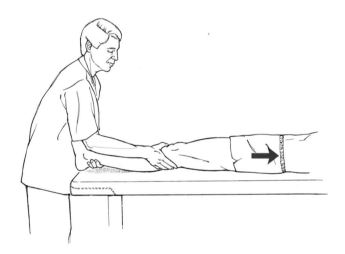

FIGURE 3–13

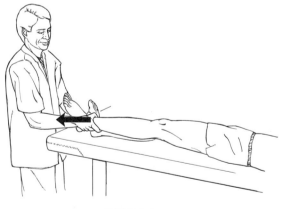

FIGURE 3–12

Grade 1 (Trace) and Grade 0 (Zero)

These grades should be avoided in the cause of clinical accuracy. The principal muscle to which pelvis elevation is attributable lies deep to the paraspinal muscle mass and can rarely be palpated. In persons who have extensive truncal atrophy or severe inanition, paraspinal muscle activity may be palpated, and possibly, but not necessarily convincingly, the Quadratus lumborum can be palpated.

Substitution

The patient may attempt to substitute with trunk lateral flexion, primarily using the abdominal muscles. The spinal extensors may be used without the Quadratus lumborum. In neither case can manual testing detect an inactive Quadratus lumborum.

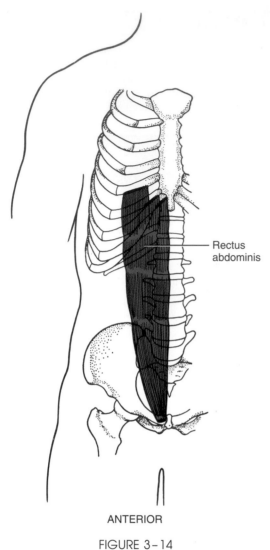

Rectus abdominis

ANTERIOR

FIGURE 3-14

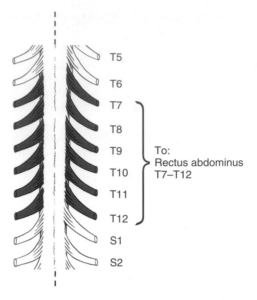

T5
T6
T7
T8
T9
T10
T11
T12
S1
S2

To:
Rectus abdominus
T7–T12

FIGURE 3-15

Range of Motion
0° to 80°

Table 3-3 TRUNK FLEXION

I.D.	Muscle	Origin	Insertion
113	Rectus abdominis (paired muscle)	Pubis Lateral fibers (tubercle on crest and pecten pubis) Medial fibers (ligamentous covering of symphysis to attach to contralateral muscle)	Ribs 5–7 (costal cartilages) Sternum (xiphoid ligaments)
110	Obliquus externus abdominis	Ribs 5–12 (interdigitating on external and inferior surfaces)	Iliac crest (outer border) Linea alba Aponeurosis from 9th costal cartilage to ASIS; both sides meet at midline to form linea alba
111	Obliquus internus abdominis	Iliac crest (anterior-2/3 of intermediate line) Thoracolumbar fascia Inguinal ligament (lateral 2/3 of upper aspect)	Ribs 9–12 (inferior border and cartilages by digitations that appear continuous with internal intercostals) Ribs 7–9 (cartilages) Aponeurosis to linea alba

Others

174	Psoas major		
175	Psoas minor		

Trunk flexion has multiple elements that include both thoracic and lumbar motion. Measurement is difficult at best and may be done in a variety of ways with considerable variability in results.

Tests for neck flexion should precede tests for trunk flexion. This will permit allowances to be made for neck weakness (should it exist), and support can be provided as required.

Grade 5 (Normal)

Position of Patient: Supine with hands clasped behind head (Fig. 3–16).

Position of Therapist: Standing at side of table at level of patient's chest to be able to ascertain whether scapulae clear table during test (see Fig. 3–16). For a patient with no other muscle weakness, the therapist does not need to touch the patient. If, however, the patient has weak hip flexors, the examiner should stabilize the pelvis by leaning across the patient on the forearms (Fig. 3–17).

Test: Patient flexes trunk through range of motion.

A curl-up is emphasized, and trunk is curled until scapulae clear table (Fig. 3–17).

Instructions to Patient: "Tuck your chin and bring your head, shoulders, and arms off the table, as in a sit-up."

Grading

Grade 5 (Normal): Patient completes range of motion until inferior angles of scapulae are off the table. (Weight of the arms serves as resistance.)

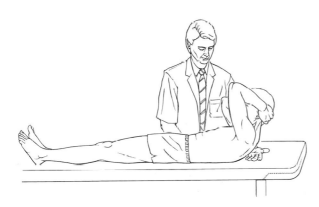

FIGURE 3–16

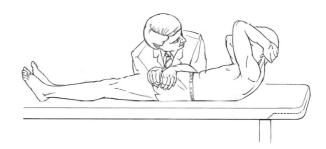

FIGURE 3–17

Grade 4 (Good)

Position of Patient: Supine with arms crossed over chest (Fig. 3–18).

Test: Other than patient's position, all other aspects of the test are the same as for Grade 5.

Grading

Grade 4 (Good): Patient completes range of motion and raises trunk until scapulae are off the table. Resistance of arms is reduced in the cross-chest position.

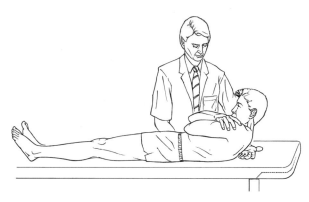

FIGURE 3–18

Grade 3 (Fair)

Position of Patient: Supine with arms outstretched in full extension above plane of body (Fig. 3–19).

Test: Other than patient's position, all other aspects of the test are the same as for Grade 5. Patient flexes trunk until inferior angles of scapulae are off the table. Position of the outstretched arms "neutralizes" resistance by bringing the weight of the arms closer to the center of gravity.

Instructions to Patient: "Raise your head, shoulders, and arms off the table."

Grading

Grade 3 (Fair): Patient completes range of motion and flexes trunk until inferior angles of scapulae are off the table.

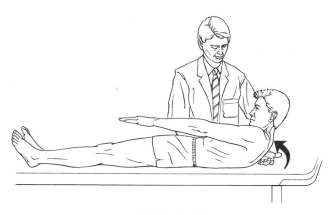

FIGURE 3–19

Grade 2 (Poor), Grade 1 (Trace), and Grade 0 (Zero)

Testing trunk flexion is rather clear-cut for Grades 5, 4, and 3. When testing Grade 2 and below, the results may be ambiguous, but observation and palpation are critical for defendable results. Sequentially from 2 to 0, the patient will be asked to raise the head (Grade 2), do an assisted forward lean (Grade 1), or cough (Grade 1).

If the abdominal muscles are weak, reverse action of the hip flexors may cause lumbar lordosis. When this occurs, the patient should be positioned with the hips flexed with feet flat on the table to disallow the hip flexors to contribute to the test motion.

Position of Patient: Supine with arms at sides. Knees flexed.

Position of Therapist: Standing at side of table. The hand used for palpation is placed at the midline of the thorax over the linea alba, and the four fingers of both hands are used to palpate the Rectus abdominis (Fig. 3–20).

Test and Instructions to Patient: The examiner tests for Grades 2, 1, and 0 in a variety of ways to make certain that muscle contractile activity that may be present is not missed.

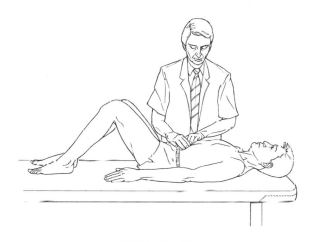

FIGURE 3–20

Grading

Sequence 1: Head raise (Fig. 3–21): Ask the patient to lift the head from the table. If the scapulae do not clear the table, the grade is 2 (Poor). If the patient cannot lift the head, proceed to Sequence 2.

Sequence 2: Assisted forward lean (Fig. 3–22): The examiner cradles the upper trunk and head off the table and asks the patient to lean forward. If there is depression of the rib cage, the grade is 2 (Poor). If there is no depression of the rib cage but visible or palpable contraction occurs, the grade assigned should be 1 (Trace). If there is no activity, the grade is 0; proceed to Sequence 3.

Sequence 3: Cough (Fig. 3–23): Ask the patient to cough. If he can cough to any degree and depression of the rib cage occurs, the grade is 2 (Poor). (If the patient coughs, regardless of its effectiveness, the abdominal muscles are automatically brought into play.) If the patient cannot cough but there is palpable Rectus abdominis activity, the grade is 1 (Trace). Lack of any demonstrable activity is grade 0 (Zero).

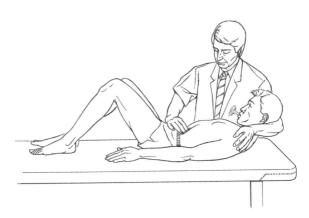

FIGURE 3–23

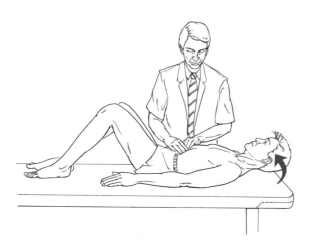

FIGURE 3–21

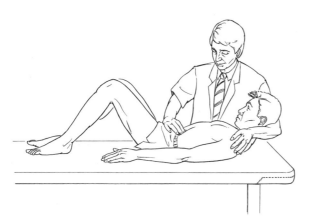

FIGURE 3–22

Helpful Hints

- In all tests observe any deviations of the umbilicus. (This is not to be confused with the response to light stroking, which elicits superficial reflex activity.) In response to muscle testing, if there is a difference in the segments of the Rectus abdominis, the umbilicus will deviate toward the stronger part (i.e., cranially if the upper parts are stronger, caudally if the lower parts are stronger).

- If the extensor muscles of the lumbar spine are weak, contraction of the abdominal muscles can cause posterior tilt of the pelvis. If this situation exists, tension of the hip flexor muscles would be useful to stabilize the pelvis; and, therefore, the examiner should position the patient in hip extension.

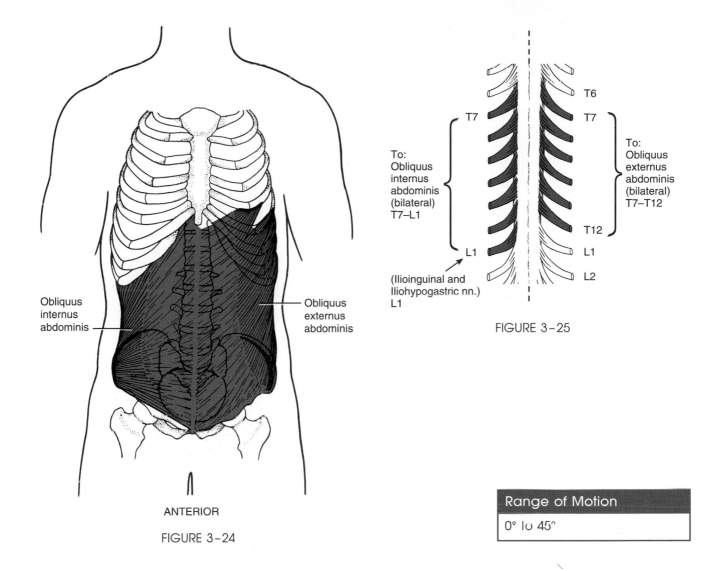

Obliquus internus abdominis

Obliquus externus abdominis

ANTERIOR

FIGURE 3–24

To:
Obliquus
internus
abdominis
(bilateral)
T7–L1

T7

L1

(Ilioinguinal and
Iliohypogastric nn.)
L1

T6
T7

To:
Obliquus
externus
abdominis
(bilateral)
T7–T12

T12

L1

L2

FIGURE 3–25

Range of Motion

0° to 45°

Table 3-4 TRUNK ROTATION

I.D.	Muscle	Origin	Insertion
110	Obliquus externus abdominis	Ribs 5–12 (interdigitating on external and inferior surfaces)	Iliac crest (outer border) Thoracolumbar fascia Linea alba Aponeurosis from 9th costal cartilage to ASIS; both sides meet at midline to form linea alba Pubic symphysis (upper border)
111	Obliquus internus abdominis	Iliac crest (anterior 2/3 of intermediate line) Thoracolumbar fascia Inguinal ligament (lateral 2/3 of upper aspect)	Ribs 9–12 (inferior border and cartilages by digitations that appear continuous with internal intercostals) Aponeurosis of Transverse abdominis to crest of pecten pubis to form falx inguinalis Inguinal ligament Linea alba Ribs 7–9 (cartilages)

Other

Deep back muscles
(one side)

Grade 5 (Normal)

Position of Patient: Supine with hands clasped behind head.

Position of Therapist: Standing at patient's waist level.

Test: Patient flexes trunk and rotates to one side. This movement is then repeated on the opposite side so that the muscles on both sides can be examined.

Right elbow to left knee tests the right external obliques and the left internal obliques (Fig. 3–26). Left elbow to right knee tests the left external obliques and the right internal obliques (Fig. 3–27). When the patient rotates to one side, the internal oblique muscle is palpated on the side toward the turn; the external oblique muscle is palpated on the side away from the direction of turning.

Substitution

If the Pectoralis major is active (inappropriately) in this test of trunk rotation at any grade, the shoulder will shrug or be raised from the table, and there is limited rotation of the trunk.

Instructions to Patient: "Lift your head and shoulders from the table, taking your right elbow toward your left knee." Then, "Lift your head and shoulders from the table, taking your left elbow toward your right knee."

Grading

Grade 5 (Normal): The scapula corresponding to the side of the external oblique function must clear the table for a Normal grade.

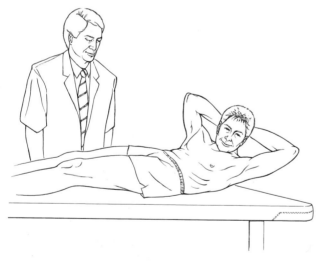

FIGURE 3–26

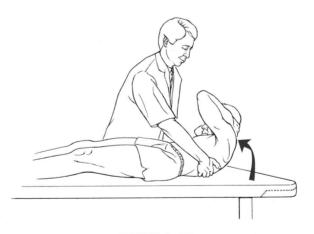

FIGURE 3–27

Grade 4 (Good)

Position of Patient. Supine with arms crossed over chest.

Test: Other than patient's position, all other aspects of the test are the same as for Grade 5. The test is done first to one side Fig. 3–28 and then to the other (Fig. 3–29).

Grade 3 (Fair)

Position of Patient: Supine with arms outstretched above plane of body.

Test: Position of therapist and instructions are the same as for Grade 5. The test is done first to the left (Fig. 3–30) and then to the right (Fig. 3–31).

Grading

Grade 3 (Fair): Patient is able to raise the scapula off the table. The therapist may use one hand to check for scapular clearance (see Fig. 3–31).

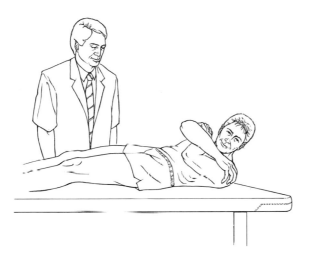

FIGURE 3–28

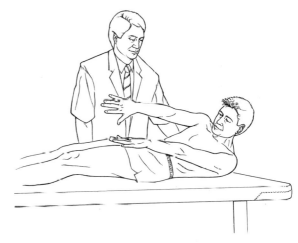

FIGURE 3–30

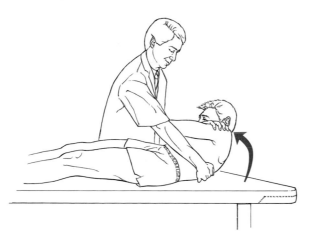

FIGURE 3–29

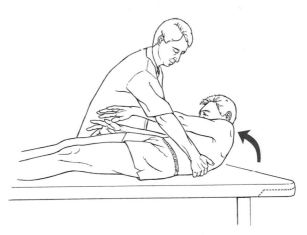

FIGURE 3–31

Grade 2 (Poor)

Position of Patient: Supine with arms outstretched above plane of body.

Position of Therapist: Standing at level of patient's waist. Therapist palpates the external oblique first on one side and then on the other, with one hand placed on the lateral part of the anterior abdominal wall distal to the rib cage (Fig. 3–32). Continue to palpate the muscle distally in the direction of its fibers until reaching the anterior superior iliac spine (ASIS).

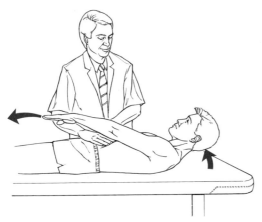

FIGURE 3–32

At the same time, the internal oblique muscle on the opposite side of the trunk is palpated. The internal oblique muscle lies under the external oblique, and its fibers run in the opposite diagonal direction.

Examiners may remember this palpation procedure better if they think of positioning their two hands as if both hands were to be in the pants pockets or grasping the abdomen in pain. (The external obliques run from out to in; the internal obliques run from in to out.)

Instructions to Patient: "Lift your head and reach toward your right knee." (Repeat to left side for the opposite muscle.)

Test: Patient attempts to raise body and turn toward the right. Repeat toward left side.

Grading

Grade 2 (Poor): Patient is unable to clear the inferior angle of the scapula from the table on the side of the external oblique being tested. The examiner must, however, be able to observe depression of the rib cage during the test activity.

Grade 1 (Trace) and Grade 0 (Zero)

Position of Patient: Supine with arms at sides. Hips flexed with feet flat on table.

Position of Therapist: Head is supported as patient attempts to turn to one side (Fig. 3–33). (Turn to the other side in a subsequent test.) Under normal conditions, the abdominal muscles stabilize the trunk when the head is lifted. In patients with abdominal weakness, the supported head permits the patient to bring in abdominal muscle activity without having to overcome the entire weight of the head.

One hand palpates the internal obliques on the side toward which the patient turns (not illustrated) and the external obliques on the side away from the direction of turning (see Fig. 3–33). The therapist assists the patient to raise the head and shoulders slightly and turn to one side. This procedure is used when abdominal muscle weakness is profound.

Instructions to Patient: "Try to lift up and turn to your right." (Repeat for turn to the left.)

Test: Patient attempts to flex trunk and turn to either side.

Grading

Grade 1 (Trace): The examiner can see or palpate muscular contraction.

Grade 0 (Zero): No response from the Obliquus internus or externus muscles.

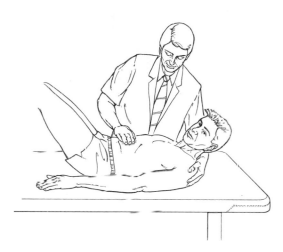

FIGURE 3–33

Helpful Hints

- In all tests observe any deviation of the umbilicus, which will move toward the strongest quadrant when there is unequal strength in the opposing oblique muscles.

- Flaring of the rib cage denotes weakness of the external oblique muscles.

- If the hip flexor muscles are weak, the examiner must stabilize the pelvis.

- To cause the abdominals to come into action automatically, the examiner may resist a downward diagonal motion of the arm or a downward and outward movement of the lower limb.

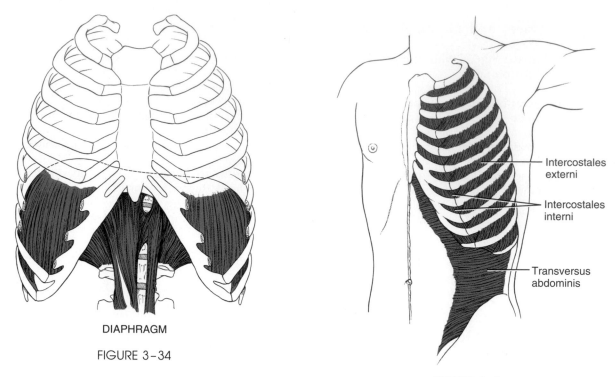

DIAPHRAGM

FIGURE 3-34

Intercostales externi

Intercostales interni

Transversus abdominis

FIGURE 3-35

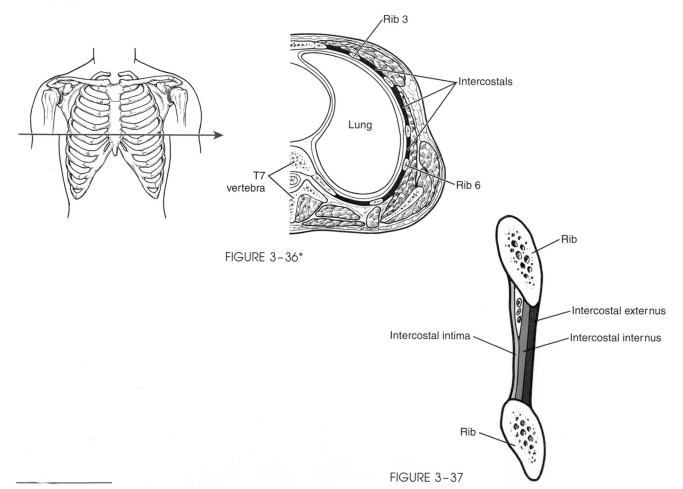

Rib 3

Intercostals

Lung

T7 vertebra

Rib 6

FIGURE 3-36*

Rib

Intercostal externus

Intercostal intima

Intercostal internus

Rib

FIGURE 3-37

* Note: Arrow indicates level of cross section.

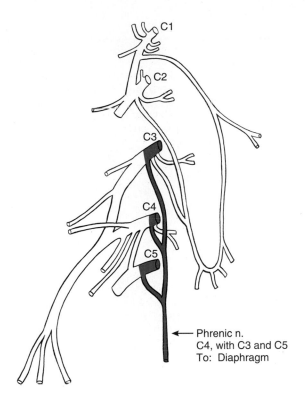

Phrenic n.
C4, with C3 and C5
To: Diaphragm

FIGURE 3–38A

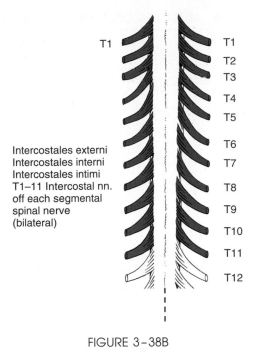

Intercostales externi
Intercostales interni
Intercostales intimi
T1–11 Intercostal nn.
off each segmental
spinal nerve
(bilateral)

FIGURE 3–38B

Range of Motion

Normal range of motion of the chest wall during quiet inspiration is about 0.75 inch (3/4"), with gender variations. Normal chest expansion in forced inspiration varies from 2.0 to 2.5 inches at the level of the xiphoid.[1]

Table 3-5 MUSCLES OF QUIET INSPIRATION

I.D.	Muscle	Origin	Insertion
101	Diaphragm (formed of 3 parts from the circumference of thoracic outlet)		Fibers all converge on central tendon of diaphragm; middle of central tendon is below and partially blended with pericardium
	Sternal	Xiphoid process (posterior)	
	Costal	Ribs 7–12 (internal surfaces of costal cartilages and ribs on each side) Interdigitates with Transversus abdominis	
	Lumbar	Medial and lateral arcuate ligaments (aponeurotic arches) L1–L2 (left crus, bodies) L1–L3 (right crus, bodies)	
102	Intercostales externi (11 pairs)	Ribs 1–11 (lower borders and tubercles; costal cartilages)	Ribs 2–12 (upper margins of rib below; last two end in free ends of the costal cartilages) External intercostal membrane
103	Intercostales interni (11 pairs)	Sternum (anterior) Ribs 1–11 (ridge on inner surface) Costal cartilages of same rib Internal intercostal membrane	Upper border of rib below Fibers run obliquely to the external intercostals
104	Intercostales intimi (innermost intercostals) Often absent	Ribs 1–11 (costal groove)	Rib below (upper margin) Fibers run in same pattern as internal intercostals
107	Levator costarum (12 pairs)	C7–T11 vertebrae (transverse processes, tip)	Rib below vertebra of origin (external surface)
80	Scalenus anterior	C3–C6 vertebrae (transverse processes, anterior tubercles)	1st rib (scalene tubercle)
81	Scalenus medius	C2 (axis)–C7 vertebrae (transverse processes, posterior tubercles) C1 (atlas) sometimes	1st rib (superior surface)
82	Scalenus posterior	C4–C6 vertebrae (transverse processes posterior tubercle, variable)	2nd rib (outer surface)

Other

Pectoralis major (arms fixed)

QUIET INSPIRATION

Diaphragm and Intercostals

Preliminary Examination
Uncover the patient's chest and abdominal areas so that the motions of the chest and abdominal walls can be observed. Watch the normal respiration pattern and observe differences in the motion of the chest wall and epigastric area and note any contraction of the neck muscles and the abdominal muscles.

Epigastric rise and flaring of the lower margin of the rib cage during inspiration indicate that the Diaphragm is active. The rise on both sides of the linea alba should be symmetrical. During quiet inspiration, epigastric rise reflects the movement of the Diaphragm descending over one intercostal space.[2,3] In deeper inspiratory efforts the Diaphragm may move across three or more intercostal spaces.

An elevation and lateral expansion of the rib cage are indicative of intercostal activity during inspiration. Exertional chest expansion measured at the level of the xiphoid process is 2.0 to 2.5 inches (the expansion may exceed 3.0 inches in more active young people and athletes).[1]

THE DIAPHRAGM

All Grades (5 to 0)

Position of Patient: Supine.

Position of Therapist: Standing next to patient at approximately waist level. One hand is placed lightly on the abdomen in the epigastric area just below the xiphoid process (Fig. 3–39). Resistance is given (by same hand) in a downward direction.

Test: Patient inhales with maximal effort and holds maximal inspiration.

Instructions to Patient: "Take a deep breath . . . as much as you can . . . hold it. Push against my hand. Don't let me push you down."

Grading

Grade 5 (Normal): Patient completes full inspiratory (epigastric) excursion and holds against maximal resistance. A Grade 5 Diaphragm takes high resistance in the range of 100 pounds.[4]

Grade 4 (Good): Completes maximal inspiratory excursion but yields against heavy resistance.

Grade 3 (Fair): Completes maximal inspiratory expansion but cannot tolerate manual resistance.

Grade 2 (Poor): Observable epigastric rise without completion of full inspiratory expansion.

Grade 1 (Trace): Palpable contraction is detected under the inner surface of the lower ribs, provided the abdominal muscles are relaxed (Fig. 3–40). Another way to detect minimal epigastric motion is by instructing the patient to "sniff" with the mouth closed.

Grade 0 (Zero): No epigastric rise and no palpable contraction of the diaphragm occur.

Substitution

Patient may attempt to substitute for an inadequate Diaphragm by hyperextending the lumbar spine in an effort to increase the response to the examiner's manual resistance.[4] The abdominal muscles also may contract, but both motions are improper attempts to follow the instruction to push up against the examiner's hand.

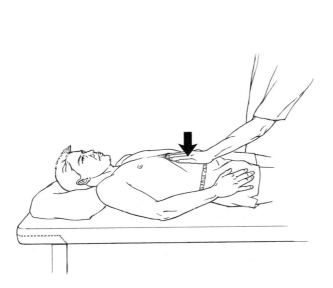

FIGURE 3–39

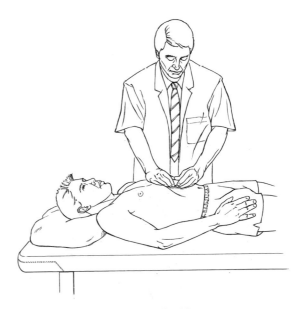

FIGURE 3–40

THE INTERCOSTALS

There is no method of direct assessment of the strength of the intercostal muscles. An indirect method measures the difference in magnitude of chest excursion between maximal inspiration and the girth of the chest at the end of full expiration.

Grades

There are no classic 5 to 0 grades given for the intercostal muscles. Instead, a flexible metal or new cloth tape is used to measure chest expansion.

Position of Patient: Supine on a firm surface. Arms at sides.

Position of Therapist: Standing at side of table. Tape measure placed lightly around thorax at level of xiphoid.

Test: Patient holds maximal inspiration for measurement and then holds maximal expiration for a second measurement. (A pneumograph may be used for the same purpose if one is available.) The difference between the two measurements is recorded as chest expansion.

Instructions to Patient: "Take a big breath in and hold it. Now blow it all out and hold it."

Coughing often is used as the clinical test for forced expiration. An effective cough requires the use of all muscles of active expiration in contrast to quiet expiration, which is the passive relaxation of the muscles of inspiration. It must be recognized, however, that a patient may not have an effective cough because of inadequate laryngeal control (refer to Chapter 7, Muscles of the Larynx) or low vital capacity.

Grades

The usual muscle test grades do not apply here, and the following scale to assess cough is used.

Functional: Normal or only slight impairment:
- Crisp or explosive expulsion of air
- Volume is sharp and clearly audible
- Able to clear airway of secretions

Weak Functional: Moderate impairment that affects the degree of active motion or endurance:
- Decreased volume and diminished air movement
- Appears labored
- May take several attempts to clear airway

Nonfunctional: Severe impairment:
- No clearance of airway
- No expulsion of air
- Cough attempt may be nothing more than an effort to clear the throat

Zero: Cough is absent.

Table 3-6 MUSCLES OF FORCED EXPIRATION

I.D.	Muscle	Origin	Insertion
110	Obliquus externus abdominis	Ribs 5–12 (interdigitating on external and inferior surfaces)	Iliac crest (outer border) Linea alba Aponeurosis from 9th costal cartilage to ASIS; both sides meet at midline to form linea alba Pubic symphysis (upper border)
111	Obliquus Internus abdominis	Iliac crest (anterior 2/3 of intermediate line) Thoracolumbar fascia Inguinal ligament (lateral 2/3 of upper aspect)	Ribs 9–12 (inferior border and cartilages by digitations that appear continuous with internal intercostals) Ribs 7–9 (cartilages) Aponeurosis to linea alba Pubic crest and pecten pubis
112	Transverse abdominis	Inguinal ligament (lateral 1/3) Iliac crest (anterior 2/3, inner lip) Thoracolumbar fascia Ribs 7–12 (costal cartilages interdigitate with diaphragm)	Linea alba (blends with broad aponeurosis) Pubic crest and pecten pubis (to form falx inguinalis)
113	Rectus abdominis	Arises via two tendons: Lateral: pubic crest (tubercle) and pecten pubis. Medial: symphysis pubis (ligamentous covering)	Ribs 5–7 (costal cartilages) Costoxiphoid ligaments
103	Intercostales interni	Ribs 1–11 (inner surface) Sternum (anterior) Internal intercostal membrane	Ribs 2–12 (upper border of rib below rib of origin)
130	Latissimus dorsi	T6–T12 and all lumbar and sacral vertebrae. (spinous processes via supraspinous ligaments) Iliac crest (posterior) Thoracolumbar fascia Ribs 9–12 (interdigitates with external abdominal oblique)	Humerus (floor of intertubercular sulcus) Deep fascia of arm

Other

| 106 | Transversus thoracis | | |

The Functional Anatomy of Coughing

Cough is an essential procedure to maintain airway patency and to clear the pharynx and bronchial tree when secretions accumulate. A cough may be a reflex or voluntary response to irritation anywhere along the airway downstream from the nose.

The cough reflex occurs as a result of stimulation of the mucous membranes of the pharynx, larynx, trachea, or bronchial tree. These tissues are so sensitive to light touch that any foreign matter or other irritation initiates the cough reflex. The sensory (afferent) limb of the reflex carries the impulses set up by the irritation via the glossopharyngeal and vagus cranial nerves to the fasciculus solitarius in the medulla, from which the motor impulses (efferent) then move out to the muscles of the pharynx, palate, tongue, and larynx and to the muscles of the abdominal wall and chest and the diaphragm. The reflex response is a deep inspiration (about 2.5 liters of air) followed quickly by a forced expiration, during which the glottis closes momentarily, trapping air in the lungs.[5] The diaphragm contracts spasmodically, as do the abdominal muscles and intercostal muscles. This raises the intrathoracic pressure (to above 200 mmHg) until the vocal cords are forced open, and the explosive outrush of air expels mucus and foreign matter. The expiratory airflow at this time may reach a velocity of 75 mph or higher.[5] Important to the reflex action is that the bronchial tree and laryngeal walls collapse because of the strong compression of the lungs, causing an invagination so that the high linear velocity of the airflow moving past and through these tissues dislodges mucus or foreign particles, thus producing an effective cough.

The three phases of cough—inspiration, compression, and forced expiration—are mediated by the muscles of the thorax and abdomen as well as those of the pharynx, larynx, and tongue. The deep inspiratory effort is supported by the Diaphragm, intercostals, and arytenoid abductor muscles (the posterior cricoarytenoids), permitting inhalation of upward of 1.5 liters of air.[6] The Palatoglossus and Styloglossus elevate the tongue and close off the oropharynx from the nasopharynx.

The compression phase requires the lateral cricoarytenoid muscles to adduct and close the glottis.

The strong expiratory movement is augmented by strong contractions of the thorax muscles, particularly the Latissimus dorsi and the oblique and transverse abdominal muscles. The abdominal muscles raise intra-abdominal pressure, forcing the relaxing Diaphragm up and drawing the lower ribs down and medially. Elevation of the Diaphragm raises the intrathoracic pressure to about 200 mmHg, and the explosive expulsion phase begins with forced abduction of the glottis.

References

Cited References

1. Carlson B. Normal chest excursion. Phys Ther 53:10–14, 1973.
2. Wade OL. Movements of the thoracic cage and diaphragm in respiration. J Physiol (Lond) 124:193–212, 1954.
3. Stone DJ, Keltz H. Effect of respiratory muscle dysfunction on pulmonary function. Am Rev Respir Dis 88:621–629, 1964.
4. Dail, CW. Muscle breathing patterns. Med Art Sci 10:2–8, 1956.
5. Guyton AC, Hall JE. Textbook of Medical Physiology, 10th ed. Philadelphia: W.B. Saunders, 2000.
6. Starr JA. Manual techniques of chest physical therapy and airway clearance techniques. *In* Zadai CC. Pulmonary Management in Physical Therapy. New York: Churchill-Livingstone, 1992.

Frownfelter DL. Chest Physical Therapy and Pulmonary Rehabilitation. Chicago: Year Book, 1987.
Frownfelter DL. Principles and Practices of Cardiopulmonary Physical Therapy, 3rd ed. St Louis: CV Mosby, 1996.
Irwin S, Tecklin JS. Cardiopulmonary Physical Therapy. St Louis: CV Mosby, 1995.
Polkey MI, Harris ML, Hughes PD, et al. The contractile properties of the elderly human diaphragm. Am J Respir Crit Care Med 155:1560–1564, 1997.
Waters RL, Morris JM. Electrical activity of muscles of the trunk during walking. J Anat 111:191–199, 1972.

Other Readings

Catton WT, Gray JE. Electromyographic study of the action of the serratus anterior in respiration. J Anat 85:412P, 1951.
Donisch EW, Basmajian JV. Electromyography of deep back muscles in man. Am J Anat 133:25–36, 1972.

CHAPTER 4

Testing the Muscles of the Upper Extremity

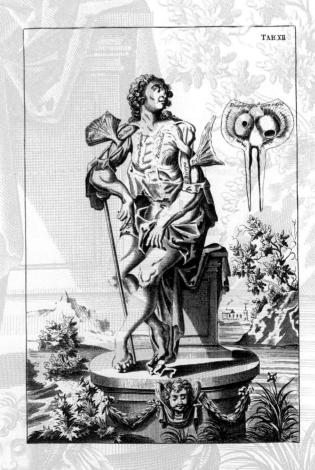

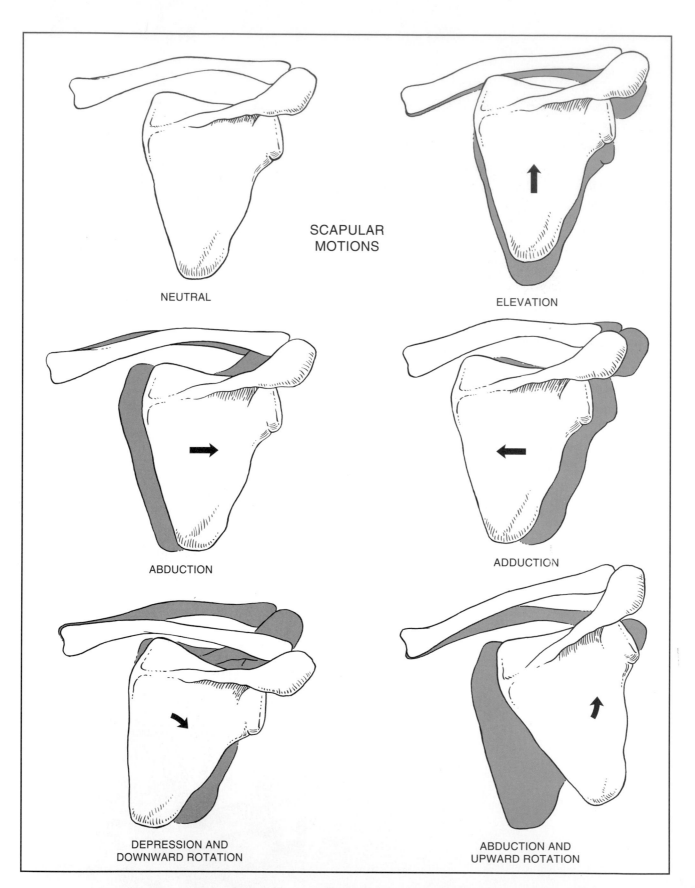

SCAPULAR MOTIONS

NEUTRAL

ELEVATION

ABDUCTION

ADDUCTION

DEPRESSION AND
DOWNWARD ROTATION

ABDUCTION AND
UPWARD ROTATION

PLATE 2

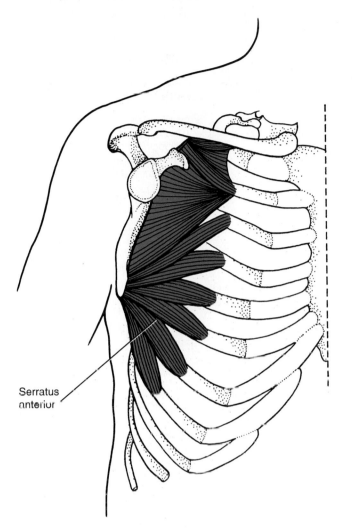

Serratus
anterior

FIGURE 4-1

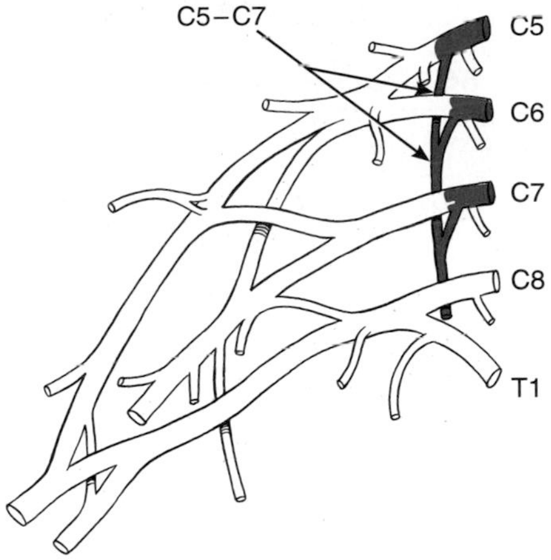

Long thoracic n.
To: Serratus anterior
C5–C7

C5
C6
C7
C8
T1

FIGURE 4-2

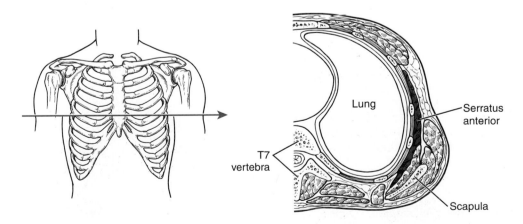

Lung

Serratus
anterior

T7
vertebra

Scapula

FIGURE 4-3

Note: arrow indicates level of cross section.

(Serratus anterior)

Table 4-1 SCAPULAR ABDUCTION AND UPWARD ROTATION

I.D.	Muscle	Origin	Insertion
128	Serratus anterior	Ribs 1–8 and often 9 and 10 (by digitations along a curved line) Intercostal fascia Aponeurosis of intercostals	Scapula (ventral surface of vertebral border) 1st digitation (superior angle) 2nd to 4th digitations (costal surface of entire vertebral border) Lower 4th or 5th digitations (costal surface of inferior angle)
Other			
129	Pectoralis minor		(See also Plate 3, page 85.)

The Serratus often is graded incorrectly, perhaps because the muscle arrangement and the bony movement are unlike those of axial structures. The test procedure here is recommended as sound in that it is in keeping with known kinesiologic and pathokinesiologic principles. The scapular muscles, however, do need further dynamic testing with electromyography (EMG), magnetic resonance imaging (MRI), and other modern technology before completely reliable functional diagnoses can be made.

The supine position, although best for isolating the Serratus, is not recommended at any grade level. The supine position allows too much substitution that may not be noticeable. The table gives added stabilization to the scapula so that it does not "wing" and protraction of the arm may be performed by the Pectoralis minor, Levator scapulae, or Rhomboids.

Preliminary Examination

Observation of the scapulae, both at rest and during active and passive shoulder flexion, is a routine part of the test. Examine the patient in short sitting position with hands in lap.

Palpate the vertebral borders of both scapulae with the thumbs; place the web of the thumb below the inferior angle; the fingers extend around the axillary borders (Fig. 4–4).

Specific Elements

1. *Position and symmetry of scapula.* Determine the position of the scapulae at rest and whether the two sides are symmetrical.

   The normal scapula lies close to the rib cage with the vertebral border nearly parallel to and from 1 to 3 inches lateral to the spinous processes. The inferior angle is tucked in. If the inferior angle of the scapula is tilted away from the rib cage, check for tightness of the Pectoralis minor, weakness of the Trapezius, and spinal deformity.

   The most prominent abnormal posture of the scapula is "winging," in which the vertebral border tilts away from the rib cage, a sign indicative of Serratus weakness. Other abnormal postures are adduction and downward rotation.

2. *Scapular range of motion.* Within the total arc of 180° of shoulder forward flexion, 120° is glenohumeral motion, and 60° is scapular motion. This

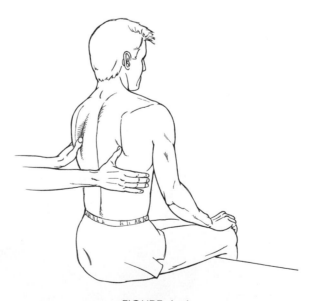

FIGURE 4-4

Preliminary Examination Continued

is true, however, if the two motions are considered as isolated functions, but they do not work as such. It would be more correct to say that the glenohumeral and scapular motions are in synchrony after 60° and up to 150°.

Passively raise the test arm in forward flexion completely above the head to determine scapular mobility. The scapula should start to rotate at about 60°, although there is considerable individual variation. Scapular rotation continues until about −20° to 30° from full flexion.

Check that the scapula basically remains in its rest position at ranges of shoulder flexion less than 60° (the position is variable among subjects). If the scapula moves as the glenohumeral joint moves below 60°, that is, if in this range they move as a unit, there is limited glenohumeral motion. Above 60° and to about 150° or 160° in both active and passive motion, the scapula moves in concert with the humerus.

3. *The Serratus always should be tested in shoulder flexion to minimize the synergy with the Trapezius.* If the scapular position at rest is normal, ask the patient to raise the test arm above the head in the sagittal plane. If the arm can be raised well above 90° (glenohumeral muscles must be at least Grade 3), observe the direction and amount of scapular motion that occurs. Normally, the scapula rotates forward in a motion that is controlled by the Serratus, and if erratic or "discoordinate" motion occurs, the Serratus is most likely weak. The normal amount of motion of the vertebral border from the start position is about the breadth of two fingers (Fig. 4-5). If the patient is able to raise the arm with simultaneous rhythmical scapular upward rotation, proceed with the test sequence for Grades 5 and 4.

4. *Scapula abnormal position at rest.* If the scapula is positioned abnormally at rest (i.e., adducted or

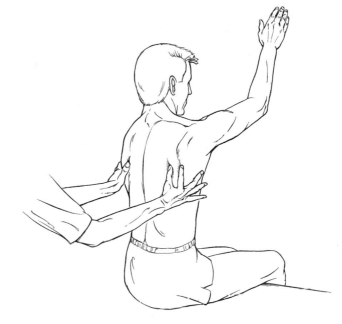

FIGURE 4-5

winging), the patient will not be able to flex the arm above 90°. Proceed to tests described for Grades 2, 1, and 0.

The Serratus anterior never can be graded higher than the grade given to shoulder flexion. If the patient has a weak Deltoid, the lever for testing is gone, and the arm cannot be used to apply resistance.

5. *Presence of a weak Triceps brachii.* If the Triceps is weak, supinate the forearm, or manually assist the elbow to maintain its extended position. In either case, do not assist humeral flexion.

(Serratus anterior)

Grade 5 (Normal) and Grade 4 (Good)

Position of Patient (All Grades): Short sitting, over end or side of table. Hands on lap.

Position of Therapist: Standing at test side of patient. Hand giving resistance is on the arm proximal to the elbow (Fig. 4–6). The other hand uses the web space along with the thumb and index finger to palpate the edges of the scapula at the inferior angle and along the vertebral and axillary borders.

Test: Patient raises arm to approximately 130° of flexion with the elbow extended. (Examiner is reminded that the arm can be elevated up to 60° without using the Serratus.) The scapula should upwardly rotate (glenoid facing up) and abduct without winging.

Instructions to Patient: "Raise your arm forward over your head. Keep your elbow straight; hold it! Don't let me push your arm down."

Grading

Grade 5 (Normal): Scapula maintains its abducted and rotated position against maximal resistance given on the arm just above the elbow in a downward direction.

Grade 4 (Good): Scapular muscles "give" or "yield" against maximal resistance given on the arm. The glenohumeral joint is held rigidly in the presence of a strong Deltoid, but the Serratus yields, and the scapula moves in the direction of adduction and downward rotation.

Grade 3 (Fair)

Positions of Patient and Therapist: Same as for Grade 5 test.

Test: Patient raises the arm to approximately 130° of flexion with elbow extended (Fig. 4–7).

Instructions to Patient: "Raise your arm forward above your head."

Grading

Grade 3 (Fair): Scapula moves through full range of motion without winging but can tolerate no resistance other than the weight of the arm.

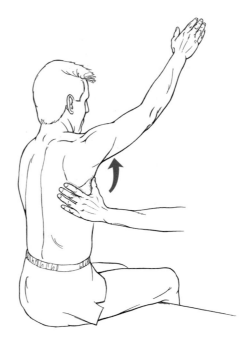

FIGURE 4–7

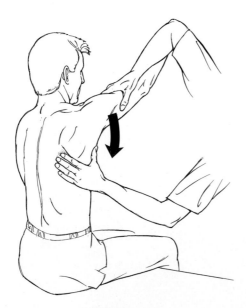

FIGURE 4–6

Alternate Test (Grades 5, 4, and 3)

Position of Patient: Short sitting with arm forward flexed to about 130° and then protracted in that plane as far as it can move.

Position of Therapist: Standing at test side of patient. Hand used for resistance grasps the forearm just above the wrist and gives resistance in a downward and backward direction. The other hand stabilizes the trunk just below the scapula on the same side; this prevents trunk rotation.

The examiner should select a spot on the wall or ceiling that can serve as a target for the patient to reach toward in line with about 130° of flexion.

Test: Patient abducts and upwardly rotates the scapula by protracting and elevating the arm to about 130° of flexion. The patient then holds against maximal resistance.

Instructions to Patient: "Bring your arm up, and reach for the target on the wall."

Grading: Same as for primary test.

Grade 2 (Poor)

Position of Patient: Short sitting with arm flexed above 90° and supported by examiner.

Position of Therapist: Standing at test side of patient. One hand supports the patient's arm at the elbow, maintaining it above the horizontal (Fig. 4–8). The other hand is placed at the inferior angle of the scapula with the thumb positioned along the axillary border and the fingers along the vertebral border (Fig. 4–8).

Test: Therapist monitors scapular motion by using a light grasp on the scapula at the inferior angle. Therapist must be sure not to restrict or resist motion. The scapula is observed to detect winging.

Instructions to Patient: "Hold your arm in this position" (i.e., above 90°). "Let it relax. Now hold your arm up again. Let it relax."

Grading

Grade 2 (Poor): If the scapula abducts and rotates upward as the patient attempts to hold the arm in the elevated position, the weakness is in the glenohumeral muscles. The Serratus is awarded a grade of 2. The Serratus is graded 2− (Poor−) if the scapula does not smoothly abduct and upwardly rotate without the weight of the arm or if the scapula moves toward the vertebral spine.

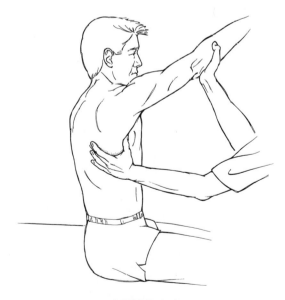

FIGURE 4–8

(Serratus anterior)

Grade 1 (Trace) and Grade 0 (Zero)

Position of Patient: Short sitting with arm forward flexed to above 90° (supported by therapist).

Position of Therapist: Standing in front of and slightly to one side of patient. Support the patient's arm at the elbow, maintaining it above 90° (Fig. 4–9). Use the other hand to palpate the Serratus with the tips of the fingers just in front of the inferior angle along the axillary border (Fig. 4–9).

Test: Patient attempts to hold the arm in the test position.

Instructions to Patient: "Try to hold your arm in this position."

Grading

Grade 1 (Trace): Muscle contraction is palpable.

Grade 0 (Zero): No contractile activity.

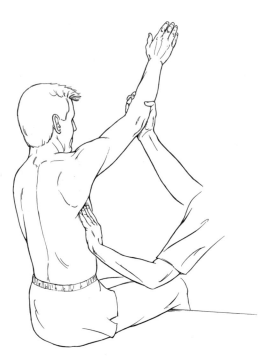

FIGURE 4–9

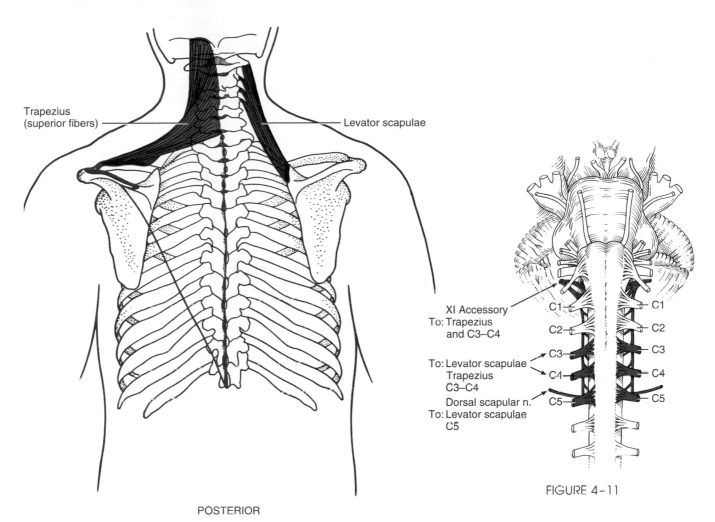

Trapezius (superior fibers)

Levator scapulae

XI Accessory
To: Trapezius
and C3–C4

To: Levator scapulae
Trapezius
C3–C4

Dorsal scapular n.
To: Levator scapulae
C5

C1   C1
C2   C2
C3   C3
C4   C4
C5   C5

FIGURE 4–11

POSTERIOR

FIGURE 4–10

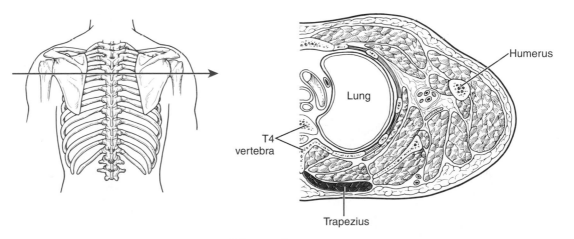

Humerus

Lung

T4
vertebra

Trapezius

FIGURE 4–12

SCAPULAR ELEVATION

(Trapezius, upper fibers)

Table 4-2 SCAPULAR ELEVATION

I.D.	Muscle	Origin	Insertion
124	Trapezius (upper fibers)	Occiput (external protuberance and superior nuchal line, medial 1/3) Ligamentum nuchae C7 vertebrae (spinous process)	Clavicle (posterior border of lateral 1/3)
127	Levator scapulae	C1–C4 vertebrae (transverse processes)	Scapula (vertebral border between superior angle and root of scapular spine)
Others			
125	Rhomboid major		
126	Rhomboid minor		(See also Plate 3, page 85.)

Grade 5 (Normal) and Grade 4 (Good)

Position of Patient: Short sitting over end or side of table. Hands relaxed in lap.

Position of Therapist: Stand behind patient. Hands contoured over top of both shoulders to give resistance in a downward direction.

Test: It is important to examine the patient's shoulders and scapula from a posterior view and to note any asymmetry of shoulder height, muscular bulk, or scapular winging. This kind of asymmetry is common and can be caused by carrying purses or briefcases habitually on one side (Fig. 4–13).

Patient elevates ("shrugs") shoulders. In the sitting position, the test is almost always performed on both sides simultaneously.

Instructions to Patient: "Shrug your shoulders" OR "Raise your shoulders toward your ears. Hold it. Don't let me push them down."

Grading

Grade 5 (Normal): Patient shrugs shoulders through available range of motion and holds against maximal resistance (Fig. 4–14).

Grade 4 (Good): Patient shrugs shoulders against strong to moderate resistance. The shoulder muscles may "give" at the end point.

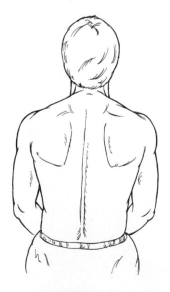

FIGURE 4–13

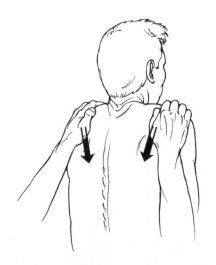

FIGURE 4–14

Grade 3 (Fair)

Position of Patient and Therapist: Same as those used for Grade 5 test except that no resistance is given (Fig. 4–15).

Test: Patient elevates shoulders through range of motion.

Instructions to Patient: "Raise your shoulders toward your ears" OR "Shrug your shoulders."

Grading

Grade 3 (Fair): Elevates shoulders through range but takes no resistance.

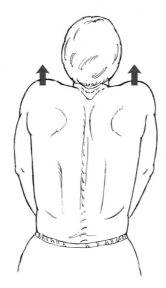

FIGURE 4–15

Grade 2 (Poor), Grade 1 (Trace), and Grade 0 (Zero)

Position of Patient: Prone or supine, fully supported on table. If prone, head is turned to one side for patient comfort (Fig. 4–16). If supine, head is in neutral position.

Position of Therapist: Stand at test side of patient. Support test shoulder in palm of one hand. The other hand palpates the upper Trapezius near its insertion above the clavicle. A second site for palpation is the upper Trapezius just adjacent to the cervical vertebrae.

Test: With the therapist supporting the shoulder, the patient elevates the shoulder (usually done unilaterally) toward the ear.

Instructions to Patient: "Raise your shoulder toward your ear."

Grading

Grade 2 (Poor): Patient completes full range of motion in gravity-eliminated position.

Grade 1 (Trace): Upper Trapezius fibers can be palpated at clavicle or neck. The Levator muscle lies deep and is more difficult to palpate in the neck (between the Sternocleidomastoid and the Trapezius). It can be felt at its insertion on the vertebral border of the scapula superior to the scapular spine.

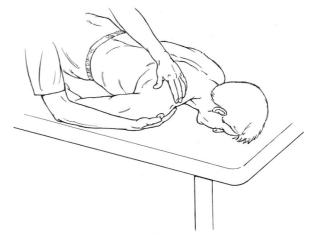

FIGURE 4–16

SCAPULAR ELEVATION

(Trapezius, upper fibers)

Alternate Test Procedure

In the sitting position, ask the patient to elevate one shoulder while the head, with the face turned away, is flexed laterally and down toward the shoulder (occiput leading). The occiput at full range will approximate the acromium. The examiner gives resistance at the shoulder in the direction of depression and simultaneously against the occiput in the anteromedial direction. If the upper Trapezius is weak, the acromium will not meet the occiput.[1]

Substitution by Rhomboids

In patients with weak shoulder elevators, the Rhomboids may attempt to substitute (whereas normally they assist). In such cases, during unsuccessful attempts to shrug the shoulder the inferior angle of the scapula will move medially toward the vertebral spine (scapular adduction), and downward motion (rotation) also may occur.

Helpful Hints

- If the sitting position for testing is contraindicated for any reason, the tests for Grade 5 and Grade 4 in the supine position will be quite inaccurate. If the Grade 3 test is done in the supine position, it will at best require manual resistance because gravity is neutralized.

- If the prone position is not comfortable, the tests for Grades 2, 1, and 0 may be performed with the patient supine, but palpation in such cases will be less than optimal.

- In the prone position the turned head offers a disadvantage. When the face is turned to either side, there is more Trapezius activity and less Levator activity on that side.

- Use the same lever (hand placement for resistance) in all subsequent scapular testing.

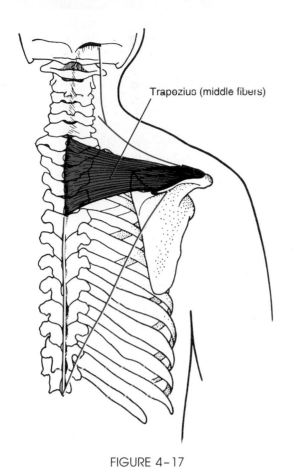

FIGURE 4-17

Trapezius (middle fibers)

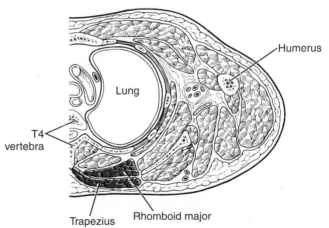

XI Accessory
To: Trapezius, middle
C3–C4

Dorsal scapular n.
To: Rhomboids
C5

C1   C1
C3   C3
C4   C4
C5   C5

FIGURF 4-18

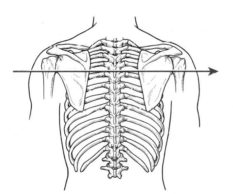

Humerus

Lung

T4
vertebra

Trapezius   Rhomboid major

FIGURE 4-19

SCAPULAR ADDUCTION

(Trapezius, middle fibers)

Range of Motion

Reliable data not available

Table 4-3 SCAPULAR ADDUCTION (RETRACTION)

I.D.	Muscle	Origin	Insertion
124	Trapezius (middle fibers)	T1–T5 vertebrae (spinous processes) Supraspinous ligaments	Scapula (medial acromial margin and superior lip of crest on scapular spine)
125	Rhomboid major	T2–T5 vertebrae (spinous processes and supraspinous ligaments)	Scapula (vertebral border between root of spine and inferior angle)
Others			
126	Rhomboid minor		
124	Trapezius (upper and lower)		
127	Levator scapulae		(See also Plate 3, page 85.)

Grade 5 (Normal), Grade 4 (Good), and Grade 3 (Fair)

Position of Patient: Prone with shoulder at edge of table. Shoulder is abducted to 90°. Elbow is flexed to a right angle (Fig. 4–20). Head may be turned to either side for comfort.

Alternatively, elbow may be fully extended provided the elbow extensor muscles are strong enough to stabilize the elbow on the humerus.

Position of Therapist: Stand at test side close to patient's arm. Stabilize the contralateral scapular area to prevent trunk rotation. There are two ways to give resistance; one does not require as much strength as the other.

1. When the posterior Deltoid is Grade 3 or better: The hand for resistance is placed over the distal end of the humerus, and resistance is directed downward toward the floor. The wrist also may be used for a longer lever, but the lever selected should be maintained consistently throughout the test.

2. When the posterior Deltoid is Grade 2 or less: Resistance is given in a downward direction (toward floor) with the hand contoured over the shoulder joint (Fig. 4–21). This placement of resistance requires less adductor muscle strength by the patient than is needed in the test described in the preceding paragraph.

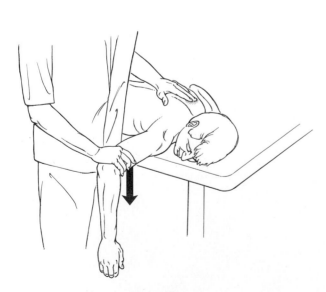

FIGURE 4-20

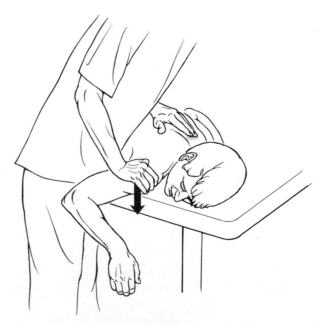

FIGURE 4-21

Grade 5 (Normal), Grade 4 (Good), and Grade 3 (Fair) Continued

The fingers of the other hand can palpate the middle fibers of the Trapezius at the spine of the scapula from the acromion to the vertebral column if necessary (Fig. 4–22).

Test: Patient horizontally abducts arm and adducts scapula.

Instructions to Patient: "Lift your elbow toward the ceiling. Hold it. Don't let me push it down."

Grading

Grade 5 (Normal): Completes available scapular adduction range and holds end position against maximal resistance.

Grade 4 (Good): Tolerates strong to moderate resistance.

Grade 3 (Fair): Completes available range but without manual resistance (see Fig. 4–22).

Grade 2 (Poor), Grade 1 (Trace), and Grade 0 (Zero)

Position of Patient and Therapist: Same as for Normal test except that the therapist uses one hand to cradle the patient's shoulder and arm, thus supporting its weight (Fig. 4–23) and the other hand for palpation.

Test: Same as that for Grades 5 to 3.

Instruction to Patient: "Try to lift your elbow toward the ceiling."

Grading

Grade 2 (Poor): Completes full range of motion without the weight of the arm.

Grade 1 (Trace) and Grade 0 (Zero): A Grade 1 (Trace) muscle exhibits contractile activity or slight movement. There will be neither motion nor contractile activity in the Grade 0 (Zero) muscle.

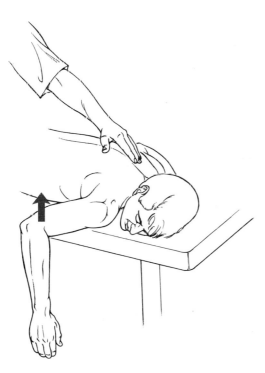

FIGURE 4–22

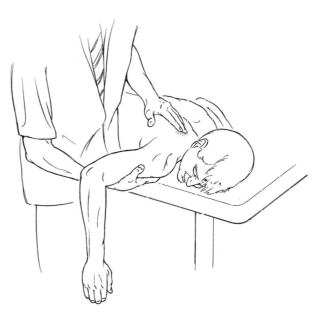

FIGURE 4–23

SCAPULAR ADDUCTION

(Trapezius, middle fibers)

Position of Patient: Prone. Place scapula in full adduction. Arm is in horizontal abduction (90°) with shoulder externally rotated and elbow fully extended.

Position of Therapist: Stand near shoulder on test side. Stabilize the opposite scapular region to avoid trunk rotation. For Grades 5 and 4 give resistance toward the floor at the distal humerus or at the wrist, maintaining consistency of location of resistance.

Instructions to Patient: "Keep your shoulder blade close to the spine. Don't let me draw it away."

Test: Patient maintains scapular adduction.

Substitutions

- By the Rhomboids: The Rhomboids can substitute for the Trapezius in adduction of the scapula. They cannot, however, substitute for the upward rotation component. When substitution by the Rhomboids occurs, the scapula will adduct and rotate downward.
- By the posterior Deltoid: If the scapular muscles are absent and the posterior Deltoid acts alone, horizontal abduction occurs at the shoulder joint but there is no scapular adduction.

Helpful Hints

When the posterior Deltoid muscle is weak, support the patient's shoulder with the palm of one hand, and allow the patient's elbow to flex. Passively move the scapula into adduction via horizontal abduction of the arm. Have the patient hold the scapula in adduction as the examiner slowly releases the shoulder support. Observe whether the scapula maintains its adducted position. If it does, it is Grade 3.

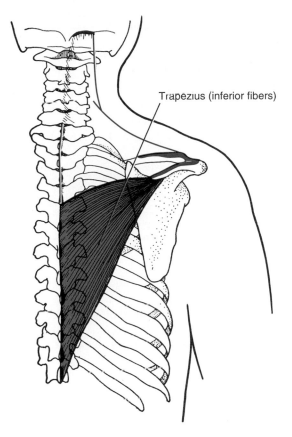

Trapezius (inferior fibers)

FIGURE 4-24

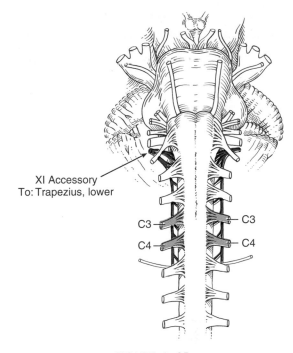

XI Accessory
To: Trapezius, lower

C3   C3
C4   C4

FIGURE 4-25

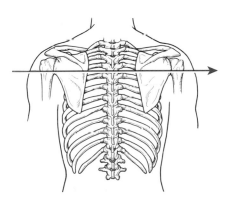

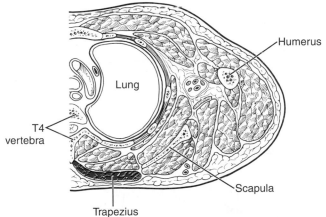

Humerus

Lung

T4
vertebra

Scapula

Trapezius

FIGURE 4-26

SCAPULAR DEPRESSION AND ADDUCTION

(Trapezius, lower fibers)

Range of Motion

Reliable data not available

Table 4-4 SCAPULAR DEPRESSION AND ADDUCTION

I.D.	Muscle	Origin	Insertion
124	Trapezius (middle and lower fibers)	T1–T5 vertebrae (spinous processes) Supraspinous ligament T6–T12 vertebrae (spinous processes)	Scapula (spine, medial end and tubercle at lateral apex via aponeurosis)

Others

130	Latissimus dorsi		
131	Pectoralis major		
129	Pectoralis minor		

Grade 5 (Normal), Grade 4 (Good), and Grade 3 (Fair)

Position of Patient: Prone with arms over head to about 145° of abduction (in line with the fibers of the lower Trapezius). Forearm is in midposition with the thumb pointing toward the ceiling. Head may be turned to either side for comfort.

Position of Therapist: Stand at test side. Hand giving resistance is contoured over the distal humerus just proximal to the elbow (Fig. 4–27). Resistance will be given straight downward (toward the floor). For a less rigorous test, resistance may be given over the axillary border of the scapula.

Fingertips of the opposite hand palpate (for Grade 3) below the spine of the scapula and across to the thoracic vertebrae, following the muscle as it curves down to the lower thoracic vertebrae.

Test: Patient raises arm from the table to at least ear level and holds it strongly against resistance. Alternatively, preposition the arm in elevation diagonally over the head and ask the patient to hold it strongly against resistance.

Instructions to Patient: "Raise your arm from the table as high as possible. Hold it. Don't let me push it down."

Grading

Grade 5 (Normal): Completes available range and holds it against maximal resistance. This is a strong muscle.

Grade 4 (Good): Takes strong to moderate resistance.

Grade 3 (Fair): Same procedure is used, but patient tolerates no manual resistance (Fig. 4–28).

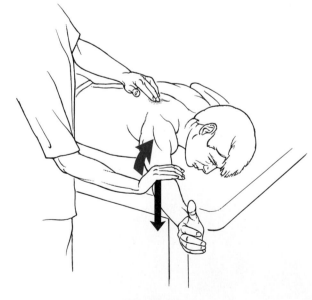

FIGURE 4–27

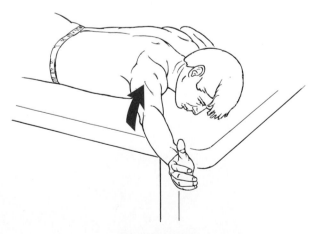

FIGURE 4–28

Grade 2 (Poor), Grade 1 (Trace), and Grade 0 (Zero)

Position of Patient: Same as for Grade 5.

Position of Therapist: Stand at test side. Support patient's arm under the elbow (Fig. 4–29).

Test: Patient attempts to lift the arm from the table. If the patient is unable to lift the arm because of a weak posterior and middle Deltoid, the examiner should lift and support the weight of the arm.

Instructions to Patient: "Try to lift your arm from the table past your ear."

Grading

Grade 2 (Poor): Completes full scapular range of motion without the weight of the arm.

Grade 1 (Trace): Contractile activity can be palpated in the triangular area between the root of the spine of the scapula and the lower thoracic vertebra (T7–T12), that is, the course of the fibers of the lower Trapezius.

Grade 0 (Zero): No palpable contractile activity.

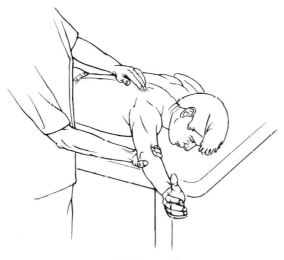

FIGURE 4–29

Helpful Hints
• If shoulder range of motion is limited in flexion and abduction, the patient's arm should be positioned over the side of the table and supported by the examiner at its maximal range of elevation as the start position.
• Examiners are reminded of the test principle that the same lever arm must be used in sequential testing (over time) for valid comparison of results.

(Rhomboids)

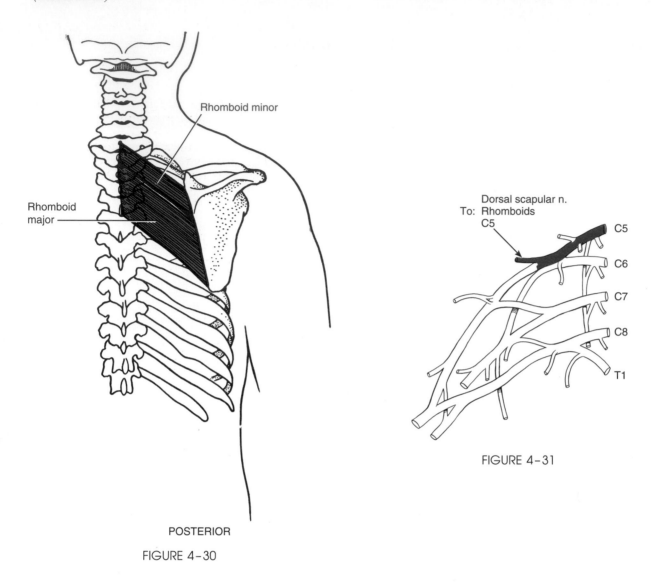

Rhomboid minor

Rhomboid major

POSTERIOR

FIGURE 4–30

Dorsal scapular n.
To: Rhomboids
C5

C5

C6

C7

C8

T1

FIGURE 4–31

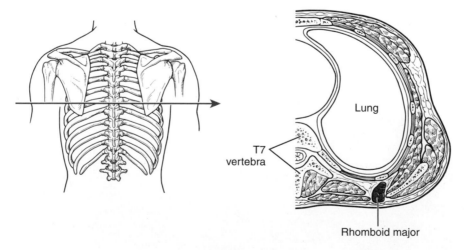

Lung

T7 vertebra

Rhomboid major

FIGURE 4–32

Range of Motion
Reliable data not available

Table 4-5 SCAPULAR ADDUCTION AND DOWNWARD ROTATION

I.D.	Muscle	Origin	Insertion
125	Rhomboid major	T2–T5 vertebrae (spinous processes) Supraspinous ligaments	Scapula (vertebral border between root of spine and inferior angle)
126	Rhomboid minor	C7–T1 vertebrae (spinous processes) Ligamentum nuchae (lower)	Scapula (vertebral margin at root of spine)
Other			
127	Levator scapulae		(See also Plate 3, page 85.)

The test for the Rhomboid muscles has become the focus of some clinical debate. Kendall and coworkers claim, with good evidence, that these muscles frequently are underrated, that is, they are too often graded at a level less than their performance.[1] At issue also is the confusion that can occur in separating the function of the Rhomboids from that of other scapular or shoulder muscles, particularly the Trapezius and the Pectoralis minor. Innervated only by C5, a test for the Rhomboids, correctly done, can confirm or rule out a cord lesion at this level. With these issues in mind, the authors present first their method and then, with the generous permission of Mrs. Kendall, her Rhomboid test as another method of assessment.

Grade 5 (Normal), Grade 4 (Good), and Grade 3 (Fair)

Position of Patient: Prone. Head may be turned to either side for comfort. Shoulder is internally rotated and the arm is adducted across the back with the elbow flexed and hand resting on the back (Fig. 4–33).

Position of Therapist: Stand at test side. When the shoulder extensor muscles are Grade 3 or above, the hand used for resistance is placed on the humerus just above the elbow, and resistance is given in a downward and outward direction (Fig. 4–34).

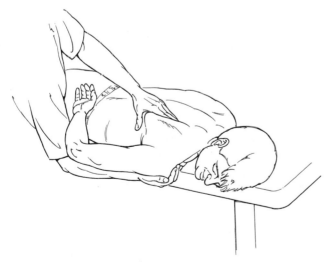

FIGURE 4–33

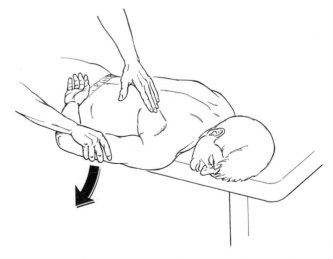

FIGURE 4–34

Grade 5 (Normal), Grade 4 (Good), and Grade 3 (Fair) Continued

When the shoulder extensors are weak, place the hand for resistance along the axillary border of the scapula (Fig. 4–35). Resistance is applied in a downward and outward direction.

The fingers of the hand used for palpation are placed deep under the vertebral border of the scapula.

Test: Patient lifts the hand off the back, maintaining the arm position across the back at the same time the examiner is applying resistance above the elbow. With strong muscle activity the therapist's fingers will "pop" out from under the edge of the scapular vertebral border. (See Fig. 4–33.)

Instructions to Patient: "Lift your hand. Hold it. Don't let me push it down."

Grading

Grade 5 (Normal): Completes available range and holds against maximal resistance (Fig. 4–36). The fingers will "pop out" from under the scapula when strong Rhomboids contract.

Grade 4 (Good): Completes range and holds against strong to moderate resistance. Fingers usually will "pop out."

Grade 3 (Fair): Completes range but tolerates no manual resistance (Fig. 4–37).

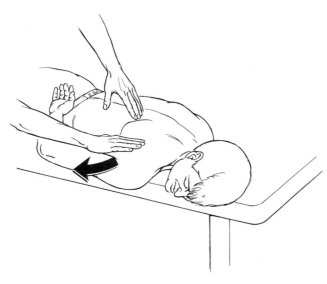

FIGURE 4–35

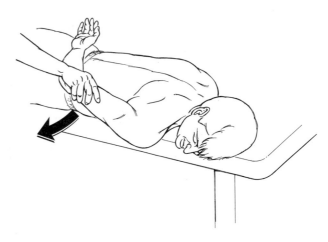

FIGURE 4–36

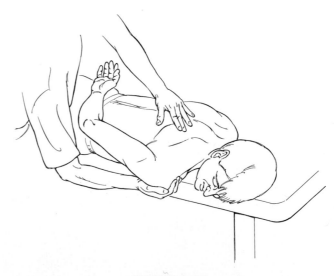

FIGURE 4–37

Grade 2 (Poor), Grade 1 (Trace), and Grade 0 (Zero)

Position of Patient: Short sitting with shoulder internally rotated and arm extended and adducted behind back (Fig. 4–38).

Position of Therapist: Stand at test side; support arm by grasping the wrist. The fingertips of one hand palpate the muscle under the vertebral border of the scapula.

Test: Patient attempts to move hand away from back.

Instructions to Patient: "Try to move your hand away from your back."

Grading

Grade 2 (Poor): Completes range of scapular motion.

Grades 1 (Trace) and 0 (Zero): A Grade 1 muscle has palpable contractile activity. A Grade 0 muscle shows no response.

Alternate Test for Grades 2, 1, and 0

Position of Patient: Prone with shoulder in about 45° of abduction and elbow at about 90° of flexion with the hand on the back.

Position of Therapist: Stand at test side and support test arm by cradling it under the shoulder (Fig. 4–39). Fingers used for palpation are placed firmly under the vertebral border of the scapula.

Test. Patient attempts to lift hand from back.

Instructions to Patient: "Try to lift your hand away from your back" OR "Lift your hand toward the ceiling."

Grading

Grade 2 (Poor): Completes partial range of scapular motion.

Grades 1 (Trace) and 0 (Zero): A Grade 1 (Trace) muscle has some palpable contractile activity. A Grade 0 muscle shows no contractile response.

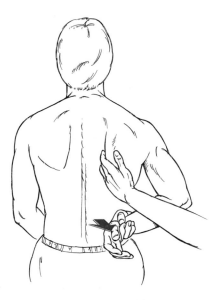

FIGURE 4–38

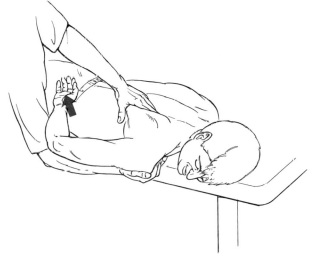

FIGURE 4–39

Alternate Rhomboid Test After Kendall[1]

As a preliminary to the Rhomboid test, the shoulder adductors should be tested and found sufficiently strong to allow the arm to be used as a lever.

Position of Patient: Prone with head turned to side of test. Nontest arm is abducted with elbow flexed.

Test arm is near the edge of the table. Arm (humerus) is fully adducted and held firm to the side of the trunk in external rotation and some extension with elbow fully flexed. In this position the scapula is in adduction, elevation, and downward rotation (glenoid down).

Position of Therapist: Stand at test side. One hand used for resistance is cupped around the flexed elbow. The resistance applied by this hand will be in the direction of scapular abduction and upward rotation (out and up; Fig. 4–40). The other hand is used to give resistance simultaneously. It is contoured over the shoulder joint and gives resistance caudally in the direction of shoulder depression.

Test: Examiner tests the ability of the patient to hold the scapula in its position of adduction, elevation, and downward rotation (glenoid down).

Instructions to Patient: "Hold your arm as I have placed it. Do not let me pull your arm forward" OR "Hold the position you are in; keep your shoulder blade against your spine as I try to pull it away."

Substitution by Middle Trapezius

The middle fibers of the Trapezius can substitute for the adduction component of the Rhomboids. The middle Trapezius cannot, however, substitute for the downward rotation component. When substitution occurs, the patient's scapula will adduct with no downward rotation (no glenoid down occurs). Only palpation can detect this substitution for sure.

Helpful Hints

When the Rhomboid test is performed with the hand behind the back, never allow the patient to lead the lifting motion with the elbow because this will activate the humeral extensors

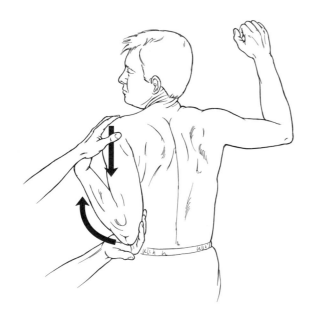

FIGURE 4–40

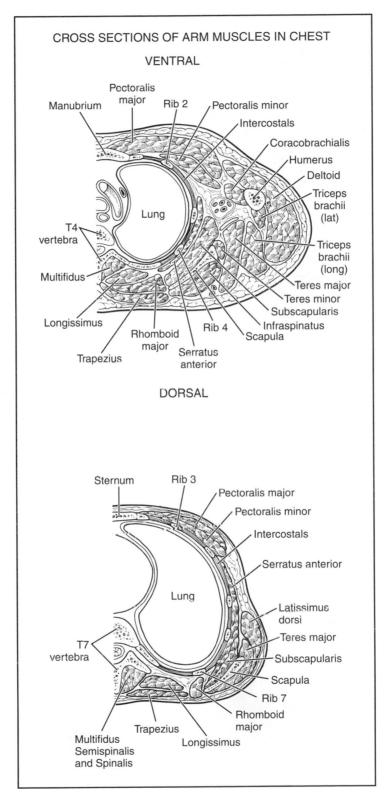

CROSS SECTIONS OF ARM MUSCLES IN CHEST

VENTRAL

Manubrium
Pectoralis major
Rib 2
Pectoralis minor
Intercostals
Coracobrachialis
Humerus
Deltoid
Triceps brachii (lat)
Triceps brachii (long)
Teres major
Teres minor
Subscapularis
Infraspinatus
Scapula
Rib 4
Rhomboid major
Serratus anterior
Trapezius
Longissimus
Multifidus
T4 vertebra
Lung

DORSAL

Sternum
Rib 3
Pectoralis major
Pectoralis minor
Intercostals
Serratus anterior
Latissimus dorsi
Teres major
Subscapularis
Scapula
Rib 7
Rhomboid major
Longissimus
Trapezius
Multifidus Semispinalis and Spinalis
T7 vertebra
Lung

PLATE 3

(Anterior Deltoid and Coracobrachialis*)

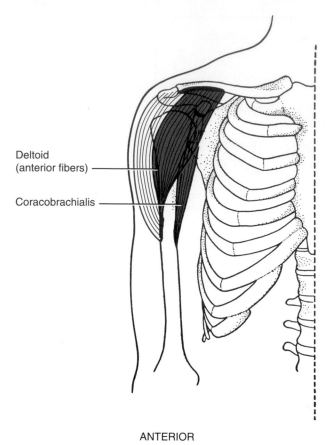

Deltoid
(anterior fibers)

Coracobrachialis

ANTERIOR

FIGURE 4–41

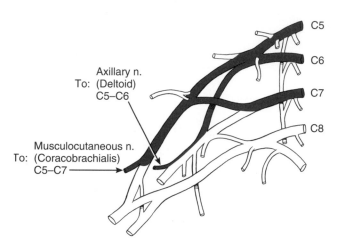

Axillary n.
To: (Deltoid)
C5–C6

Musculocutaneous n.
To: (Coracobrachialis)
C5–C7

C5

C6

C7

C8

FIGURE 4–42

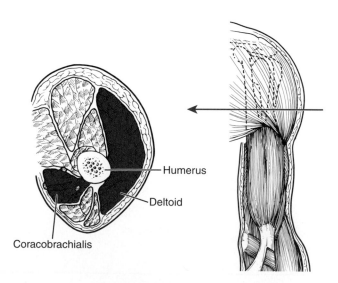

Humerus

Deltoid

Coracobrachialis

FIGURE 4–43

---

*The Coracobrachialis muscle cannot be isolated, nor is it readily palpable. It has no unique function. It is included here because classically it is considered a shoulder flexor and adductor.

Range of Motion
0° to 80°

Table 4-6 SHOULDER FLEXION

I.D.	Muscle	Origin	Insertion
133	Deltoid (anterior)	Clavicle (anterior superior border of lateral 1/3 of shaft)	Humerus (deltoid tuberosity on shaft)
139	Coracobrachialis	Scapula (coracoid process at apex)	Humerus (shaft, medial surface at middle 1/3)

Others

131	Pectoralis major (upper)	
133	Deltoid (middle)	
128	Serratus anterior (via upwardly rotating scapula and preventing scapular adduction)	

Grade 5 (Normal) and Grade 4 (Good)

Position of Patient: Short sitting with arms at sides, elbow slightly flexed, forearm pronated.

Position of Therapist: Stand at test side. Hand giving resistance is contoured over the distal humerus just above the elbow. The other hand may stabilize the shoulder (Fig. 4–44).

Test: Patient flexes shoulder to 90° without rotation or horizontal movement (Fig. 4–44). The scapula should be allowed to abduct and upwardly rotate.

Instructions to Patient: "Raise your arm forward to shoulder height. Hold it. Don't let me push it down."

Grading

Grade 5 (Normal): Holds end position (90°) against maximal resistance.

Grade 4 (Good): Holds end position against strong to moderate resistance.

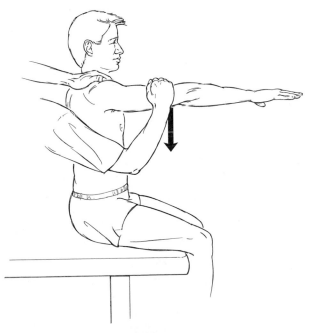

FIGURE 4-44

*The Coracobrachialis muscle cannot be isolated, nor is it readily palpable. It has no unique function. It is included here because classically it is considered a shoulder flexor and adductor.

SHOULDER FLEXION

(Anterior Deltoid and Coracobrachialis*)

Grade 3 (Fair)

Position of Patient: Short sitting, arm at side with elbow slightly flexed and forearm pronated

Position of Therapist: Stand at test side.

Test: Patient flexes shoulder to 90° (Fig. 4–45).

Instructions to Patient: "Raise your arm forward to shoulder height."

Grading

Grade 3 (Fair): Completes test range (90°) but tolerates no resistance.

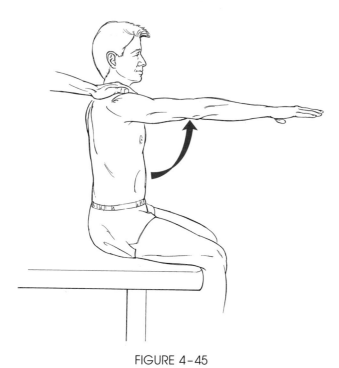

FIGURE 4–45

Grade 2 (Poor), Grade 1 (Trace), and Grade 0 (Zero)

Position of Patient: Short sitting with arm at side and elbow slightly flexed.

Position of Therapist: Stand at test side. Fingers used for palpation are placed on the anterior surface of the Deltoid over the shoulder joint (Fig. 4–46).

Test: Patient attempts to flex shoulder to 90°.

Instructions to Patient: "Try to raise your arm."

Grading

Grade 2 (Poor): Completes partial range of motion as this is against gravity.

Grade 1 (Trace): Examiner feels or sees contractile activity in the anterior Deltoid, but no motion occurs.

Grade 0 (Zero): No contractile activity.

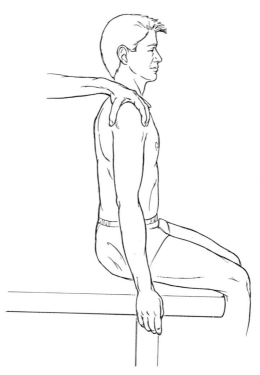

FIGURE 4–46

---

*The Coracobrachialis muscle cannot be isolated, nor is it readily palpable. It has no unique function. It is included here because classically it is considered a shoulder flexor and adductor.

Alternate Test for Grades 2, 1, and 0

If for any reason the patient is unable to sit, the test can be conducted in the side-lying position (test side up). In this posture, the examiner cradles the test arm at the elbow before asking the patient to flex the shoulder. For Grade 2 (Poor) the patient must complete full range of motion.

Helpful Hints

Although the Coracobrachialis is a minor contributor to shoulder flexion, it is deep-lying and may be difficult or impossible to palpate within a reasonable range of comfort for the patient.

Substitutions

- In the absence of a Deltoid the patient may attempt to flex the shoulder with the Biceps brachii by first externally rotating the shoulder (Fig. 4–47). To avoid this, the arm should be kept in the midposition between internal and external rotation.
- Attempted substitution by the upper Trapezius results in shoulder elevation.
- Attempted substitution by the Pectoralis major results in horizontal adduction.
- The patient may lean backward or try to elevate the shoulder girdle to assist in flexion.

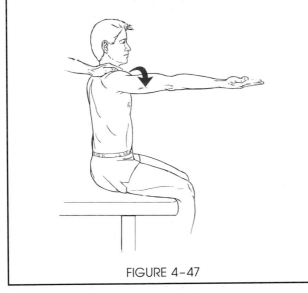

FIGURE 4–47

---

*The Coracobrachialis muscle cannot be isolated, nor is it readily palpable. It has no unique function. It is included here because classically it is considered a shoulder flexor and adductor.

SHOULDER EXTENSION

(Latissimus dorsi, Teres major*, Posterior Deltoid)

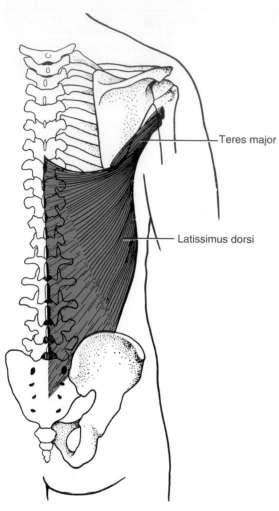

Teres major

Latissimus dorsi

POSTERIOR

FIGURE 4-48

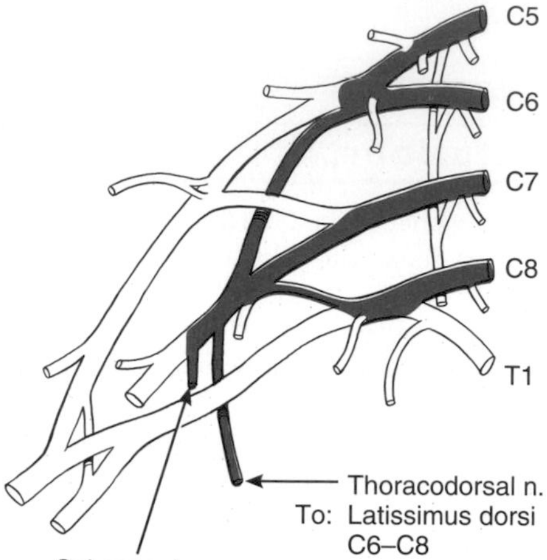

C5

C6

C7

C8

T1

Thoracodorsal n.
To: Latissimus dorsi
C6–C8

Subscapular n.
(lower)
To: Teres major
C5–C6

FIGURE 4-49

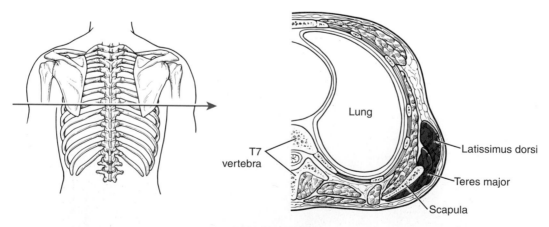

Lung

T7
vertebra

Latissimus dorsi

Teres major

Scapula

FIGURE 4-50

*The role of the Teres major is often disputed as a shoulder extensor and EMG studies vary but it has long been considered to move the humerus posteriorly.

Range of Motion
0° to 45° (up to 60°)

Table 4-7 SHOULDER EXTENSION

I.D.	Muscle	Origin	Insertion
130	Latissimus dorsi	T6–T12, L1–L5, and sacral vertebrae (spinous processes) Supraspinous ligaments Ribs 9–12 (by slips interdigitating with Obliquus abdominis externus) Ilium (crest, posterior) Thoracolumbar fascia	Humerus (intertubercular sulcus, floor) Deep fascia of arm
133	Deltoid (posterior)	Scapula (spine on lower lip of lateral and posterior borders)	Humerus (deltoid tuberosity on midshaft via humeral tendon)
138	Teres major	Scapula (dorsal surface of inferior angle)	Humerus (intertubercular sulcus, medial lip)
Other			
142	Triceps brachii (long head)		

Grade 5 (Normal) and Grade 4 (Good)

There are three tests for Grades 5 and 4 that should be used routinely. The first is the traditional way of testing shoulder extension in the prone position. The other two tests are used to isolate the Latissimus dorsi to the extent possible and to simulate a more functional movement.

Test 1: Generic Shoulder Extension

Position of Patient: Prone with arms at sides and shoulder internally rotated (palm up) (Fig. 4–51).

Position of Therapist: Stand at test side. Hand used for resistance is contoured over the posterior arm just above the elbow.

Test: Patient raises arm off the table, keeping the elbow straight (Fig. 4–52).

Instructions to Patient: "Lift your arm as high as you can. Hold it. Don't let me push it down."

Grading

Grade 5 (Normal): Completes available range and holds against maximal resistance.

Grade 4 (Good): Completes available range but yields against strong resistance.

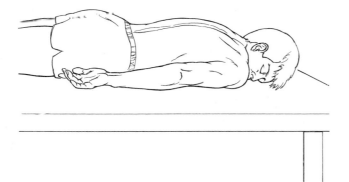

FIGURE 4-51

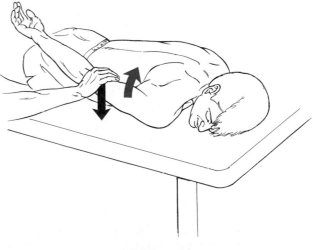

FIGURE 4-52

SHOULDER EXTENSION

(Latissimus dorsi, Teres major,* Posterior Deltoid)

Grade 5 (Normal) and Grade 4 (Good) Continued

Test 2: To Isolate Latissimus dorsi

Position of Patient: Prone with head turned to test side; arms are at sides and shoulder is internally rotated (palm up). Test shoulder is "hiked" to the level of the chin.

Position of Therapist: Stand at test side. Grasp forearm above patient's wrist with both hands (Fig. 4–53).

Test: Patient depresses arm caudally and in so doing approximates the rib cage to the pelvis.

Instructions to Patient: "Reach toward your feet. Hold it. Don't let me push your arm upward toward your head."

Grading

Grade 5 (Normal): Patient completes available range against maximal resistance. If the therapist is unable to push the arm upward using both hands for resistance, test the patient in the sitting position as described in Test 3.

Grade 4 (Good): Patient completes available range of motion, but the shoulder yields at end point against strong resistance.

Test 3: To Isolate Latissimus dorsi

Position of Patient: Short sitting, with hands flat on table adjacent to hips (Fig. 4–54).

If the patient's arms are too short to assume this position, provide a push-up block for each hand.

Position of Therapist: Stand behind patient. Fingers are used to palpate fibers of the Latissimus dorsi on the lateral aspects of the thoracic wall (bilaterally) just above the waist (Fig. 4–54). (In this test the sternal head of the Pectoralis major is equally active.)

Test: Patient pushes down on hands (or blocks) and lifts buttocks from table (Fig. 4–54).

Instructions to Patient: "Lift your bottom off the table."

Grading

Grade 5 (Normal): Patient is able to lift buttocks clear of table.

Grade 4 (Good): There is no Grade 4 in this sequence because the prone test (Test 2) determines a grade of less than 5.

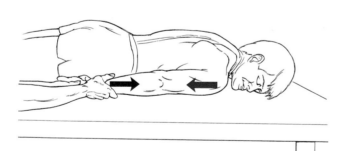

FIGURE 4–53

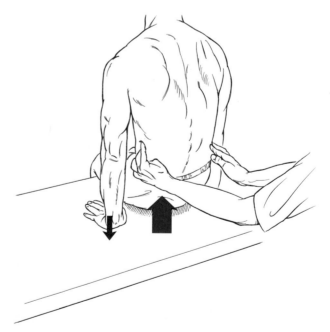

FIGURE 4–54

---

*The role of the Teres major is often disputed as a shoulder extensor and EMG studies vary, but it has long been considered to move the humerus posteriorly.

Grade 3 (Fair) and Grade 2 (Poor)

Position of Patient: Prone with head turned to one side. Arms at sides; test arm is internally rotated (palm up) (Fig. 4–55).

Position of Therapist: Stand at test side.

Test: Test 1 (generic extension): Patient raises arm off table (Fig. 4–55). Test 2 (isolation of Latissimus): Patient pushes arm toward feet.

Instructions to Patient: Test 1: "Lift your arm as high as you can." Test 2 (Latissimus): "Reach down toward your feet."

Grading

Grade 3 (Fair): Completes available range of motion with no manual resistance.

Grade 2 (Poor): Completes partial range of motion.

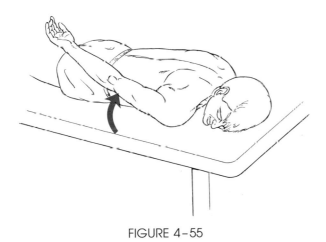

FIGURE 4–55

Grade 1 (Trace) and Grade 0 (Zero)

Position of Patient: Prone with arms at sides and shoulder internally rotated (palm up).

Position of Therapist: Stand at test side. Fingers for palpation (Latissimus) are placed on the side of the thoracic wall (Fig. 4–56) below and lateral to the inferior angle of the scapula.

Palpate over the posterior shoulder just superior to the axilla for posterior Deltoid fibers. Palpate the Teres major on the lateral border of the scapula just below the axilla. The Teres major is the lower of the two muscles that enter the axilla at this point; it forms the lower posterior rim of the axilla.

Test and Instructions to Patient: Patient attempts to lift arm from table on request.

Grading

Grade 1 (Trace): Palpable contractile activity in any of the participating muscles but no movement of the shoulder.

Grade 0 (Zero): No contractile response in participating muscles.

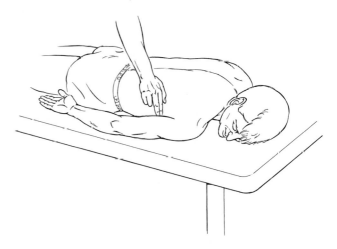

FIGURE 4–56

---

*The role of the Teres major is often disputed as a shoulder extensor and EMG studies vary, but it has long been considered to move the humerus posteriorly.

SHOULDER SCAPTION

(Deltoid and Supraspinatus)

Range of Motion
0° to 170°

Table 4-8 SCAPTION

I.D.	Muscle	Origin	Insertion
133	Deltoid		
	Anterior fibers	Clavicle (shaft; anterior-superior border, lateral 1/3)	Humerus (deltoid tuberosity via humeral tendon)
	Middle fibers	Scapula (crest of spine and acromium, lateral superior margin)	
135	Supraspinatus	Scapula (supraspinous fossa) Supraspinatus fascia	Humerus (greater tubercle, highest facet) Articular capsule of glenohumeral joint

This recently minted motion is arm elevation in the plane of the scapula, that is, 30° to 45° anterior to the coronal plane about halfway between shoulder flexion and shoulder abduction.[2] This movement, called scaption, is more functional than either forward flexion or abduction.

Grade 5 (Normal) to Grade 0 (Zero)

Position of Patient (All Grades): Short sitting.

Position of Therapist: Stand in front of and slightly to the test side of patient. Hand used for resistance is contoured over the arm above the elbow (Grades 5 and 4 only).

Test: Patient elevates arm halfway between flexion and abduction (30° to 45° anterior to coronal plane) (Fig. 4–57).

Instructions to Patient: "Raise your arm to shoulder height halfway between straight-ahead and out to the side. Hold it. Don't let me push your arm down." (Demonstrate this motion to the patient.)

Grading

Grade 5 (Normal): Completes available range of motion and holds against maximal resistance.

Grade 4 (Good): Completes available range and holds against strong resistance but there will be some yielding at the end of the range.

Grade 3 (Fair): Completes available range but tolerates no resistance other than the weight of the arm.

Grade 2 (Poor): Moves only through partial range of motion. The therapist's fingers for palpation are positioned on the anterior and medial aspect of the shoulder (for Grades 2 and below).

Grade 1 (Trace) and Grade 0 (Zero): Palpable or visible contractile activity for Grade 1; no activity detected for Grade 0.

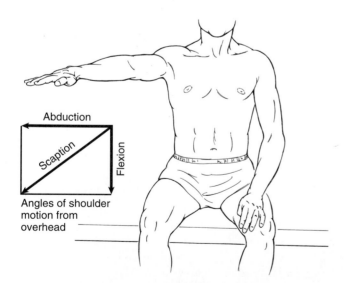

Abduction

Scaption

Flexion

Angles of shoulder motion from overhead

FIGURE 4–57

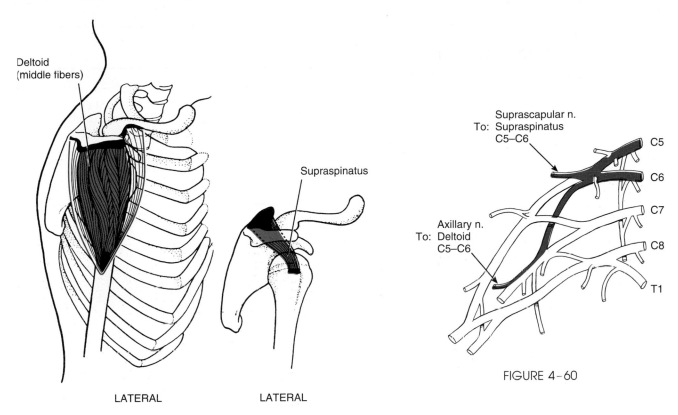

Deltoid
(middle fibers)

Supraspinatus

Suprascapular n.
To: Supraspinatus
C5–C6

C5

C6

C7

C8

T1

Axillary n.
To: Deltoid
C5–C6

LATERAL

LATERAL

FIGURE 4-58 AND FIGURE 4-59

FIGURE 4-60

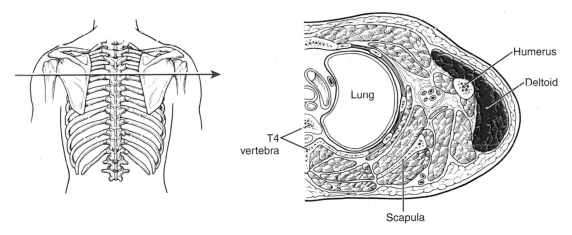

Humerus

Deltoid

Lung

T4
vertebra

Scapula

FIGURE 4-61

SHOULDER ABDUCTION

(Middle Deltoid and Supraspinatus)

Range of Motion
0° to 180°

Table 4-9 SHOULDER ABDUCTION

I.D.	Muscle	Origin	Insertion
133	Deltoid (middle fibers)	Scapula (acromium, lateral margin, superior surface, and crest of spine)	Humerus (deltoid tuberosity on shaft via humeral tendon)
135	Supraspinatus	Scapula (supraspinous fossa, medial 2/3) Supraspinatus fascia	Humerus (greater tubercle, highest facet) Articular capsule of glenohumeral joint

Grade 5 (Normal), Grade 4 (Good), and Grade 3 (Fair)

Preliminary Evaluation: Examiner should check for full range of shoulder motion in all planes and should observe scapula for stability and smoothness of movement. (Refer to test for Scapular abduction and upward rotation.)

Position of Patient: Short sitting with arm at side and elbow slightly flexed.

Position of Therapist: Stand behind patient. Hand giving resistance is contoured over arm just above elbow (Fig. 4–62).

Test: Patient abducts arm to 90°.

Instructions to Patient: "Lift your arm out to the side to shoulder level. Hold it. Don't let me push it down."

Grading

Grade 5 (Normal): Holds end test position against maximal downward resistance.

Grade 4 (Good): Holds end test position against strong to moderate downward resistance.

Grade 3 (Fair): Completes range of motion to 90° with no manual resistance (Fig. 4–63).

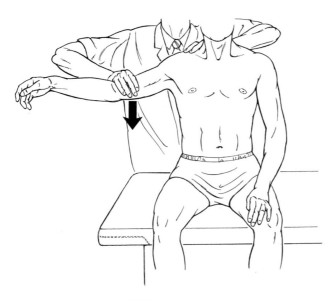

FIGURE 4–62

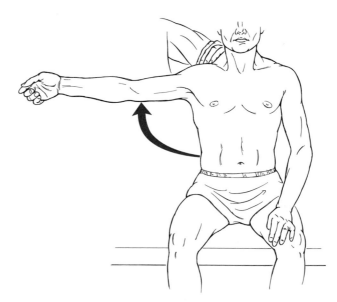

FIGURE 4–63

Grade 2 (Poor)

Position of Patient: Short sitting with arm at side and slight elbow flexion.

Position of Therapist: Stand behind patient to palpate muscles on test side. Palpate the Deltoid (Fig. 4–64) lateral to the acromial process on the superior aspect of the shoulder. The Supraspinatus can be palpated by placing the fingers deep under the Trapezius in the supraspinous fossa of the scapula.

Test: Patient attempts to abduct arm.

Instructions to Patient: "Try to lift your arm out to the side."

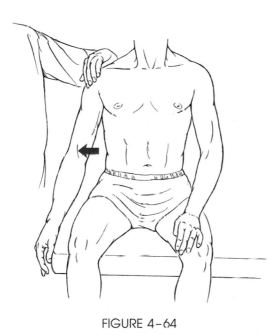

FIGURE 4–64

Alternate Test for Grade 2

Position of Patient: Supine. Arm at side supported on table (Fig. 4–65).

Position of Therapist: Stand at test side of patient. (Fig. 4–65 shows therapist on opposite side to avoid obstructing test procedure illustrated.) Hand used for palpation is positioned as described for Grade 2 test.

Test: Patient attempts to abduct shoulder by sliding arm on table without rotating it (see Fig. 4–65).

Instructions to Patient: "Take your arm out to the side."

Grading

Grade 2 (Poor): Completes partial range of motion for sitting test and full range for supine test.

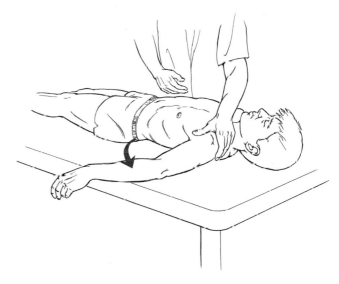

FIGURE 4–65

SHOULDER ABDUCTION

(Middle Deltoid and Supraspinatus)

Grade 1 (Trace) and Grade 0 (Zero)

Position of Patient: Short sitting.

Position of Therapist: Stand behind and to the side of patient. Therapist cradles test arm with the shoulder in about 90° of abduction providing limb support at the elbow (Fig. 4–66).

Test: Patient tries to maintain the arm in abduction.

Instructions to Patient: "Try to hold your arm in this position."

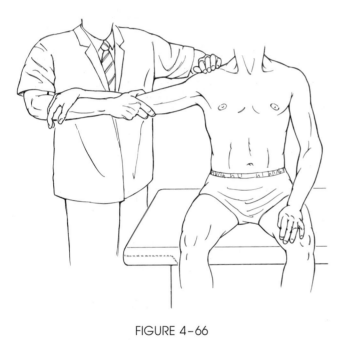

FIGURE 4–66

Alternate Test for Grade 1 and Grade 0 (Supine)

Position of Patient: Supine with arm at side and elbow slightly flexed.

Position of Therapist: Stand at side of table at a place where the Deltoid can be reached. Palpate the Deltoid on the lateral surface of the upper one-third of the arm (Fig. 4–67).

Grading

Grade 1 (Trace): Palpable or visible contraction of Deltoid with no movement.

Grade 0 (Zero): No contractile activity.

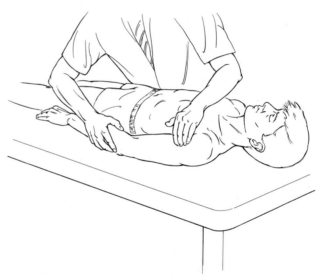

FIGURE 4–67

Helpful Hints

- Turning the face to the opposite side and extending the neck will put the Trapezius on slack and make the Supraspinatus more accessible for palpation.

- The Deltoid and Supraspinatus work in tandem, and when one is active in abduction the other also will be active. Only when Supraspinatus weakness is suspected is it necessary to palpate.

- Do not allow shoulder elevation or lateral flexion of the trunk to the opposite side because these movements can create an illusion of abduction.

Substitution by Biceps Brachii

When a patient uses the Biceps to substitute, the shoulder will externally rotate and the elbow will flex. The arm will be raised but not by the action of the abductor muscles. To avoid this substitution begin the test with the arm in a few degrees of elbow flexion, but do not allow active contraction of the Biceps during the test.

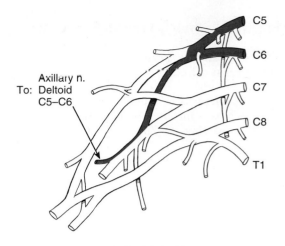

FIGURE 4-69

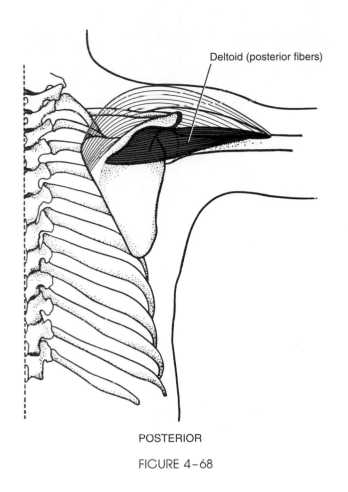

POSTERIOR

FIGURE 4-68

Range of Motion

When starting from a position of 90° of forward flexion: 0° to 90° (range, 90°)

When starting with the arm in full horizontal adduction: −40° to 90° (range, 130°)

Table 4-10 SHOULDER HORIZONTAL ABDUCTION

I.D.	Muscle	Origin	Insertion
133	Deltoid (posterior fibers)	Scapula (spine on lower lip of crest)	Humerus (deltoid tuberosity via humeral tendon)
Others			
136	Infraspinatus		
137	Teres minor		

SHOULDER HORIZONTAL ABDUCTION

(Posterior Deltoid)

Grade 5 (Normal), Grade 4 (Good), and Grade 3 (Fair)

Position of Patient: Prone. Shoulder abducted to 90° and forearm off edge of table with elbow flexed.

Position of Therapist: Stand at test side. Hand giving resistance is contoured over posterior arm just above the elbow (Fig. 4–70).

Test: Patient horizontally abducts shoulder against maximal resistance.

Instructions to Patient: "Lift your elbow up toward the ceiling. Hold it. Don't let me push it down."

Grading

Grade 5 (Normal): Completes range and holds end position against maximal resistance.

Grade 4 (Good): Completes range and holds end position against strong to moderate resistance.

Grade 3 (Fair): Completes range of motion with no manual resistance (Fig. 4–71).

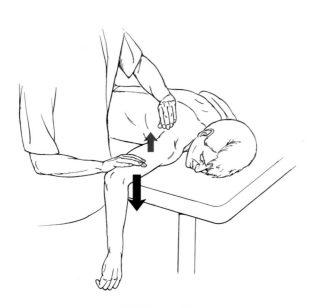

FIGURE 4–70

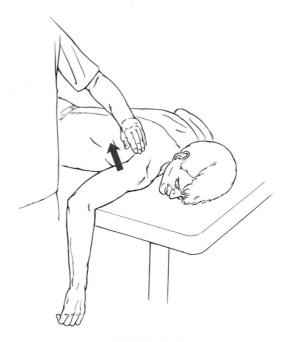

FIGURE 4–71

Grade 2 (Poor), Grade 1 (Trace), Grade 0 (Zero)

Position of Patient: Short sitting over end or side of table.

Position of Therapist: Stand at test side. Support forearm under distal surface (Fig. 4–72) and palpate over the posterior surface of the shoulder just superior to the axilla.

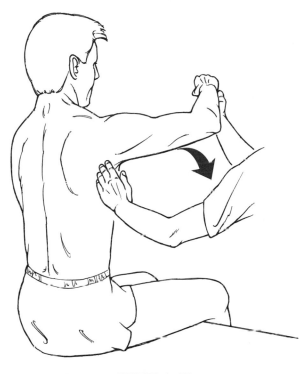

FIGURE 4–72

Alternate Test for Grades 2, 1, and 0

Position of Patient: Short sitting with arm supported on table (smooth surface) in 90° of abduction; elbow partially flexed.

Position of Therapist: Stand behind patient. Stabilize by contouring one hand over the superior aspect of the shoulder and the other over the scapula (Fig. 4–73). Palpate the fibers of the posterior Deltoid below and lateral to the spine of the scapula and on the posterior aspect of the proximal arm adjacent to the axilla.

Test: Patient slides (or tries to move) the arm across the table in horizontal abduction.

Instructions to Patient: "Slide your arm backward."

Grading

Grade 2 (Poor): Moves through full range of motion.

Grade 1 (Trace): Palpable contraction; no motion.

Grade 0 (Zero): No contractile activity.

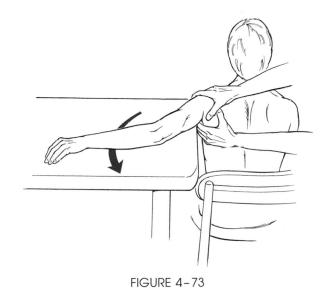

FIGURE 4–73

Helpful Hints

If the scapular muscles are weak, the examiner must manually stabilize the scapula to avoid scapular abduction.

Substitution by Triceps Brachii (Long Head)

Maintain the elbow in flexion to avoid substitution by the long head of the Triceps.

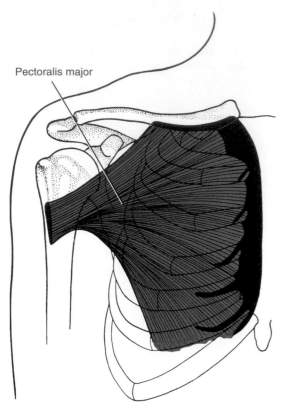

FIGURE 4–74

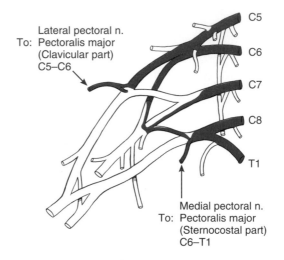

Lateral pectoral n.
To: Pectoralis major
(Clavicular part)
C5–C6

C5

C6

C7

C8

T1

Medial pectoral n.
To: Pectoralis major
(Sternocostal part)
C6–T1

FIGURE 4–75

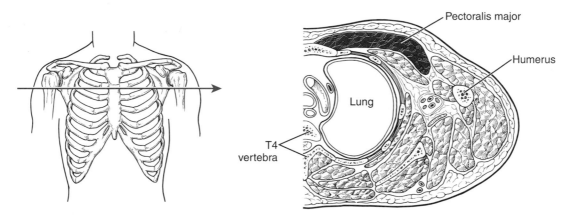

FIGURE 4–76

Range of Motion
0° to 130°
When starting from a position of 90° of forward flexion: 0° to − 40° (range, 40°)
When starting with the arm in full horizontal abduction: 0° passing across the midline to − 40° (range, 130°)

Table 4-11 SHOULDER HORIZONTAL ADDUCTION

I.D.	Muscle	Origin	Insertion
131	Pectoralis major		
	Clavicular part	Clavicle (sternal half of anterior surface)	Humerus (intertubercular sulcus, lateral lip)
	Sternal part	Sternum (anterior surface down to rib 6) Ribs 2–7 (costal cartilages) Aponeurosis of Obliquus externus abdominis	Both parts converge on a bilaminar common tendon
Other			
133	Deltoid (anterior fibers)		

Preliminary Examination

The examiner begins with the patient supine and checks the range of motion and then tests both heads of the Pectoralis major simultaneously. The patient is asked to move the arm in horizontal adduction, keeping it parallel to the floor without rotation.

If the arm moves across the body in a diagonal motion, test the sternal and clavicular heads of the muscle separately. Testing both heads of the Pectoralis major separately should be routine in any patient with cervical spinal cord injury because of their different nerve root innervation.

Grade 5 (Normal) and Grade 4 (Good)

Position of Patient
Whole Muscle: Supine. Shoulder abducted to 90°; elbow flexed to 90° (Fig. 4–77).

Clavicular Head: Patient begins test with shoulder in 60° of abduction with elbow flexed. Patient then is asked to horizontally adduct the shoulder.

Sternal Head: Patient begins test with shoulder in about 120° of abduction with elbow flexed.

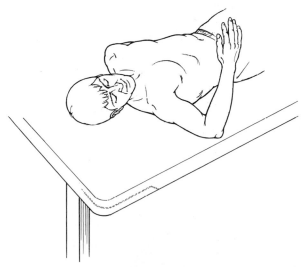

FIGURE 4–77

(Pectoralis major)

Grade 5 (Normal) and Grade 4 (Good) Continued

Position of Therapist: Stand at side of shoulder to be tested. Hand used for resistance is contoured around the forearm just proximal to the wrist. The other hand is used to check the activity of the Pectoralis major on the upper aspect of the chest just medial to the shoulder joint (Fig. 4–78). (Palpation is not needed in a Grade 5 test, but it is prudent to assess activity in the muscle being tested.)

Palpate the clavicular fibers of the Pectoralis major up under the medial half of the clavicle (Fig. 4–79). Palpate the sternal fibers on the chest wall at the lower anterior border of the axilla (Fig. 4–80).

Test: When the *whole muscle* is tested, the patient horizontally adducts the shoulder through the available range of motion.

To test the *clavicular head*, the patient's motion begins at 60° of abduction and moves up and in

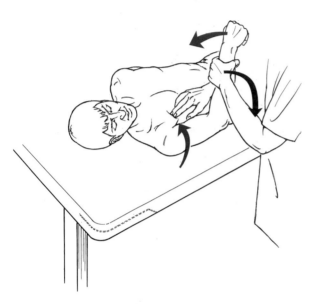

FIGURE 4–78

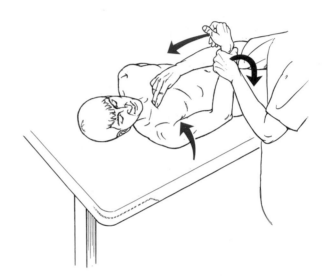

FIGURE 4–79

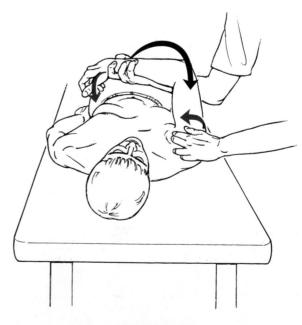

FIGURE 4–80

Grade 5 (Normal) and Grade 4 (Good) Continued

across the body. The examiner applies resistance above the wrist in a downward direction (toward floor) and outward (i.e., opposite to the direction of the fibers of the clavicular head, which moves the arm diagonally up and inward (see Fig. 4–79).

To test the *sternal head,* the motion begins at 120° of shoulder abduction and moves diagonally down and in toward patient's opposite hip. Resistance is given above the wrist in an up and outward direction (i.e., opposite to the motion of the sternal head, which is diagonally down and inward (see Fig. 4–80).

Instructions to Patient
Both Heads: "Move your arm across your chest. Hold it. Don't let me pull it back."

Clavicular Head: "Move your arm up and in."

Sternal Head: "Move your arm down and in."

Grading

Grade 5 (Normal): Complete range of motion and takes maximal resistance.

Grade 4 (Good): Completes range of motion and takes strong to moderate resistance, but muscle exhibits some "give" at end of range.

Grade 3 (Fair)

Position of Patient: Supine. Shoulder at 90° of abduction and elbow at 90° of flexion.

Position of Therapist: Same as for Grade 5.

Test
Both Heads: Patient horizontally adducts extremity across chest in a straight pattern with no diagonal motion (Fig. 4–81).

Clavicular Head: Direction of motion by the patient is diagonally up and inward.

Sternal Head: Direction of motion is diagonally down and inward.

Instructions to Patient: Same as for the Grade 5 (Normal) test, but no resistance is offered.

Grading

Grade 3 (Fair): Patient completes available range of motion in all three tests with no resistance other than the weight of the extremity.

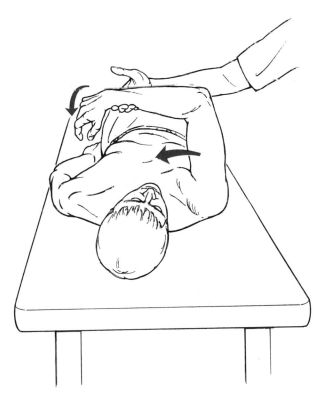

FIGURE 4–81

(Pectoralis major)

Grade 2 (Poor), Grade 1 (Trace), and Grade 0 (Zero)

Position of Patient: Supine. Arm is supported in 90° of abduction with elbow flexed to 90°.

Alternate Position: Patient is seated with test arm supported on table (at level of axilla) with arm in 90° of abduction (or in scaption) and elbow slightly flexed (Fig. 4–82). Friction of the table surface should be minimized.

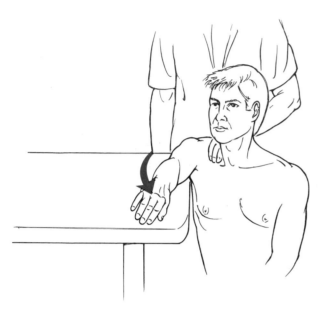

FIGURE 4-82

Position of Therapist: Stand at side of shoulder to be tested or behind the sitting patient. When the patient is supine, support the full length of the forearm and hold the limb at the wrist (see Fig. 4–80).

For both tests palpate the Pectoralis major muscle on the anterior aspect of the chest medial to the shoulder joint (see Fig. 4–78.)

Test: Patient attempts to horizontally adduct the shoulder. The use of the alternate test position, in which the arm moves across the table, precludes individual testing for the two heads.

Instructions to Patient: "Try to move your arm across your chest." In seated position: "Move your arm forward."

Grading

Grade 2 (Poor): Patient horizontally adducts shoulder through available range of motion with the weight of the arm supported by the examiner or the table.

Grade 1 (Trace): Palpable contractile activity.

Grade 0 (Zero): No contractile activity.

Helpful Hints

This test requires resistance on the forearm, which in turn requires that the elbow flexors be strong. If they are weak, provide resistance on the arm just proximal to the elbow.

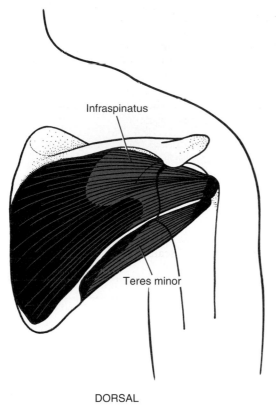

Infraspinatus
Teres minor
DORSAL

FIGURE 4-83

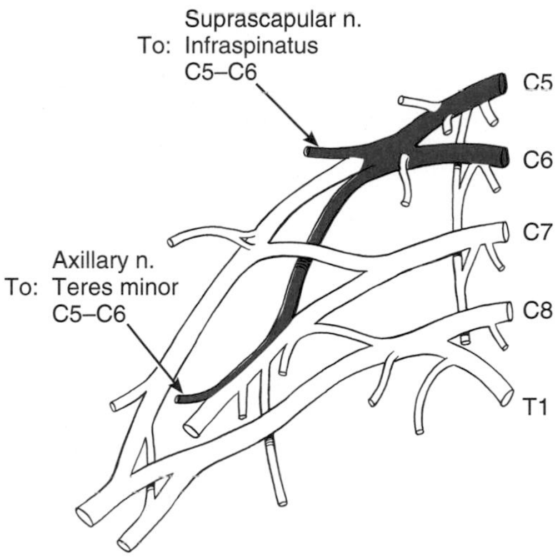

Suprascapular n.
To: Infraspinatus
C5–C6
Axillary n.
To: Teres minor
C5–C6
C5
C6
C7
C8
T1

FIGURE 4-84

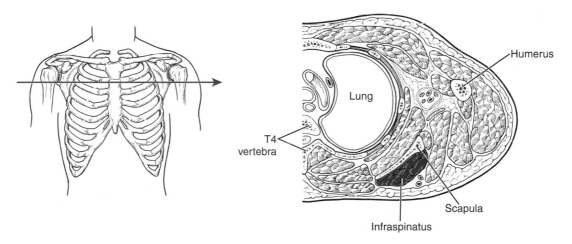

Humerus
Lung
T4
vertebra
Scapula
Infraspinatus

FIGURE 4-85

SHOULDER EXTERNAL ROTATION

(Infraspinatus and Teres minor)

<table>
<tr><td colspan="2">**Range of Motion**</td></tr>
<tr><td colspan="2">0° to 60°</td></tr>
<tr><td colspan="2">(In literature, range varies between 0° and 90°. Range also varies with elevation of arm.)</td></tr>
</table>

Table 4-12 SHOULDER EXTERNAL ROTATION

I.D.	Muscle	Origin	Insertion
136	Infraspinatus	Scapula (infraspinous fossa, medial 2/3) Infraspinous fascia	Humerus (greater tubercle, middle facet)
137	Teres minor	Scapula (lateral border, superior 2/3)	Humerus (greater tubercle, lowest facet) Humerus (shaft, distal to lowest facet) Capsule of glenohumeral joint

Other

133	Deltoid (posterior)		

Grade 5 (Normal), Grade 4 (Good), and Grade 3 (Fair)

Position of Patient: Prone with head turned toward test side. Shoulder abducted to 90° with arm fully supported on table; forearm hanging vertically over edge of table. Place a folded towel under the arm at the edge of the table if it has a sharp edge.

Alternate Position: Short sitting with elbow flexed to 90°. The amount of resistance tolerated in this position may be much greater for Grades 5 and 4.

Position of Therapist: Stand at test side at level of patient's waist (Fig. 4–86). Two fingers of one hand are used to give resistance at the wrist for Grades 5 and 4. The other hand supports the elbow to provide some counterpressure at the end of the range.

Test: Patient moves forearm upward through the range of external rotation.

Instructions to Patient: "Raise your arm to the level of the table. Hold it. Don't let me push it down." Therapist may need to demonstrate the desired motion.

Grading

Grade 5 (Normal): Completes available range of motion and holds firmly against two-finger resistance.

Grade 4 (Good): Completes available range, but the muscle at end range yields or gives way.

Grade 3 (Fair): Completes available range of motion but is unable to take any manual resistance (Fig. 4–87).

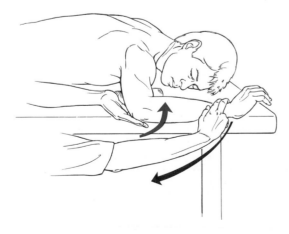

FIGURE 4-86

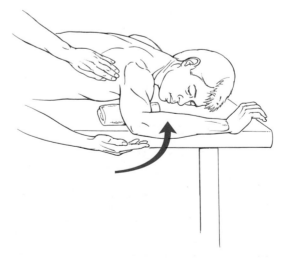

FIGURE 4-87

Grade 2 (Poor), Grade 1 (Trace), and Grade 0 (Zero)

Position of Patient: Prone with head turned to test side, trunk at edge of table. The entire limb hangs down loosely from the shoulder in neutral rotation, palm facing table (Fig. 4–88).

Position of Therapist: Stand or sit on a low stool at test side of patient at shoulder level. Palpate the Infraspinatus over the body of the scapula below the spine in the infraspinous fossa (see Fig. 4–87). Palpate the Teres minor on the inferior margin of the axilla and along the axillary border of the scapula (see Fig. 4–88).

Test: Patient attempts to externally rotate the shoulder. Alternatively, place the patient's arm in external rotation and ask the patient to hold the end position (Fig. 4–89).

Instructions to Patient: "Turn your palm outward."

Grading

Grade 2 (Poor): Completes available range (i.e., palm faces forward) in this gravity-eliminated position.

Grade 1 (Trace): Palpation of either or both muscles reveals contractile activity but no motion.

Grade 0 (Zero): No palpable or visible activity.

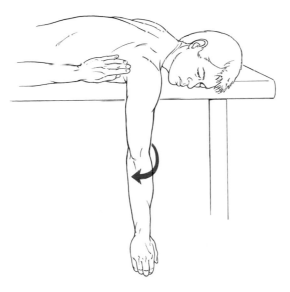

FIGURE 4–88

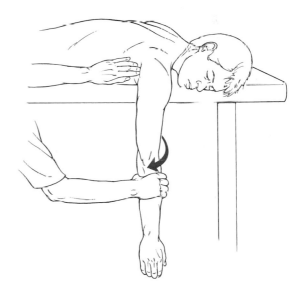

FIGURE 4–89

Helpful Hints

- Resistance in tests of shoulder rotation should be administered gradually and slowly, with great care taken to prevent injury which can occur readily because the shoulder lacks inherent stability. This is particularly important for the elderly patient.

- The therapist must be careful to discern whether supination occurs instead of the requested external rotation during the testing of Grades 2 and 1 muscles because this motion can be mistaken for lateral rotation.

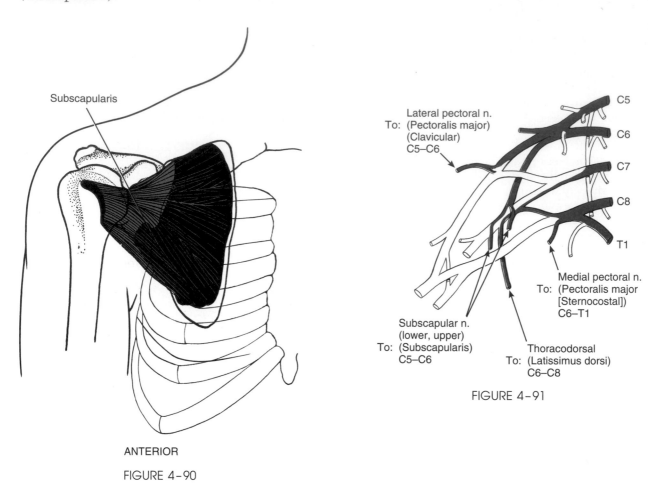

Subscapularis

ANTERIOR

FIGURE 4–90

Lateral pectoral n.
To: (Pectoralis major)
(Clavicular)
C5–C6

C5
C6
C7
C8
T1

Medial pectoral n.
To: (Pectoralis major
[Sternocostal])
C6–T1

Subscapular n.
(lower, upper)
To: (Subscapularis)
C5–C6

Thoracodorsal
To: (Latissimus dorsi)
C6–C8

FIGURE 4–91

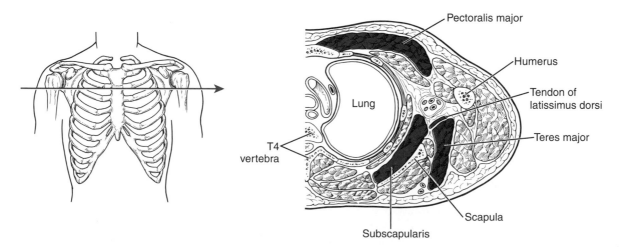

Pectoralis major

Humerus

Tendon of
latissimus dorsi

Teres major

Lung

T4
vertebra

Scapula

Subscapularis

FIGURE 4–92

Range of Motion
0° to 80°
(In literature, range varies from 0° to 45° and to as high as 90°. Range also varies with elevation of arm.)

Table 4-13 SHOULDER INTERNAL ROTATION

I.D.	Muscle	Origin	Insertion
134	Subscapularis	Scapula (fills fossa on costal surface) Intermuscular septa Aponeurosis of subscapularis	Humerus (lesser tubercle) Capsule of glenohumeral joint (anterior)
131	Pectoralis major		
	Clavicular part	Clavicle (sternal half of anterior surface)	Humerus (intertubercular sulcus, lateral lip)
	Sternal part	Sternum (anterior surface down to rib 6) Ribs 2–7 costal cartilages Aponeurosis of Obliquus externus abdominis	Both parts converge on a bilaminar common tendon
130	Latissimus dorsi	T6–T12; L1–L5 and sacral vertebrae (spinous processes) Supraspinous ligaments Ribs 9–12 (by slips which interdigitate with Obliquus externus abdominus) Ilium (crest, posterior) Thoracolumbar fascia	Humerus (floor of intertubercular sulcus) Deep fascia of arm
138	Teres major	Scapula (dorsal surface of inferior angle)	Humerus (intertubercular sulcus, medial lip)
Other			
133	Deltoid (anterior)		

Grade 5 (Normal), Grade 4 (Good), and Grade 3 (Fair)

Position of Patient: Prone with head turned toward test side. Shoulder is abducted to 90° with folded towel placed under distal arm and forearm hanging vertically over edge of table. Short sitting is a common alternate position.

Position of Therapist: Stand at test side. Hand giving resistance is placed on the volar side of the forearm just above the wrist. The other hand provides counterforce at the elbow (Fig. 4–93). The resistance hand applies resistance in a downward and forward direction; the counterforce is applied backward and slightly upward. Stabilize the scapular region if muscles are weak.

Test: Patient moves arm through available range of internal rotation (backward and upward).

Instructions to Patient: "Move your forearm up and back. Hold it. Don't let me push it down." Demonstrate the desired motion to the patient.

Grading

Grade 5 (Normal): Completes available range and holds firmly against strong resistance.

Grade 4 (Good): Completes available range, but there is a "spongy" feeling against strong resistance.

Grade 3 (Fair): Completes available range with no manual resistance (Fig. 4–94).

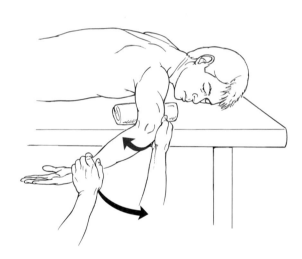

FIGURE 4–93

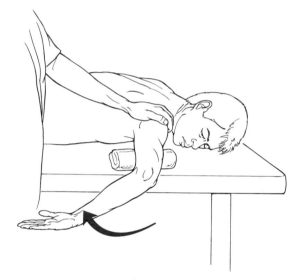

FIGURE 4–94

Grade 2 (Poor), Grade 1 (Trace), and Grade 0 (Zero)

Position of Patient: Prone with head turned toward test side. Patient must be near the edge of the table on test side so that entire arm can hang down freely over the edge (Fig. 4–95). Arm is in neutral with palm facing the table.

Position of Therapist: Stand at test side or sit on low stool. Hand used for palpation must find the tendon of the Subscapularis deep in the central area of the axilla (Fig. 4–96). Therapist may have to stabilize test arm at the shoulder.

Test: Patient internally rotates arm with thumb leading so that the palm faces out or away from the table.

Instructions to Patient: "Turn your arm so that the palm faces away from the table" (not shown).

Grading

Grade 2 (Poor): Completes available range.

Grade 1 (Trace): Palpable contraction occurs.

Grade 0 (Zero): No palpable contraction.

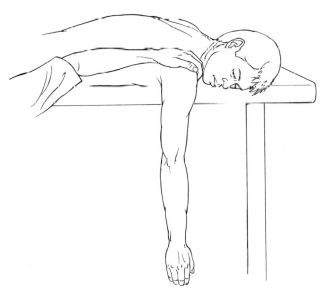

FIGURE 4–95

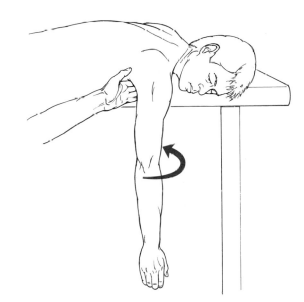

FIGURE 4–96

Helpful Hints

- The therapist should be wary of pronation in this test. Forearm pronation is rather easily mistaken for internal rotation.

- Internal rotation is a stronger motion than external rotation. This is largely a factor of differing muscle mass.

- If you cannot palpate the Subscapularis, try the Pectoralis major, which, as a surface muscle, is more readily felt.

- The hand of the examiner may substitute for a towel roll under the distal arm, the purpose being to protect the patient from the discomfort of moving against a hard table and to keep the arm horizontal to the floor.

- The prone position is preferred to the supine or sitting position in tests for Grades 2, 1, and 0 because a weak patient has a tendency to use trunk rotation as a substitute.

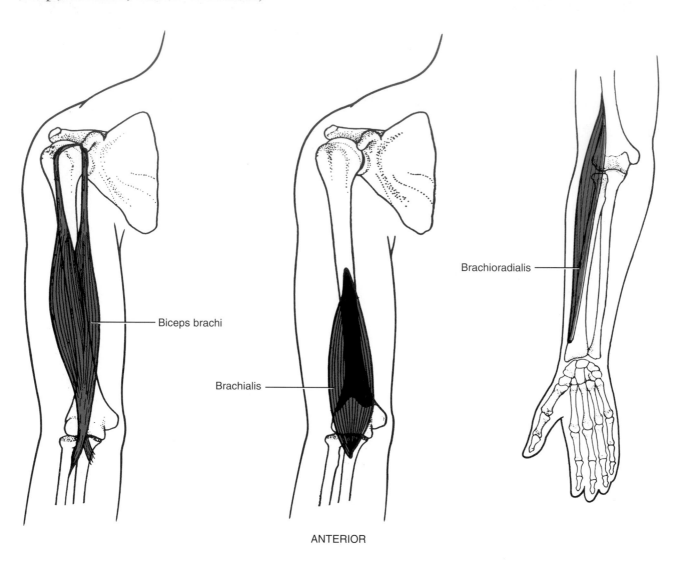

Biceps brachi

Brachialis

Brachioradialis

ANTERIOR

FIGURES 4–97, 98, 99

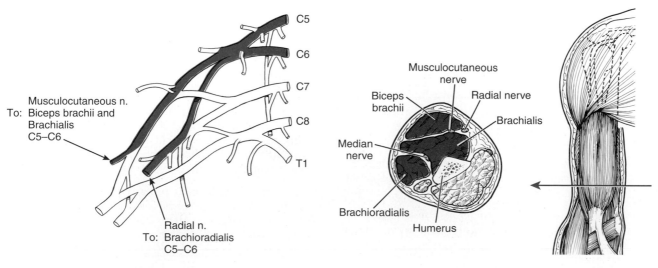

Musculocutaneous n.
To: Biceps brachii and
Brachialis
C5–C6

Radial n.
To: Brachioradialis
C5–C6

C5
C6
C7
C8
T1

FIGURE 4–100

Musculocutaneous
nerve

Biceps
brachii

Radial nerve

Brachialis

Median
nerve

Brachioradialis

Humerus

FIGURE 4–101

Range of Motion
0° to 150°

Table 4-14 ELBOW FLEXION

I.D.	Muscle	Origin	Insertion
140	Biceps brachii		
	Short head	Scapula (coracoid process, apex)	Radius (radial tuberosity)
	Long head	Scapula (supraglenoid tubercle)	Bicipital aponeurosis
		Capsule of glenohumeral joint and glenoid labrum	
141	Brachialis	Humerus (shaft anterior, distal 1/2) Intermuscular septa (medial)	Ulna (tuberosity and coronoid process)
143	Brachioradialis	Humerus (lateral supracondylar ridge, proximal 2/3) Lateral intermuscular septum	Radius (distal end just proximal to styloid process)
Others			
146	Pronator teres		
148	Extensor carpi radialis longus		
151	Flexor carpi radialis		
153	Flexor carpi ulnaris		(See also Plate 4, page 127)

Grade 5 (Normal), Grade 4 (Good), and Grade 3 (Fair)

Position of Patient: Short sitting with arms at sides. The following are the positions of choice, but it is doubtful whether the individual muscles can be separated when strong effort is used. The Brachialis in particular is independent of forearm position.

Biceps brachii: forearm in supination (Fig. 4–102)
Brachialis: forearm in pronation (Fig. 4–103)
Brachioradialis: forearm in midposition between pronation and supination (Fig. 4–104)

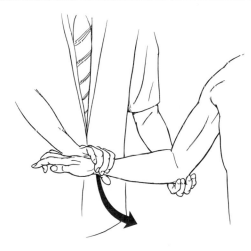

FIGURE 4–103

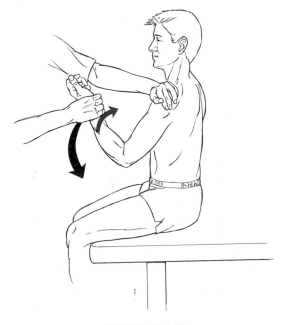

FIGURE 4–102

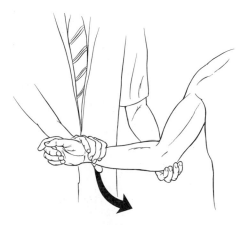

FIGURE 4–104

(Biceps, Brachialis, and Brachioradialis)

Grade 5 (Normal), Grade 4 (Good), and Grade 3 (Fair) Continued

Position of Therapist: Stand in front of patient toward the test side. Hand giving resistance is contoured over the flexor surface of the forearm proximal to the wrist (see Fig. 4–102). The other hand applies counterforce by cupping the palm over the anterior superior surface of the shoulder.

No resistance is given in a Grade 3 test, but the test elbow is cupped by the examiner's hand (Fig. 4–105, Biceps illustrated at end range).

Test (All Three Forearm Positions): Patient flexes elbow through range of motion.

Instructions to Patient (All Three Tests)
Grades 5 and 4: "Bend your elbow. Hold it. Don't let me pull it down."

Grade 3: "Bend your elbow."

Grading

Grade 5 (Normal): Completes available range and holds firmly against maximal resistance.

Grade 4 (Good): Completes available range against strong to moderate resistance, but the end point may not be firm.

Grade 3 (Fair): Completes available range with each forearm position with no manual resistance.

Grade 2 (Poor)

Position of Patient
All Elbow Flexors: Short sitting with arm abducted to 90° and supported by examiner (Fig. 4–106). Forearm is supinated (Biceps), pronated (Brachialis), and in midposition (Brachioradialis).

Alternate Position for Patients Unable to Sit: Supine. Elbow is flexed to about 45° with forearm supinated (for Biceps) (Fig. 4–106), pronated (for Brachialis), and in midposition (for Brachioradialis) (Fig. 4–107), Biceps illustrated.

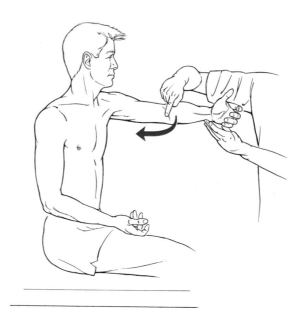

FIGURE 4–106

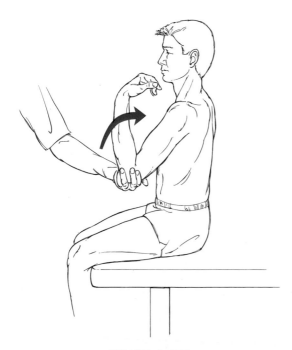

FIGURE 4–105

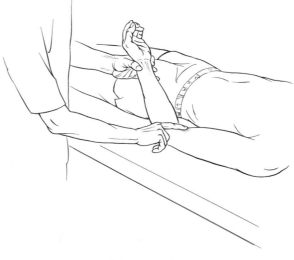

FIGURE 4–107

Grade 5 (Normal), Grade 4 (Good), and Grade 3 (Fair) Continued

Position of Therapist

All Three Flexors: Stand in front of patient and support abducted arm under the elbow and wrist if necessary (see Fig. 4–106). Palpate the tendon of the Biceps in the antecubital space (see Fig. 4–107). On the arm the muscle fibers may be felt on the anterior surface of the middle two-thirds with the short head lying medial to the long head.

Palpate the Brachialis in the distal arm medial to the tendon of the Biceps. Palpate the Brachioradialis on the proximal volar surface of the forearm, where it forms the lateral border of the cubital fossa (Fig. 4–108).

Test: Patient attempts to flex the elbow.

Instructions to Patient: "Try to bend your elbow."

Grading

Grade 2 (Poor): Completes range of motion (in each of the muscles tested).

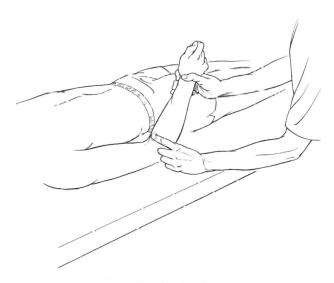

FIGURE 4–108

Grade 1 (Trace) and Grade 0 (Zero)

Positions of Patient and Therapist: Supine for all three muscles with therapist standing at test side (see Fig. 4–108). All other aspects are the same as Grade 2 test.

Test: Patient attempts to bend elbow with hand supinated, pronated, and in midposition.

Grading

Grade 1 (Trace): Examiner can palpate a contractile response in each of the three muscles for which a Trace grade is given.

Grade 0 (Zero): No palpable contractile activity.

Helpful Hints

- The patient's wrist flexor muscles should remain relaxed throughout the test because strongly contracting wrist flexors may assist in elbow flexion.

- If the sitting position is contraindicated for any reason, all tests for these muscles may be performed in the supine position, but in that case manual resistance should be part of the Grade 3 test (gravity compensation).

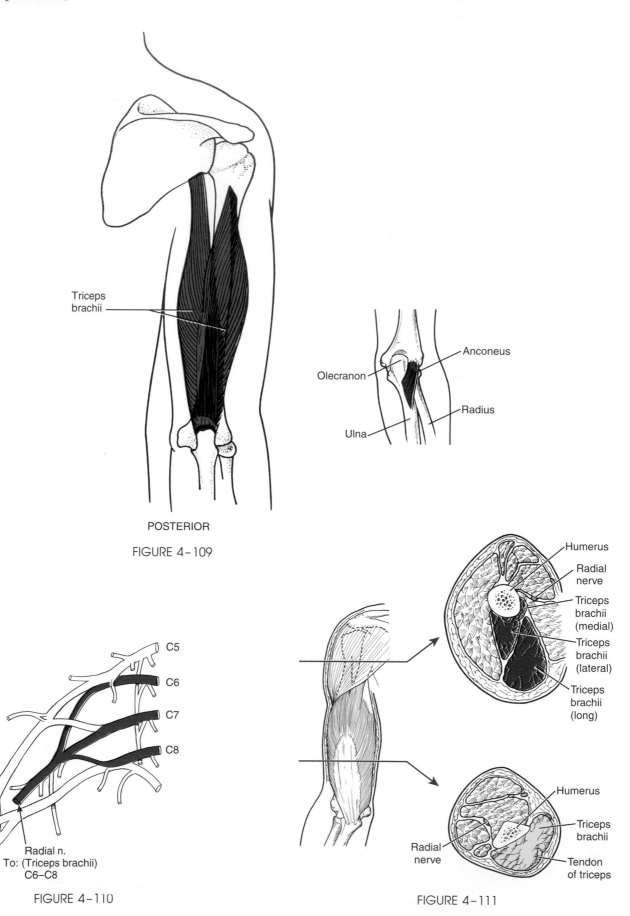

Triceps
brachii

POSTERIOR

FIGURE 4-109

Olecranon

Anconeus

Ulna

Radius

C5

C6

C7

C8

Radial n.
To: (Triceps brachii)
C6–C8

FIGURE 4-110

Humerus

Radial
nerve

Triceps
brachii
(medial)

Triceps
brachii
(lateral)

Triceps
brachii
(long)

Humerus

Triceps
brachii

Radial
nerve

Tendon
of triceps

FIGURE 4-111

Range of Motion

150° to 0°

Table 4-15 ELBOW EXTENSION

I.D.	Muscle	Origin	Insertion
142	Triceps brachii		All heads have a common tendon to:
	Long head	Scapula (infraglenoid tuberosity and capsule of glenohumeral joint)	Ulna (olecranon process, upper surface)
	Lateral head	Humerus (shaft, oblique ridge, posterior surface)	Blends with antebrachial fascia
		Lateral intermuscular septum	Capsule of elbow joint
	Medial head	Humerus (shaft: entire length of posterior surface) Medial and lateral intermuscular septa	
Other			
144	Anconeus		(See also Plate 4, page 127.)

ELBOW EXTENSION

(Triceps brachii)

Grade 5 (Normal), Grade 4 (Good), and Grade 3 (Fair)

Position of Patient: Prone on table. The patient starts the test with the arm in 90° of abduction and the forearm flexed and hanging vertically over the side of the table (Fig. 4–112).

Position of Therapist: For the prone patient the therapist provides support just above the elbow. The other hand is used to apply downward resistance on the dorsal surface of the forearm (Fig. 4–113) illustrates end position).

Test: Patient extends elbow to end of available range or until the forearm is horizontal to the floor.

Instructions to Patient: "Straighten your elbow. Hold it. Don't let me bend it." Do not allow hyperextension.

Grading

Grade 5 (Normal): Completes available range and holds firmly against maximal resistance.

Grade 4 (Good): Completes available range against strong resistance, but there is a "give" to the resistance at the end range.

Grade 3 (Fair): Completes available range with no manual resistance (Fig. 4–114).

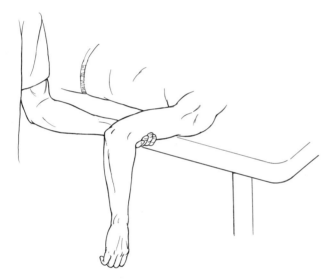

FIGURE 4–112

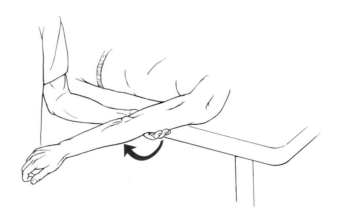

FIGURE 4–114

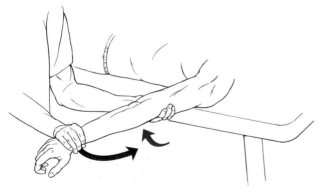

FIGURE 4–113

Grade 2 (Poor), Grade 1 (Trace), and Grade 0 (Zero)

Position of Patient: Short sitting. The arm is abducted to 90° with the shoulder in neutral rotation and the elbow flexed to about 45°. The entire limb is horizontal to the floor (Fig. 4–115).

Position of Therapist: Stand at test side of patient. For the Grade 2 test, support the limb at the elbow. For a Grade 1 or 0 test, support the limb under the forearm and palpate the Triceps on the posterior surface of the arm just proximal to the olecranon process (Fig. 4–116).

Test: Patient attempts to extend the elbow.

Instructions to Patient: "Try to straighten your elbow."

Grading

Grade 2 (Poor): Completes available range in the absence of gravity.

Grade 1 (Trace): Examiner can feel tension in the Triceps tendon just proximal to the olecranon (see Fig. 4–116) or contractile activity in the muscle fibers on the posterior surface of the arm.

Grade 0 (Zero): No evidence of any muscle activity.

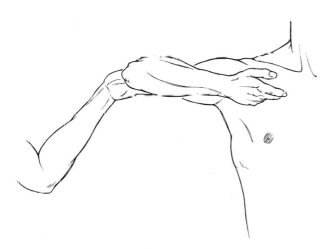

FIGURE 4–115

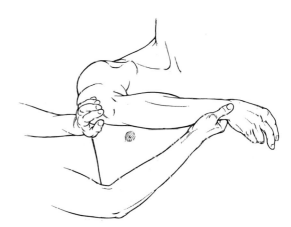

FIGURE 4–116

Substitutions

- Via external rotation. When the patient is sitting with the arm abducted, elbow extension can be accomplished with a Grade 0 Triceps (Fig. 4–117). This can occur when the patient externally rotates the shoulder, thus dropping the arm below the forearm. As a result, the elbow literally falls into extension.

- Via horizontal adduction. This substitution can accomplish elbow extension and is done purposefully by patients with a cervical cord injury and a Grade 0 Triceps. With the distal segment fixed (as when the examiner stabilizes the hand or wrist), the patient horizontally adducts the arm, and the thrust pulls the elbow into extension (Fig. 4–118). The therapist, therefore, should provide support at the elbow for testing purposes rather than at the wrist.

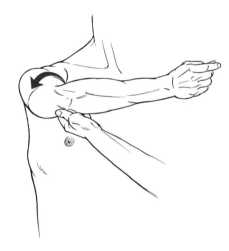

FIGURE 4–117

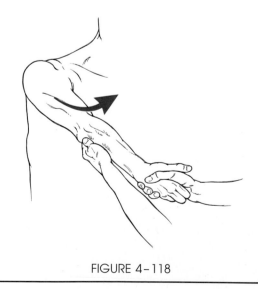

FIGURE 4–118

Helpful Hints

- The therapist should confirm that muscle activity is seen and felt (i.e.. Triceps activity is actually present) because patients can become very adept at substituting. In fact, patients frequently are taught substitution, encouraged to use it as a functional movement, but are not allowed to do so for the purpose of testing.

- Give resistance in Grades 5 and 4 tests with the elbow slightly flexed to avoid enabling the patient to "lock" the elbow joint by hyperextending it.

- While elbow extension is tested in the prone position there must be awareness that with the shoulder horizontally abducted, the two-joint muscle is less effective, and the test grade well may be lower than it should be.[1]

- An alternate position for Grades 5, 4, and 3 is with the patient short sitting. The examiner stands behind the patient, supporting the arm in 90° of abduction just above the flexed elbow (Fig. 4–119). The patient straightens the elbow against the resistance given at the wrist.

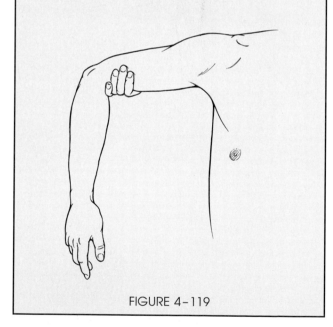

FIGURE 4–119

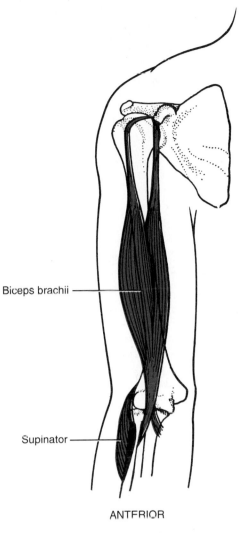

Biceps brachii

Supinator

ANTERIOR

FIGURE 4-120

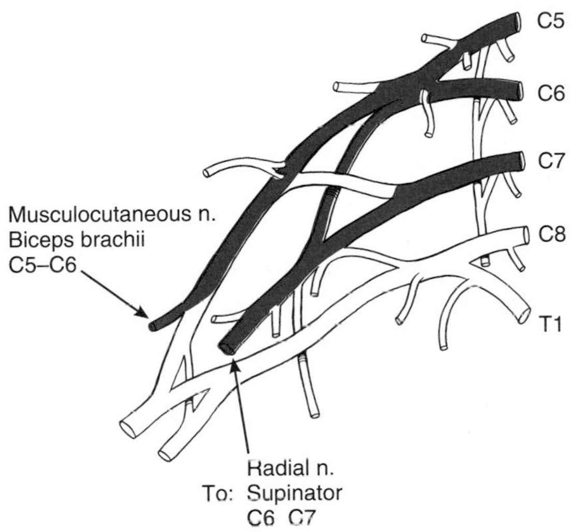

Musculocutaneous n.
Biceps brachii
C5–C6

Radial n.
To: Supinator
C6 C7

C5

C6

C7

C8

T1

FIGURE 4-121

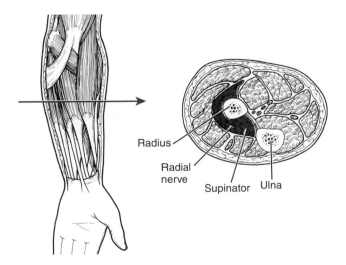

Radius

Radial nerve

Supinator   Ulna

FIGURE 4-122

FOREARM SUPINATION

(Supinator and Biceps brachii)

Range of Motion

0° to 80°

Table 4-16 FOREARM SUPINATION

I.D.	Muscle	Origin	Insertion
145	Supinator	Humerus (lateral epicondyle) Ulna (supinator crest) Radial collateral ligament of elbow joint Annular ligament of radioulnar joint Aponeurosis of supinator	Radius (shaft, lateral aspect of proximal 1/3)
140	Biceps brachii Short head Long head	 Scapula (coracoid apex) Scapula (supraglenoid tubercle) Capsule of glenohumeral joint and glenoid labrum	 Radius (radial tuberosity) Bicipital aponeurosis (See also Plate 4, page 127.)

Grade 5 (Normal), Grade 4 (Good), and Grade 3 (Fair)

Position of Patient: Short sitting; arm at side and elbow flexed to 90°; forearm in pronation (Fig. 4–123, showing end range). Alternatively, patient may sit at a table.

Position of Therapist: Stand at side or in front of patient. One hand supports the elbow (see Fig. 4–123). For resistance, grasp the forearm on the volar surface at the wrist.

Test: Patient begins in pronation and supinates the forearm until the palm faces the ceiling. Therapist resists motion in the direction of pronation. (No resistance is given for Grade 3.)

Alternate Test: Grasp patient's hand as if shaking hands; cradle the elbow and resist via the hand grip (Fig. 4–124). This test is used if the patient has Grade 5 or 4 wrist and hand strength. If wrist flexion is painful, give resistance at the wrist a more difficult level, but less painful.

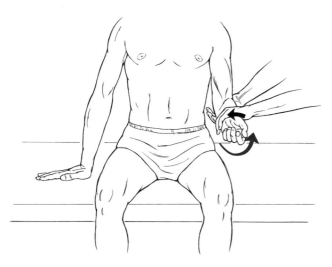

FIGURE 4–123

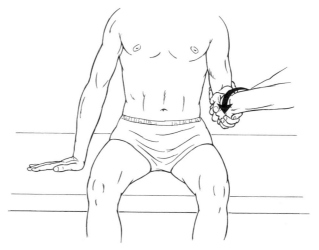

FIGURE 4–124

Grade 5 (Normal), Grade 4 (Good), and Grade 3 (Fair) Continued

Instructions to Patient: "Turn your palm up. Hold it. Don't let me turn it down. Keep your wrist and fingers relaxed."

For Grade 3: "Turn your palm up."

Grading

Grade 5 (Normal): Completes full available range of motion and holds against maximal resistance.

Grade 4 (Good): Completes full range of motion against strong to moderate resistance.

Grade 3 (Fair): Completes available range of motion without resistance (Fig. 4–125, showing end range).

Grade 2 (Poor)

Position of Patient: Short sitting with shoulder flexed between 45° and 90° and elbow flexed to 90°. Forearm in neutral.

Position of Therapist: Support the test arm by cupping the hand under the elbow.

Test: Patient supinates forearm (Fig. 4–126) through partial range of motion.

Instructions to Patient: "Turn your palm toward your face."

Grading

Grade 2 (Poor): Completes a full range of motion.

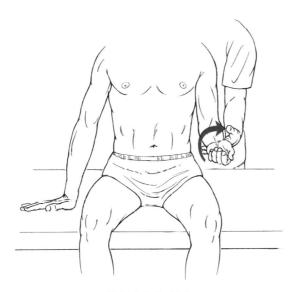

FIGURE 4-125

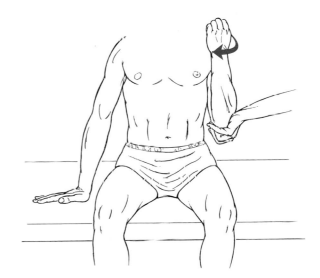

FIGURE 4-126

FOREARM SUPINATION

(Supinator and Biceps brachii)

Grade 1 (Trace) and Grade 0 (Zero)

Position of Patient: Short sitting. Arm and elbow are flexed as for the Grade 3 test.

Position of Therapist: Support the forearm just distal to the elbow. Palpate the Supinator distal to the head of the radius on the dorsal aspect of the forearm (Fig. 4–127).

Test: Patient attempts to supinate the forearm.

Instructions to Patient: "Try to turn your palm so it faces the ceiling."

Grading

Grade 1 (Trace): Slight contractile activity but no limb movement.

Grade 0 (Zero): No contractile activity.

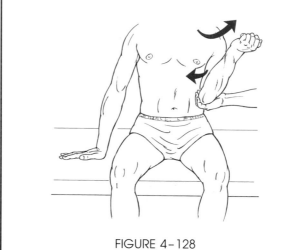

Substitution

- Patient may externally rotate and adduct the arm across the body (Fig. 4–128) as forearm supination is attempted. When this occurs, the forearm rolls into supination with no activity of the Supinator muscle.
- Patient should be instructed to keep the wrist and fingers as relaxed as possible to avoid substitution by the wrist extensors.

FIGURE 4–128

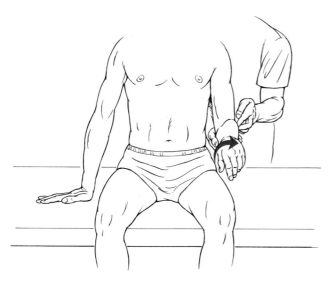

FIGURE 4–127

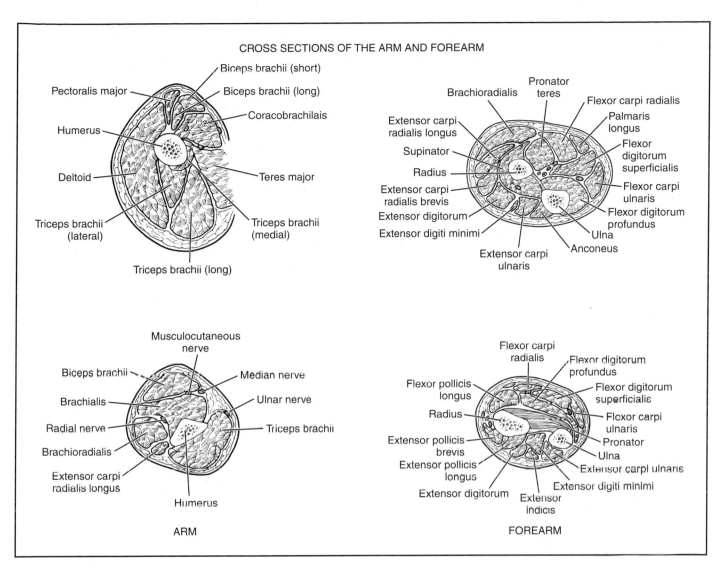

CROSS SECTIONS OF THE ARM AND FOREARM

ARM

FOREARM

PLATE 4

(Pronator teres and Pronator quadratus)

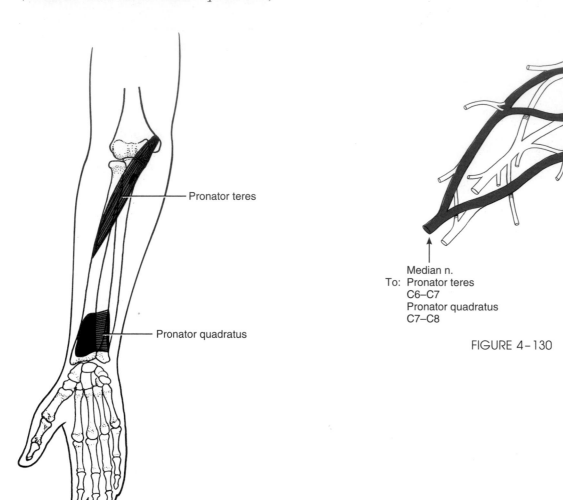

Pronator teres

Pronator quadratus

FIGURE 4-129

C5
C6
C7
C8
T1

Median n.
To: Pronator teres
C6–C7
Pronator quadratus
C7–C8

FIGURE 4-130

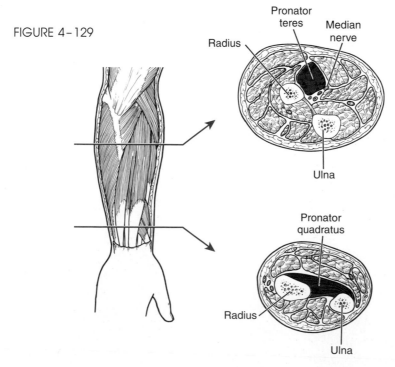

Pronator
teres

Median
nerve

Radius

Ulna

Pronator
quadratus

Radius

Ulna

FIGURE 4-131

FOREARM PRONATION

(Pronator teres and Pronator quadratus)

Table 4-17 FOREARM PRONATION

I.D.	Muscle	Origin	Insertion
146	Pronator teres		Radius (midshaft, lateral surface)
	Humeral head	Humerus (shaft proximal to medial epicondyle) Common tendon of origin of flexor muscles Intermuscular septum Antebrachial fascia	
	Ulnar head	Ulna (coronoid process, medial) Joins humeral head in common tendon	
147	Pronator quadratus	Ulna (oblique ridge on distal 1/4 of anterior surface) Muscle aponeurosis	Radius (shaft, anterior surface distally; also area above ulnar notch)
Other			
151	Flexor carpi radialis		(See also Plate 4, page 127.)

Grade 5 (Normal), Grade 4 (Good), and Grade 3 (Fair)

Position of Patient: Short sitting or may sit at a table. Arm at side with elbow flexed to 90° and forearm in supination.

Position of Therapist: Standing at side or in front of patient. Support the elbow (Fig. 4–132, showing end range). Hand used for resistance grasps the forearm over the dorsal surface at the wrist.

Test: Patient pronates the forearm until the palm faces downward. Therapist resists motion at the wrist in the direction of supination for Grades 4 and 5. (No resistance is given for Grade 3.)

Alternate Test: Grasp patient's hand as if to shake hands, cradling the elbow with the other hand and resisting pronation via the hand grip. This alternate test may be used if the patient has Normal or Good wrist and hand strength.

Instructions to Patient: "Turn your palm down. Hold it. Don't let me turn it up. Keep your wrist and fingers relaxed."

Grading

Grade 5 (Normal): Completes available range of motion and holds against maximal resistance.

Grade 4 (Good): Completes all available range against strong to moderate resistance.

Grade 3 (Fair): Completes available range without resistance (Fig. 4–133, showing end range).

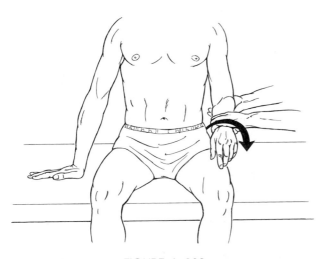

FIGURE 4-132

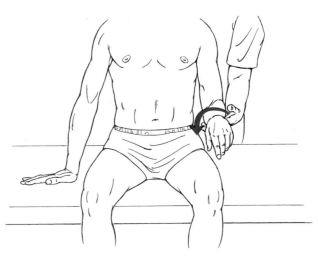

FIGURE 4-133

FOREARM PRONATION

(Pronator teres and Pronator quadratus)

Grade 2 (Poor)

Position of Patient: Short sitting with shoulder flexed between 45° and 90° and elbow flexed to 90°. Forearm in neutral (not illustrated).

Position of Therapist: Support the test arm by cupping the hand under the elbow.

Test: Patient pronates forearm.

Instructions to Patient: "Turn your palm facing outward away from your face."

Grading

Grade 2 (Poor): Completes range of motion (Fig. 4–134, showing end range).

Grade 1 (Trace) and Grade 0 (Zero)

Position of Patient: Short sitting. Arm is positioned as for the Grade 3 test.

Position of Therapist: Support the forearm just distal to the elbow. The fingers of the other hand are used to palpate the Pronator teres over the upper third of the volar surface of the forearm on a diagonal line from the medial condyle of the humerus to the lateral border of the radius (Fig. 4–135).

Test: Patient attempts to pronate the forearm.

Instructions to Patient: "Try to turn your palm down."

Grading

Grade 1 (Trace): Visible or palpable contractile activity with no motion of the part.

Grade 0 (Zero): No contractile activity.

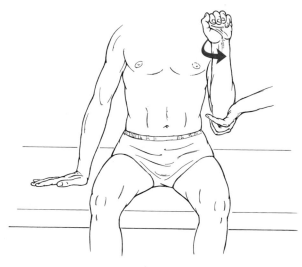

FIGURE 4–134

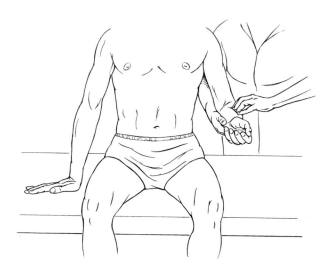

FIGURE 4–135

Substitution

Patient may internally rotate the shoulder or abduct it during attempts at pronation (Fig. 4–136). When this occurs, the forearm rolls into pronation without the benefit of activity by the pronator muscles.

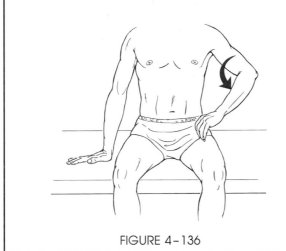

FIGURE 4–136

Helpful Hints

Patient should be instructed to keep the wrist and fingers relaxed to avoid substitution by the Flexor carpi radialis and the finger flexors.

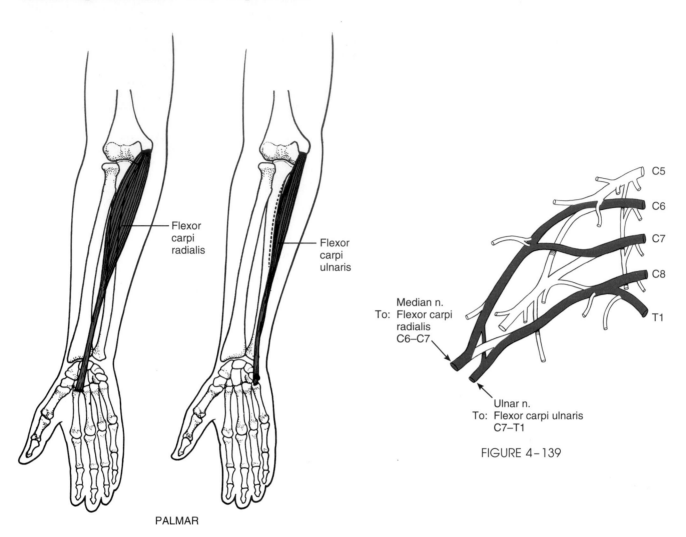

Flexor carpi radialis

Flexor carpi ulnaris

Median n.
To: Flexor carpi radialis
C6–C7

Ulnar n.
To: Flexor carpi ulnaris
C7–T1

FIGURE 4–139

PALMAR

FIGURES 4–137,138

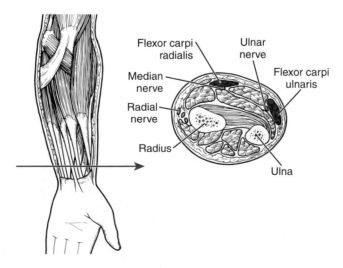

Flexor carpi radialis

Ulnar nerve

Median nerve

Flexor carpi ulnaris

Radial nerve

Radius

Ulna

FIGURE 4–140

(Flexor carpi radialis and Flexor carpi ulnaris)

Range of Motion
0° to 80°

Table 4-18 WRIST FLEXION

I.D.	Muscle	Origin	Insertion
151	Flexor carpi radialis	Humerus (medial epicondyle via common flexor tendon) Antebrachial fascia Intermuscular septum	2nd and 3rd metacarpals (base, palmar surface)
153	Flexor carpi ulnaris Two heads	Humeral head (medial epicondyle via common flexor tendon) Ulnar head (olecranon, medial margin; shaft, proximal 2/3 posterior via an aponeurosis) Intermuscular septum	Pisiform bone Hamate bone 5th metacarpal, base

Others

152	Palmaris longus		
156	Flexor digitorum superficialis		
157	Flexor digitorum profundus		
166	Abductor pollicis longus		
169	Flexor pollicis longus		(See also Plate 4, page 127.)

Grade 5 (Normal) and Grade 4 (Good)

Position of Patient (All Tests): Short sitting. Forearm is supported on its dorsal surface on a table. To start, forearm is supinated (Fig. 4–141). Wrist is in neutral or slightly extended.

Position of Therapist: One hand supports the patient's forearm under the wrist (Fig. 4–141).

Test: Patient flexes the wrist, keeping the digits and thumb relaxed.

To Test Both Wrist Flexors: The examiner applies resistance to the palm of the test hand with the thumb circling around to the dorsal surface (Fig. 4–142). Resistance is given evenly across the hand in a straight-down direction into wrist extension.

To Test the Flexor carpi radialis: Resistance is focused over the 2nd metacarpal (radial side of the hand) in the direction of extension and ulnar deviation.

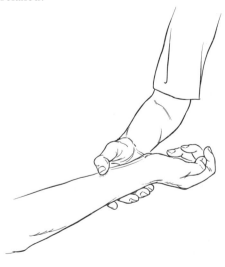

FIGURE 4–141

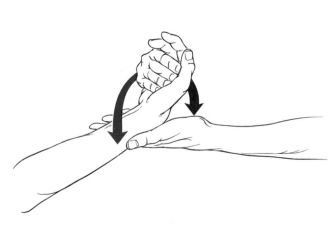

FIGURE 4–142

(Flexor carpi radialis and Flexor carpi ulnaris)

Grade 5 (Normal) and Grade 4 (Good) Continued

To Test the Flexor carpi ulnaris: Resistance is focused over the 5th metacarpal (ulnar side of the hand) in the direction of extension and radial deviation.

Instructions to Patient (All Tests): "Bend your wrist. Hold it. Don't let me pull it down. Keep your fingers relaxed."

Grading

Grade 5 (Normal): Completes available range of wrist flexion and holds against maximal resistance.

Grade 4 (Good): Completes available range and holds against strong to moderate resistance.

Grade 3 (Fair)

Position of Patient: Starting position with forearm supinated and wrist neutral as in Grade 5 and 4 tests.

Position of Therapist: Support the patient's forearm under the wrist.

Test

For Both Wrist Flexors: Patient flexes the wrist straight up without resistance and without radial or ulnar deviation.

For Flexor carpi radialis: Patient flexes the wrist in radial deviation (Fig. 4–143).

For Flexor carpi ulnaris: Patient flexes the wrist in ulnar deviation (Fig. 4–144).

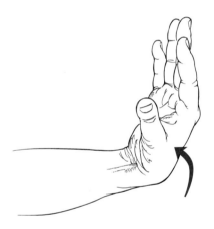

FIGURE 4–143

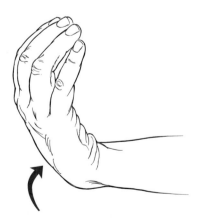

FIGURE 4–144

Grade 3 (Fair) Continued

Instructions to Patient
For Both Wrist Flexors: "Bend your wrist. Keep it straight with your fingers relaxed."

For Flexor carpi radialis: "Bend your wrist leading with the thumb side."

For Flexor carpi ulnaris: "Bend your wrist leading with the little finger."

Grading

Grade 3 (Fair) (All Tests): Completes available range without resistance.

Grade 2 (Poor)

Position of Patient: Short sitting with elbow supported on table. Forearm in midposition with hand resting on ulnar side (Fig. 4–145).

Position of Therapist: Support patient's forearm proximal to the wrist.

Test: Patient flexes wrist with the ulnar surface gliding across or not touching the table (Fig. 4–145). To test the two wrist flexors separately, hold the forearm so that the wrist does not lie on the table and ask the patient to perform the flexion motion while the wrist is in ulnar and then radial deviation.

Instructions to Patient: "Bend your wrist, keeping your fingers relaxed."

Grading

Grade 2 (Poor): Completes available range of wrist flexion without assistance of gravity.

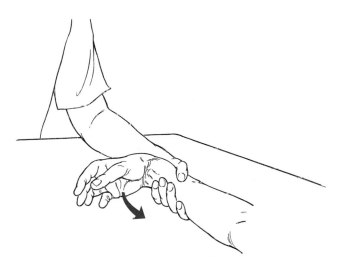

FIGURE 4–145

(Flexor carpi radialis and Flexor carpi ulnaris)

Grade 1 (Trace) and Grade 0 (Zero)

Position of Patient: Supinated forearm supported on table.

Position of Therapist: Support the wrist in flexion; the index finger of the other hand is used to palpate the appropriate tendons.

Palpate the tendons of the Flexor carpi radialis (Fig. 4–146) and the Flexor carpi ulnaris (Fig. 4–147) in separate tests.

The Flexor carpi radialis lies on the lateral palmar aspect of the wrist (Fig. 4–146) lateral to the Palmaris longus, if the patient has one!

The tendon of the Flexor carpi ulnaris (Fig. 4–147) lies on the medial palmar aspect of the wrist.

Test: Patient attempts to flex the wrist.

Instructions to Patient: "Try to bend your wrist. Relax. Bend it again." Patient should be asked to repeat the test so the examiner can feel the tendons during both relaxation and contraction.

Grading

Grade 1 (Trace): One or both tendons may exhibit visible or palpable contractile activity, but the part does not move.

Grade 0 (Zero): No contractile activity.

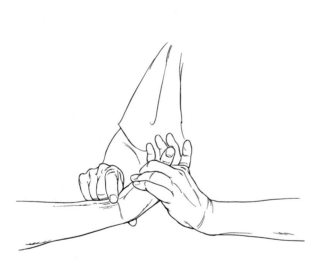

FIGURE 4–146

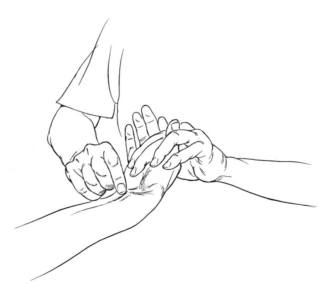

FIGURE 4–147

(Extensor carpi radialis longus, Extensor carpi radialis brevis, and Extensor carpi ulnaris)

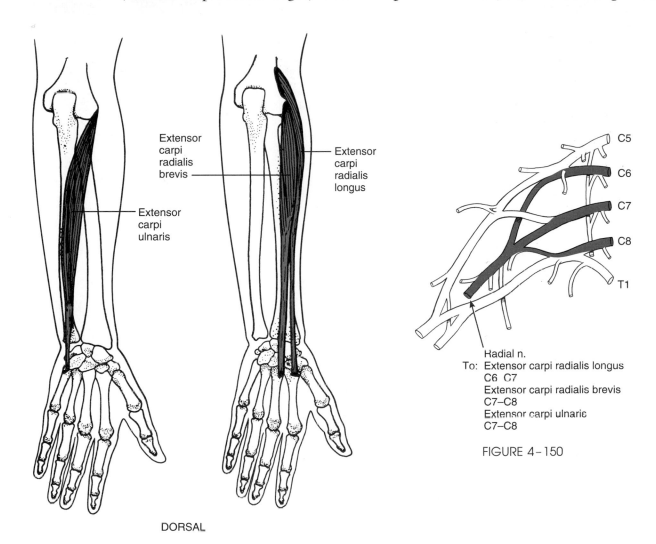

Extensor
carpi
radialis
brevis

Extensor
carpi
ulnaris

Extensor
carpi
radialis
longus

C5
C6
C7
C8
T1

Radial n.
To: Extensor carpi radialis longus
C6–C7
Extensor carpi radialis brevis
C7–C8
Extensor carpi ulnaris
C7–C8

FIGURE 4–150

DORSAL

FIGURES 4–148,149

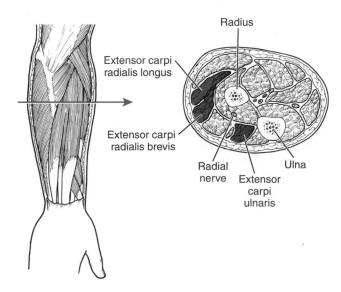

Radius

Extensor carpi
radialis longus

Extensor carpi
radialis brevis

Radial
nerve

Extensor
carpi
ulnaris

Ulna

FIGURE 4–151

WRIST EXTENSION

(Extensor carpi radialis longus, Extensor carpi radialis brevis, and Extensor carpi ulnaris)

Range of Motion

0° to 70°

Table 4–19 WRIST EXTENSION

I.D.	Muscle	Origin	Insertion
148	Extensor carpi radialis longus	Humerus (lateral supracondylar ridge, distal 1/3) Common forearm extensor tendon Lateral intermuscular septum	2nd metacarpal bone (base on radial side of dorsal aspect)
149	Extensor carpi radialis brevis	Humerus (lateral epicondyle via common forearm extensor tendon) Radial collateral ligament of elbow joint Aponeurosis of muscle	3rd metacarpal bone (base of dorsal surface on radial side) 2nd metacarpal (occasionally)
150	Extensor carpi ulnaris	Humerus (lateral epicondyle via common extensor tendon) Ulna (posterior border by an aponeurosis)	5th metacarpal bone (tubercle on medial side of base)
Others			
154	Extensor digitorum		
158	Extensor digiti minimi		
155	Extensor indicis		(See also Plate 4, page 127.)

Grade 5 (Normal), Grade 4 (Good), and Grade 3 (Fair)

Position of Patient: Short sitting. Elbow is flexed, forearm is fully pronated, and both are supported on the table.

Position of Therapist: Sit or stand at a diagonal in front of patient. Support the patient's forearm. The hand used for resistance is placed over the dorsal surface of the metacarpals.

To test all three muscles, the patient extends the wrist without deviation. Resistance for Grades 4 and 5 is given in a forward and downward direction over the 2nd to 5th metacarpals (Fig. 4–152).

To test the Extensor carpi radialis longus and brevis (for extension with radial deviation), resistance is given on the dorsal surface of the 2nd and 3rd metacarpals (radial side of hand) in the direction of flexion and ulnar deviation.

To test the Extensor carpi ulnaris (for extension and ulnar deviation), resistance is given on the dorsal surface of the 5th metacarpal (ulnar side of hand) in the direction of flexion and radial deviation.

Test: For the combined test of the three wrist extensor muscles, the patient extends the wrist straight up through the full available range. Do not permit extension of the fingers.

To test the two radial extensors, the patient extends the wrist, leading with the thumb side of the hand. The wrist may be prepositioned in some extension and radial deviation to direct the patient's motion.

To test the Extensor carpi ulnaris, the patient extends the wrist, leading with the ulnar side of the hand. The therapist may preposition the wrist in this attitude to direct the movement ulnarward.

Instructions to Patient: "Bring your wrist up. Hold it. Don't let me push it down." For Grade 3: "Bring your wrist up."

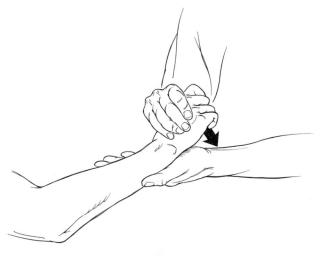

FIGURE 4–152

(Extensor carpi radialis longus, Extensor carpi radialis brevis, and Extensor carpi ulnaris)

Grade 5 (Normal), Grade 4 (Good), and Grade 3 (Fair) Continued

Grading

Grade 5 (Normal): Completes full wrist extension (when testing all three muscles) against maximal resistance. Full extension is not required for the tests of radial and ulnar deviation.

Grade 4 (Good): Completes full wrist extension against strong to moderate resistance when all muscles are being tested. When testing the individual muscles, full wrist extension will not be achieved.

Grade 3 (Fair): Completes full range of motion with no resistance in the test for all three muscles. In the separate tests for the radial and ulnar extensors, the deviation required precludes a large range of motion.

Grade 2 (Poor)

Position of Patient: Forearm supported on table in neutral position.

Position of Therapist: Support the patient's wrist. This elevates the hand from the table and removes friction (Fig. 4–153).

Test: Patient extends the wrist.

Instructions to Patient: "Bend your wrist back."

Grading

Grade 2 (Poor): Completes full range with gravity eliminated.

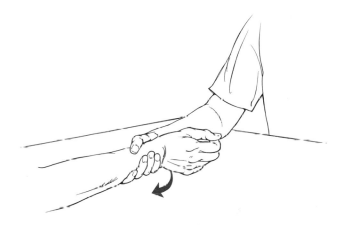

FIGURE 4–153

(Extensor carpi radialis longus, Extensor carpi radialis brevis, and Extensor carpi ulnaris)

Grade 1 (Trace) and Grade 0 (Zero)

Position of Patient: Hand and forearm supported on table with hand fully pronated.

Position of Therapist: Support the patient's wrist in extension. The other hand is used for palpation. Use one finger to palpate one muscle in a given test.

Extensor carpi radialis longus: Palpate this tendon on the dorsum of the wrist in line with the 2nd metacarpal (Fig. 4–154).

Extensor carpi radialis brevis: Palpate this tendon on the dorsal surface of the wrist in line with the 3rd metacarpal bone (Fig. 4–155).

Extensor carpi ulnaris: Palpate this tendon on the dorsal wrist surface proximal to the 5th metacarpal and just distal to the ulnar styloid process (Fig. 4–156).

Test: Patient attempts to extend the wrist.

Instructions to Patient: "Try to bring your wrist back."

Grading

Grade 1 (Trace): For any given muscle there is visible or palpable contractile activity, but no wrist motion ensues.

Grade 0 (Zero): No contractile activity.

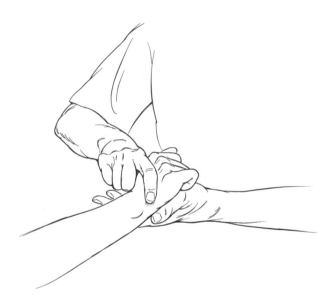

FIGURE 4–156

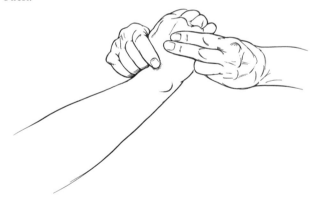

FIGURE 4–154

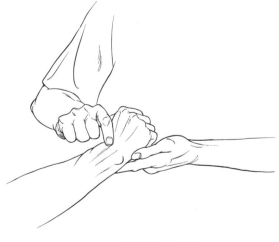

FIGURE 4–155

Substitution

The most common substitution occurs when the finger extensors are allowed to participate. This can be avoided to a large extent by ensuring that the fingers are relaxed and are not permitted to extend.

Helpful Hints

- The radial wrist extensors are considerably stronger than the Extensor carpi ulnaris.

- A patient with complete quadriplegia at C5–C6 will have only the radial wrist extensors remaining. Radial deviation during extension is therefore the prevailing extensor motion at the wrist.

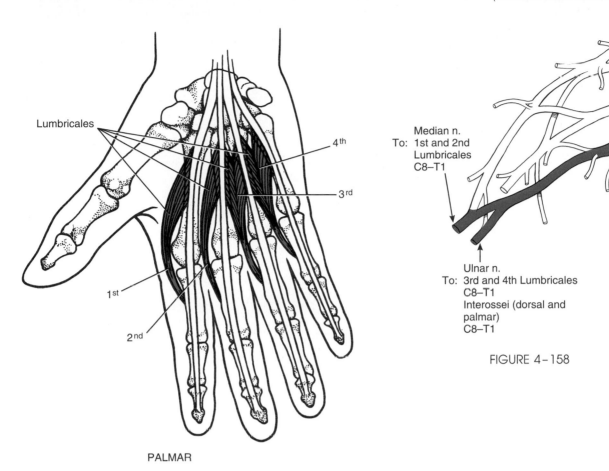

Lumbricales

4th

3rd

1st

2nd

PALMAR

FIGURE 4–157

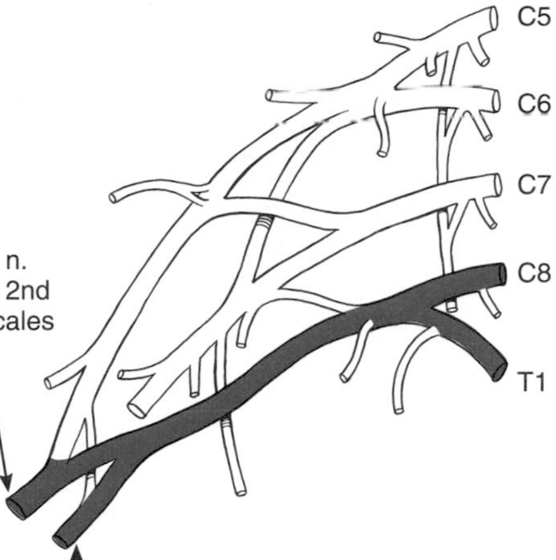

Median n.
To: 1st and 2nd
Lumbricales
C8–T1

Ulnar n.
To: 3rd and 4th Lumbricales
C8–T1
Interossei (dorsal and
palmar)
C8–T1

C5

C6

C7

C8

T1

FIGURE 4–158

FINGER MP FLEXION

(Lumbricales and Interossei)

Range of Motion

MP joints: 0° to 90°

Table 4-20 MP FLEXION OF FINGERS

I.D.	Muscle	Origin	Insertion
163	Lumbricales (4 in number)	Tendons of flexor digitorum profundus:	Extensor digitorum expansion. Each muscle runs distally to the *radial* side of its corresponding digit, attaches to the dorsal digital expansion
	1st Lumbrical	Index finger (radial side, palmar surface)	1st Lumbrical to index finger
	2nd Lumbrical	Middle finger (radial side, palmar surface)	2nd Lumbrical to long finger
	3rd Lumbrical	Middle and ring fingers (double heads from adjacent sides of tendons)	3rd Lumbrical to ring finger 4th Lumbrical to little finger
	4th Lumbrical	Ring and little fingers (adjacent sides of tendons)	
164	Dorsal Interossei (Four bipennate muscles) 1st Dorsal Interosseus (often named *Abductor indicis*)	Metacarpal bones (each muscle arises by two heads from adjacent sides of metacarpals between which each lies) 1st dorsal: between thumb and index finger 2nd dorsal: between index and long finger 3rd dorsal: between long and ring finger 4th dorsal: between ring and little finger	All: Dorsal expansion Proximal phalanges (bases) 1st dorsal: index finger (radial side) 2nd dorsal: long finger (radial side) 3rd dorsal: long finger (ulnar side) 4th dorsal: ring finger (ulnar side)
165	Palmar Interossei three muscles (a 4th muscle often is described)	Metacarpal bones 2, 4, and 5. (muscles lie on palmar surfaces of metacarpals rather than between them) No palmar Interosseous on long finger All muscles lie on aspect of metacarpal facing the long finger. 1st palmar: 2nd metacarpal (ulnar side) 2nd palmar: 4th metacarpal (radial side) 3rd palmar: 5th metacarpal (radial side)	All: Dorsal expansion Proximal phalanges 1st palmar: index finger (ulnar side) 2nd palmar: ring finger (radial side) 3rd palmar: little finger (radial side)

Others

156	Flexor digitorum superficialis
157	Flexor digitorum profundus
160	Flexor digiti minimi
161	Opponens digiti minimi

Grade 5 (Normal), Grade 4 (Good), and Grade 3 (Fair)

Position of Patient: Short sitting or supine with forearm in supination. Wrist is maintained in neutral. The metacarpophalangeal (MP) joints should be fully extended; all interphalangeal (IP) joints are flexed (Fig. 4–159).

Position of Therapist: Stabilize the metacarpals proximal to the MP joint. Resistance is given on the palmar surface of the proximal row of phalanges in the direction of MP extension (Fig. 4–160).

Test: Patient simultaneously flexes the MP joints and extends the IP joints. Fingers may be tested separately. Do not allow fingers to curl; they must remain extended.

Instructions to Patient: "Uncurl your fingers while flexing your knuckles. Hold it. Don't let me straighten your knuckles." The final position is a right angle at the MP joints. Demonstrate motion to patient and insist on practice to get the motions performed correctly simultaneously.

Grading

Grade 5 (Normal): Patient completes simultaneous MP flexion and finger extension and holds against maximal resistance. Resistance is given to fingers individually because of the variant strength of the different Lumbricales. The Lumbricales also have different innervations.

Grade 4 (Good): Patient completes range of motion against moderate to strong resistance.

Grade 3 (Fair): Patient completes both motions correctly and simultaneously without resistance.

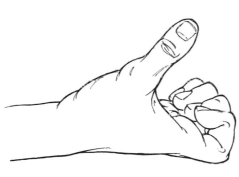

FIGURE 4–159

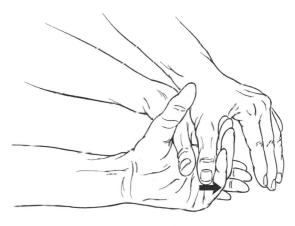

FIGURE 4–160

(Lumbricales and Interossei)

Grade 2 (Poor), Grade 1 (Trace), and Grade 0 (Zero)

Position of Patient: Forearm and wrist in midposition to remove influence of gravity. MP joints are fully extended; all IP joints are flexed.

Position of Therapist: Stabilize metacarpals.

Test: Patient attempts to flex MP joints through full available range while extending IP joints (Fig. 4–161).

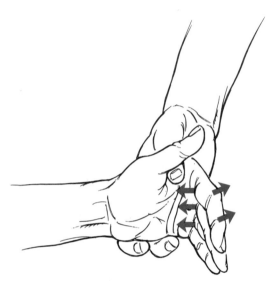

FIGURE 4–161

Instructions to Patient: "Try to uncurl your fingers while bending your knuckles." Demonstrate motion to patient and allow practice.

Grading

Grade 2 (Poor): Completes full range of motion in gravity-eliminated position.

Grade 1 (Trace): Except in the hand that is markedly atrophied, the Lumbricales cannot be palpated. A grade of 1 is given for minimal motion.

Grade 0 (Zero): A grade of Zero is given in the absence of any movement.

Substitution

The long finger flexors may substitute for the Lumbricales. To avoid this pattern, make sure that the IP joints fully extend.

 ### Hand Testing Requires Judgment and Experience

When evaluating the muscles of the hand, care must be taken to use graduated resistance that takes into consideration the relatively small mass of the muscles. In general, the examiner should not use the full thrust of the fist, wrist, or arm but rather one or two fingers to resist hand motions.

The degree of resistance offered to hand muscles is an issue, particularly when testing a postoperative hand. Similarly, the amount of motion allowed or encouraged should be monitored. Sudden or excessive excursions could "tear out" a surgical reconstruction.

Applying resistance in a safe fashion requires experience in assessing hand injuries or repair and a large amount of clinical judgment to avoid dislodging a tendon transfer or other surgical reconstruction. The neophyte examiner would be wise to err in the direction of caution.

Considerable practice in testing normal hands and comparing injured hands with their normal contralateral sides should give some of the necessary judgment with which to approach the fragile hand.

This text remains true to the principles of testing in the ranges of 5, 4, and 3 with respect to gravity. It is admitted, however, that the influence of gravity on the fingers is inconsequential, so the gravity and antigravity positions are not considered in valid muscle tests of the hand.

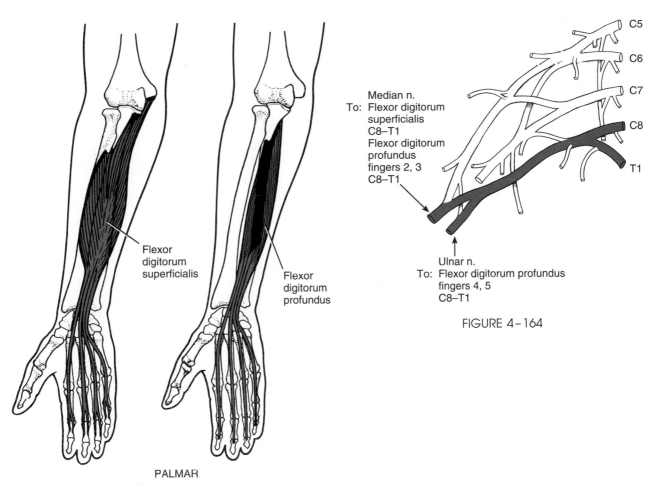

Flexor digitorum superficialis

Flexor digitorum profundus

PALMAR

FIGURE 4–162,163

Median n.
To: Flexor digitorum superficialis
C8–T1
Flexor digitorum profundus
fingers 2, 3
C8–T1

Ulnar n.
To: Flexor digitorum profundus
fingers 4, 5
C8–T1

C5
C6
C7
C8
T1

FIGURE 4–164

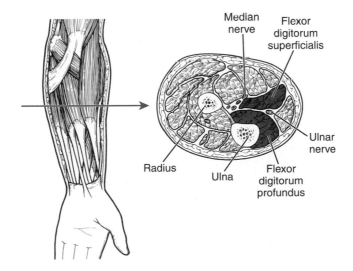

Median nerve

Flexor digitorum superficialis

Radius

Ulna

Flexor digitorum profundus

Ulnar nerve

FIGURE 4–165

FINGER PIP AND DIP FLEXION

(Flexor digitorum superficialis and Flexor digitorum profundus)

Range of Motion
PIP joints: 0° to 100°
DIP joints: 0° to 90°

Table 4-21 PIP AND DIP FINGER FLEXION

I.D.	Muscle	Origin	Insertion
156	Flexor digitorum superficialis (2 heads)	*Humero-ulnar head:* humerus (medial epicondyle via common flexor tendon) Ulna (medial collateral ligament of elbow joint); coronoid process (medial side) Intermuscular septum *Radial head:* radius (oblique line on anterior shaft)	Four tendons arranged in two pairs: Superficial pair: middle and ring fingers (sides of middle phalanges) Deep pair: index and little fingers (sides of middle phalanges)
157	Flexor digitorum profundus	Ulna (proximal 3/4 of anterior and medial shaft; medial coronoid process) Interosseous membrane (ulnar)	Four tendons to: Digits 2–5 (distal phalanges, at base of palmar surface)

PIP TESTS
(Flexor digitorum superficialis)

Grade 5 (Normal), Grade 4 (Good), and Grade 3 (Fair)

Position of Patient: Forearm supinated, wrist in neutral. Finger to be tested is in slight flexion at the MP joint (Fig. 4–166).

Position of Therapist: Hold all fingers (except the one being tested) in extension at all joints (see Fig. 4–166). Isolation of the index finger may not be complete. The other hand is used to resist the head (distal end) of the middle phalanx of the test finger in the direction of extension (not illustrated).

Test: Each of the four fingers is tested separately. Patient flexes the PIP joint without flexing the DIP joint. Do not allow motion of any joints of the other fingers.

Flick the terminal end of the finger being tested with the thumb to make certain that the Flexor digitorum profundus is not active; that is, the DIP joint goes into extension. The distal phalanx should be floppy.

Instructions to Patient: "Bend your index [then long, ring, or little] finger; hold it. Don't let me straighten it. Keep your other fingers relaxed."

Grading

Grade 5 (Normal): Completes range of motion and holds against maximal finger resistance.

Grade 4 (Good): Completes range against moderate resistance.

Grade 3 (Fair): Completes range of motion with no resistance (Fig. 4–167).

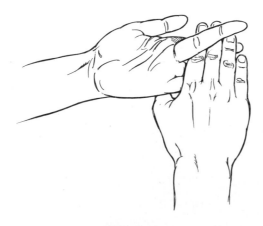

FIGURE 4–166

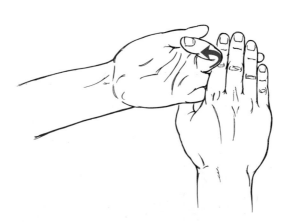

FIGURE 4–167

Grade 2 (Poor), Grade 1 (Trace), and Grade 0 (Zero)

Position of Patient: Forearm is in midposition to eliminate the influence of gravity on finger flexion.

Position of Therapist: Same as for Grades 5, 4, and 3.

Palpate the Flexor digitorum superficialis on the palmar surface of the wrist between the Palmaris longus and the Flexor carpi ulnaris (Fig. 4–168).

Test: Patient flexes the PIP joint.

Instructions to Patient: "Bend your middle finger." (Select other fingers individually.)

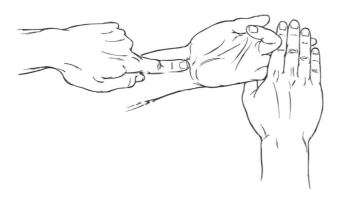

FIGURE 4–168

Grading

Grade 2 (Poor): Completes range of motion.

Grade 1 (Trace): Palpable or visible contractile activity, which may or may not be accompanied by a flicker of motion.

Grade 0 (Zero): No contractile activity.

Substitutions

- The major substitution for this motion is offered by the Flexor digitorum profundus, and this will occur if the DIP joint is allowed to flex.
- If the wrist is allowed to extend, tension increases in the long finger flexors, and may result in passive flexion of the IP joints. This is referred to as a "tenodesis" action.
- Relaxation of IP extension will result in passive IP flexion.

Helpful Hints

Many persons cannot isolate the little finger. When this is the case, test the little and ring fingers at the same time.

(Flexor digitorum superficialis and Flexor digitorum profundus)

DIP TESTS
(Flexor digitorum profundus)

Grade 5 (Normal), Grade 4 (Good), and Grade 3 (Fair)

Position of Patient: Forearm in supination, wrist in neutral, and proximal PIP joint in extension.

Position of Therapist: Stabilize the middle phalanx in extension by grasping it on either side (Fig. 4–169). Resistance is provided on the distal phalanx in the direction of extension (not illustrated).

Test: Test each finger individually. Patient flexes distal phalanx of each finger.

Instructions to Patient: "Bend the tip of your finger. Hold it. Don't let me straighten it."

Grading

Grade 5 (Normal): Completes available range against a carefully assessed maximal level of resistance (See Sidebar, p. 144).

Grade 4 (Good): Completes maximal available range against some resistance.

Grade 3 (Fair): Completes maximum available range with no resistance (see Fig. 4–169).

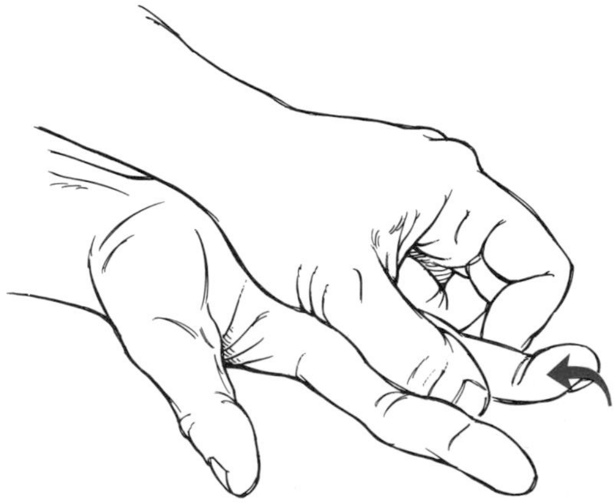

Grade 2 (Poor), Grade 1 (Trace), and Grade 0 (Zero)

All aspects of testing these grades are the same as those used for the higher grades except that the position of the forearm is in neutral to eliminate the influence of gravity.

Grades are assigned as for the PIP tests.

The tendon of the Flexor digitorum profundus can be palpated on the palmar surface of the middle phalanx of each finger.

Substitutions

- The wrist must be kept in a neutral position and must not be allowed to extend to rule out the tenodesis effect of the wrist extensors.
- Don't be fooled if the patient extends the DIP joint and then relaxes, which can give the impression of active finger flexion.

FIGURE 4–169

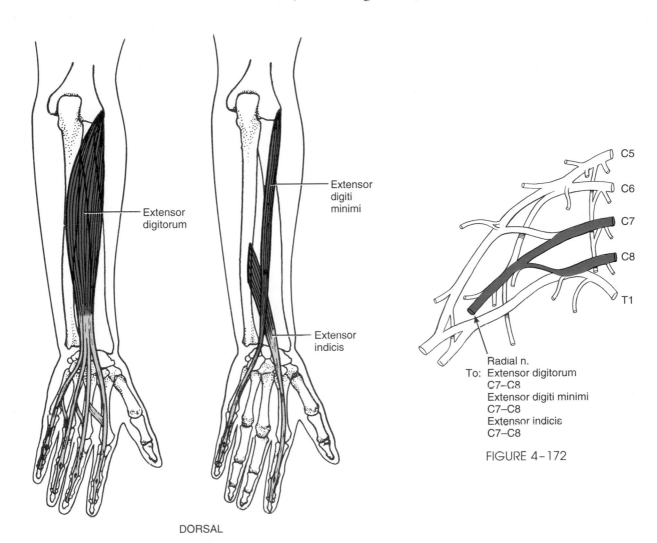

Extensor digitorum

Extensor digiti minimi

Extensor indicis

Radial n.
To: Extensor digitorum
C7–C8
Extensor digiti minimi
C7–C8
Extensor indicis
C7–C8

FIGURE 4–172

DORSAL

FIGURES 4–170,171

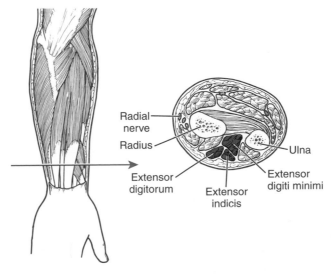

Radial nerve

Radius

Ulna

Extensor digitorum

Extensor indicis

Extensor digiti minimi

FIGURE 4–173

(Extensor digitorum, Extensor indicis, Extensor digiti minimi)

Range of Motion
0° to 45°

Table 4-22 MP FINGER EXTENSION

I.D.	Muscle	Origin	Insertion
154	Extensor digitorum	Humerus (lateral epicondyle via common extensor tendon) Intermuscular septum Antebrachial fascia	Via 4 tendons to digits 2–5 (via the extensor expansion, to dorsum of middle and distal phalanges; one tendon to each finger)
155	Extensor indicis	Ulna (posterior surface of shaft) Interosseous membrane	2nd digit (via tendon of Extensor digitorum into extensor hood)
158	Extensor digiti minimi	Humerus (lateral epicondyle via common extensor tendon) Intermuscular septa	5th digit (extensor hood)

Grade 5 (Normal), Grade 4 (Good), and Grade 3 (Fair)

Position of Patient: Forearm in pronation, wrist in neutral. MP joints and IP joints are in relaxed flexion posture.

Position of Therapist: Stabilize the wrist in neutral. Place the index finger of the resistance hand across the dorsum of all proximal phalanges just distal to the MP joints. Give resistance in the direction of flexion.

Test

Extensor digitorum: Patient extends MP joints (all fingers simultaneously), allowing the IP joints to be in slight flexion (Fig. 4–174).

Extensor indicis: Patient extends the MP joint of the index finger.

Extensor digiti minimi: Patient extends the MP joint of the 5th digit.

Instructions to Patient: "Bend your knuckles back as far as they will go." Demonstrate motion to patient and instruct to copy.

Grading

Grade 5 (Normal): Completes active extension range of motion with appropriate level of strong resistance.

Grade 4 (Good): Completes active range with some resistance.

Grade 3 (Fair): Completes active range with no resistance.

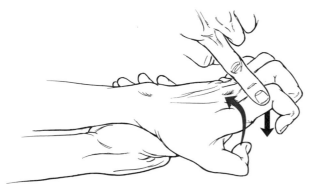

FIGURE 4–174

Grade 2 (Poor), Grade 1 (Trace), and Grade 0 (Zero)

Procedures: Test is the same as that for Grades 5, 4, and 3 except that the forearm is in the midposition.

The tendons of the Extensor digitorum (n = 4), the Extensor indicis (n = 1), and the Extensor digiti minimi (n = 1) are readily apparent on the dorsum of the hand as they course in the direction of each finger.

Grading

Grade 2 (Poor): Completes range.

Grade 1 (Trace): Visible tendon activity but no joint motion.

Grade 0 (Zero): No contractile activity.

Substitution
Flexion of the wrist will produce IP extension through a tenodesis action.

Helpful Hints
• MP extension of the fingers is not a strong motion, and only slight resistance is required to "break" the end position.   • It is usual for the active range of motion to be considerably less than the available passive range. In this test, therefore, the "full available range" is not used, and the active range is accepted.   • Another way to check whether there is functional extensor strength in the fingers is to "flick" the proximal phalanx of each finger downward; if the finger rebounds, it is functional.

(Dorsal interossei)

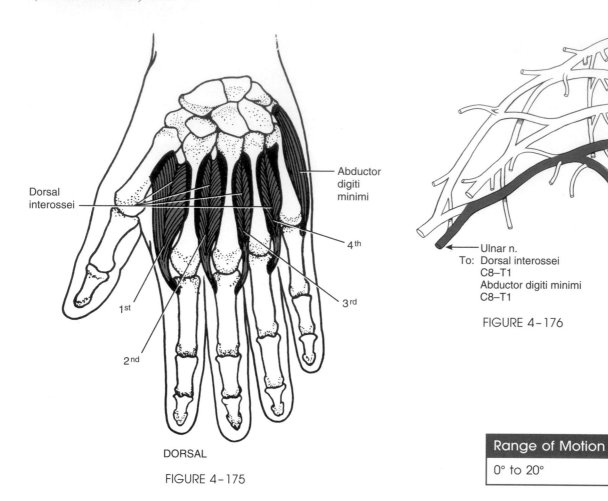

Dorsal interossei

Abductor digiti minimi

4th

1st

2nd

3rd

DORSAL

FIGURE 4–175

Ulnar n.
To: Dorsal interossei
C8–T1
Abductor digiti minimi
C8–T1

FIGURE 4–176

Range of Motion
0° to 20°

Table 4-23 FINGER ABDUCTION

I.D.	Muscle	Origin	Insertion
164	Dorsal interossei Four bipennate muscles (1st dorsal Interosseous, often named *Abductor indicis*)	Metacarpal bones (each muscle arises by 2 heads from adjacent sides of metacarpals between which each lies) 1st dorsal: between thumb and index finger 2nd dorsal: between index and long finger 3rd dorsal: between long and ring fingers 4th dorsal: between ring and little finger	All: Dorsal extensor expansion: proximal phalanges (bases) 1st dorsal: index finger (radial side) 2nd dorsal: long finger (radial side) 3rd dorsal: long finger (ulnar side) 4th dorsal: ring finger (ulnar side)
159	Abductor digiti minimi	Pisiform bone Tendon of Flexor carpi ulnaris Pisohamate ligament	5th digit (base of proximal phalanx, ulnar side) Dorsal expansion of Extensor digiti minimi

Others

154	Extensor digitorum (no action on long finger)		
158	Extensor digiti minimi (little finger)		

Grade 5 (Normal) and Grade 4 (Good)

Position of Patient: Forearm pronated, wrist in neutral. Fingers start in extension and adduction. MP joints in neutral and avoid hyperextension.

Position of Therapist: Support the wrist in neutral. The fingers of the other hand are used to give resistance on the distal phalanx, on the radial side of the finger and the ulnar side of the adjacent finger (i.e., they are squeezed together). The direction of resistance will cause any pair of fingers to approximate (Fig. 4–177).

Test: Abduction of fingers (individual tests):

Dorsal Interossei:
    Abduction of ring finger toward little finger
    Abduction of middle finger toward ring finger
    Abduction of middle finger toward index finger
    Abduction of index finger toward thumb

The long (middle) finger (digit 3, finger 2) will move one way when tested with the index finger and the opposite way when tested with the ring finger (see Fig. 4–175, which shows a dorsal Interosseus on either side). When testing the little finger with the ring finger, the Abductor digiti minimi is being tested along with the 4th dorsal Interosseus.

Abductor digiti minimi: Patient abducts 5th digit away from ring finger.

Instructions to Patient: "Spread your fingers. Hold them. Don't let me push them together."

Grading

Grade 5 (Normal) and Grade 4 (Good): Neither the dorsal Interossei nor the Abductor digiti minimi will tolerate much resistance. Grading between a 5 and a 4 muscle is a judgment call based on possible comparison with the contralateral side as well as on clinical experience. Figure 4–178 illustrates the test for 2nd and 4th dorsal Interossei.

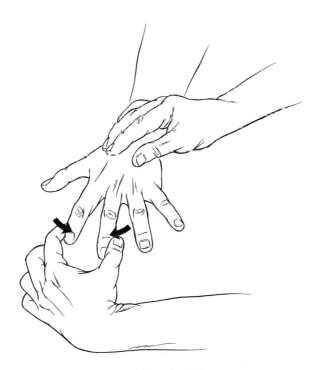

FIGURE 4–177

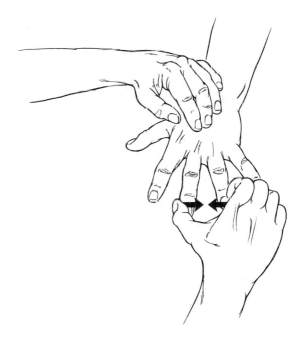

FIGURE 4–178

FINGER ABDUCTION

(Dorsal Interossei)

Grade 3 (Fair)

Grade 3 (Fair): Patient can abduct any given finger. Remember that the long finger has two dorsal Interossei and therefore must be tested as it moves away from the midline in both directions (Fig. 4–179).

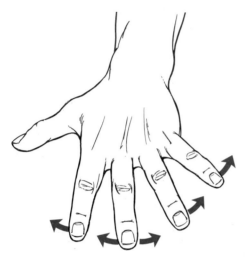

FIGURE 4–179

Grade 2 (Poor), Grade 1 (Trace), and Grade 0 (Zero)

Procedures and Grading: Same as for higher grades in this test. A Grade 2 should be assigned if the patient can complete only a partial range of abduction for any given finger. The only dorsal Interosseus that is readily palpable is the 1st at the base of the proximal phalanx (Fig. 4–180).

The Abductor digiti minimi is palpable on the ulnar border of the hand.

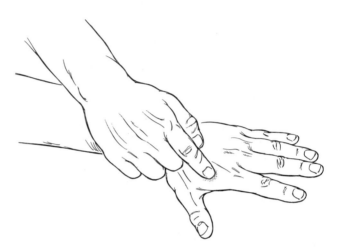

FIGURE 4–180

Helpful Hints

Provide resistance for a Grade 5 test by flicking each finger toward adduction; if the finger tested rebounds, the grade is Normal.

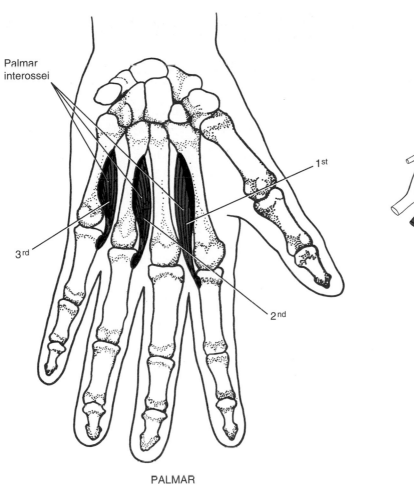

Palmar interossei

1st

3rd

2nd

PALMAR

FIGURE 4–181

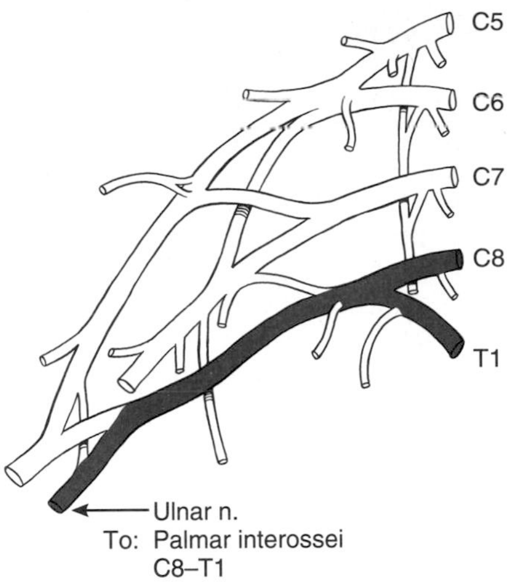

C5
C6
C7
C8
T1

Ulnar n.
To: Palmar interossei
C8–T1

FIGURE 4–182

Range of Motion
20° to 0°

Table 4-24 FINGER ADDUCTION

I.D.	Muscle	Origin	Insertion
165	Palmar Interossei Three muscles (a 4th muscle often is described)	Metacarpal bones 2, 4, and 5 Muscles lie on palmar surfaces of metacarpals rather than between them. No palmar Interosseous on long finger All muscles lie on aspect of a metacarpal facing the long finger 1st palmar: 2nd metacarpal (ulnar side) 2nd palmar: 4th metacarpal (radial side) 3rd palmar: 5th metacarpal (radial side)	All: dorsal extensor expansion 1st palmar: index finger (proximal phalanx, ulnar side) 2nd palmar: ring finger (proximal phalanx, radial side) 3rd palmar: little finger (proximal phalanx, radial side)
Other			
155	Extensor indicis		

(Palmar Interossei)

Grade 5 (Normal) and Grade 4 (Good)

Position of Patient: Forearm pronated (palm down), wrist in neutral, and fingers extended and adducted. MP joints are neutral; avoid flexion.

Position of Therapist: Examiner grasps the middle phalanx on each of two adjoining fingers (Fig. 4–183). Resistance is given in the direction of abduction for each finger tested. The examiner is trying to "pull" the fingers apart. Each finger should be resisted separately.

Test: Adduction of fingers (individual tests):

Adduction of little finger toward ring finger
Adduction of ring finger toward long finger
Adduction of index finger toward long finger
Adduction of thumb toward index finger

Occasionally there is a 4th palmar Interosseus (not illustrated in Fig. 4–181) that some consider a separate muscle from the Adductor pollicis. In any event, the two muscles cannot be clinically separated.

Because the middle finger (also called the long finger, digit 3, or finger 2) has no palmar Interosseus, it is not tested in adduction.

Instructions to Patient: "Hold your fingers together. Don't let me spread them apart."

Grading

Grade 5 (Normal) and Grade 4 (Good): These muscles are notoriously weak in the sense of not tolerating much resistance. Distinguishing between Grades 5 and 4 is an exercise in futility, and the grade awarded will depend on the amount of the examiner's experience with normal hands.

Grade 3 (Fair): Patient can adduct fingers toward middle finger but cannot hold against resistance (Fig. 4–184)

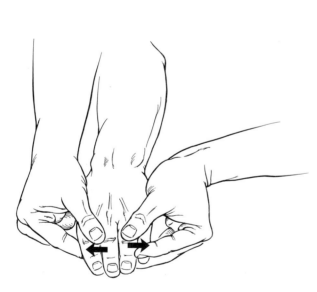

FIGURE 4–183

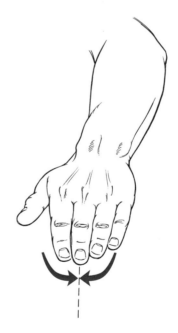

FIGURE 4–184

Grade 2 (Poor), Grade 1 (Trace), and Grade 0 (Zero)

Procedures: Same as for Grades 5, 4, and 3.

For Grade 2, the patient can adduct each of the fingers tested through a partial range of motion. The test for Grade 2 is begun with the fingers abducted.

Palpation of the palmar Interossei is rarely feasible. By placing the examiner's finger against the side of a finger to be tested, the therapist may detect a slight outward motion for a muscle less than Grade 2.

Substitution

Caution must be used to ensure that finger flexion does not occur because the long finger flexors can contribute to adduction.

Helpful Hints

The fingers can be judged quickly by grasping the distal phalanx and flicking the finger in the direction of abduction. If the finger rebounds or snaps back, that Interosseous is functional.

THUMB MP AND IP FLEXION

(Flexor pollicis brevis and Flexor pollicis longus)

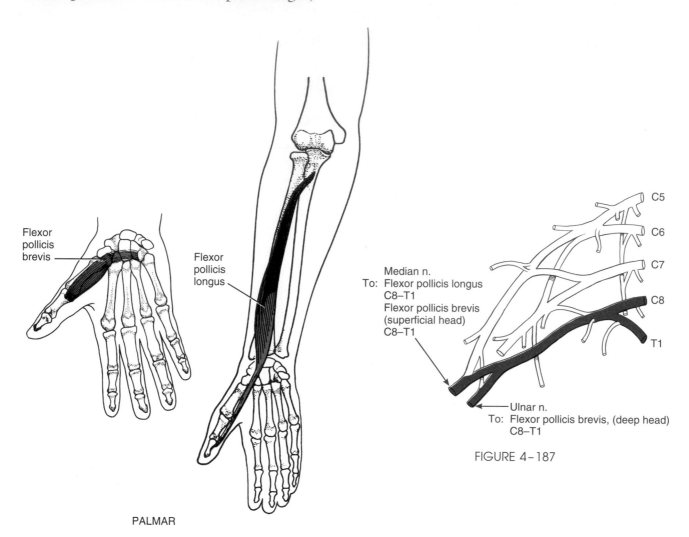

Flexor
pollicis
brevis

Flexor
pollicis
longus

Median n.
To: Flexor pollicis longus
C8–T1
Flexor pollicis brevis
(superficial head)
C8–T1

C5

C6

C7

C8

T1

Ulnar n.
To: Flexor pollicis brevis, (deep head)
C8–T1

FIGURE 4–187

PALMAR

FIGURES 4–185,186

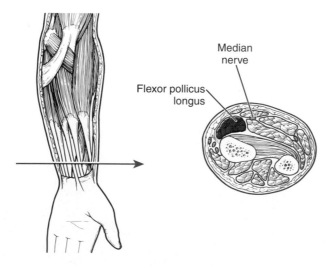

Median
nerve

Flexor pollicus
longus

FIGURE 4–188

(Flexor pollicis brevis and Flexor pollicis longus)

Range of Motion
MP flexion: 0° to 50°
IP flexion: 0° to 80°

Table 4–25 THUMB MP AND IP FLEXION

I.D.	Muscle	Origin	Insertion
MP Flexion			
170	Flexor pollicis brevis *Superficial head* (often blended with Opponens pollicis)	Flexor retinaculum (distal) Trapezium bone (tubercle, distal)	Thumb (base of proximal phalanx, radial side)
	Deep head	Trapezoid bone Capitate bone Palmar ligaments of distal carpal bones	
IP Flexion			
169	Flexor pollicis longus	Radius (anterior surface of middle 1/2) and adjacent Interosseous membrane Ulna (coronoid process, lateral border (variable)) Humerus (medial epicondyle (variable))	Thumb (base of distal phalanx, palmar surface)

THUMB MP AND IP FLEXION

(Flexor pollicis brevis and Flexor pollicis longus)

THUMB MP AND IP FLEXION TESTS
(Flexor pollicis brevis)

Grade 5 (Normal) to Grade 0 (Zero)

Position of Patient: Forearm in supination, wrist in neutral. Carpometacarpal (CMC) joint is at 0°; IP joint is at 0°. Thumb in adduction, lying relaxed and adjacent to the 2nd metacarpal (Fig. 4–189).

Position of Therapist: Stabilize the 1st metacarpal firmly to avoid any wrist or CMC motion. The other hand gives one-finger resistance to MP flexion on the proximal phalanx in the direction of extension (Fig. 4–190).

Test: Patient flexes the MP joint of the thumb, keeping the IP joints straight (see Fig. 4–190).

Instructions to Patient: "Bring your thumb across the palm of your hand. Keep the thumb in touch with your palm. Don't bend the end joint. Hold it. Don't let me pull it back."

   Demonstrate thumb flexion and have patient practice the motion.

Grading

Grade 5 (Normal): Completes range of motion against maximal thumb resistance.

Grade 4 (Good): Tolerates strong to moderate resistance.

Grade 3 (Fair): Completes full range of motion with perhaps a slight amount of resistance because gravity is eliminated.

Grade 2 (Poor): Completes range of motion.

Grade 1 (Trace): Palpate the muscle by initially locating the tendon of the Flexor pollicis longus in the thenar eminence (Fig. 4–191). Then palpate the muscle belly of the Flexor pollicis brevis on the ulnar side of the longus tendon in the thenar eminence.

Grade 0 (Zero): No visible or palpable contractile activity.

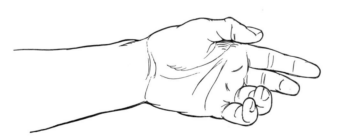

FIGURE 4–189

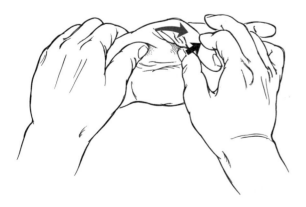

FIGURE 4–190

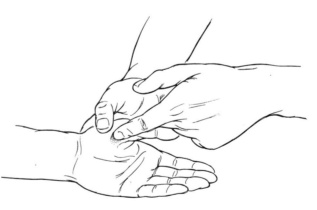

FIGURE 4–191

Substitution by Flexor Pollicis Longus

The long thumb flexor can substitute but only after flexion of the IP joint begins. To avoid this substitution, do not allow flexion of the distal joint of the thumb.

(Flexor pollicis brevis and Flexor pollicis longus)

THUMB IP FLEXION TESTS
(Flexor pollicis longus)

Grade 5 (Normal) to Grade 0 (Zero)

Position of Patient: Forearm supinated with wrist in neutral and MP joint of thumb in extension.

Position of Therapist: Stabilize the MP joint of the thumb firmly in extension by grasping the patient's thumb across that joint. Give resistance with the other hand against the palmar surface of the distal phalanx of the thumb in the direction of extension (Fig. 4–192).

Test: Patient flexes the IP joint of the thumb.

Instructions to Patient: "Bend the end of your thumb. Hold it. Don't let me straighten it."

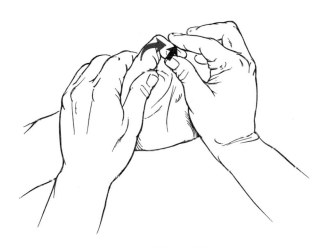

FIGURE 4–192

Grading

Grade 5 (Normal) and Grade 4 (Good): Patient tolerates maximal finger resistance from examiner for Grade 5. This muscle is very strong, and a Grade 4 muscle will tolerate strong resistance. Full range always should be completed.

Grade 3 (Fair): Completes a full range of motion with minimal resistance because gravity is eliminated.

Grade 2 (Poor): Completes range of motion.

Grade 1 (Trace) and Grade 0 (Zero): Palpate the tendon of the Flexor pollicis longus on the palmar surface of the proximal phalanx of the thumb. Palpable activity is graded 1; no activity is graded 0.

Substitution

Do not allow the distal phalanx of the thumb to extend at the beginning of the test. If the distal phalanx is extended and then relaxes, the examiner may think active flexion has occurred.

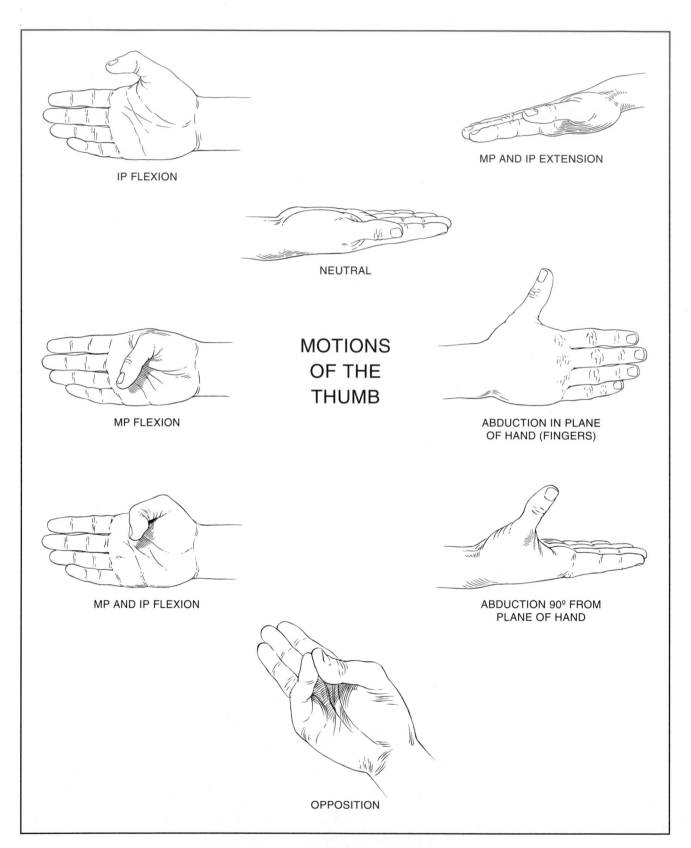

IP FLEXION

MP AND IP EXTENSION

NEUTRAL

MP FLEXION

MOTIONS
OF THE
THUMB

ABDUCTION IN PLANE
OF HAND (FINGERS)

MP AND IP FLEXION

ABDUCTION 90º FROM
PLANE OF HAND

OPPOSITION

PLATE 5

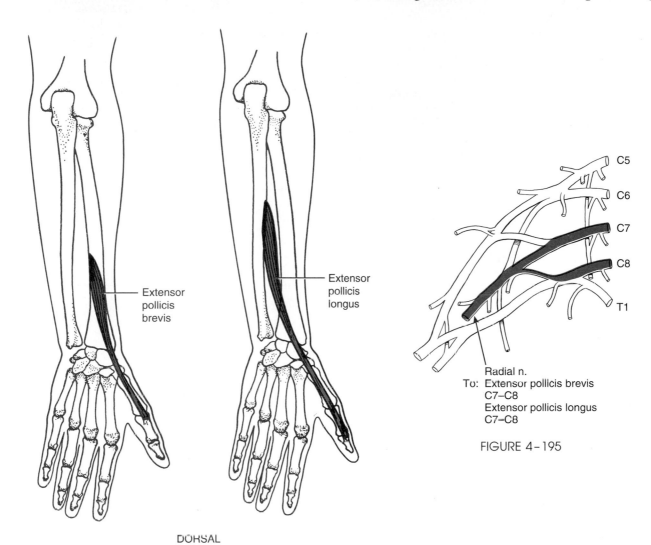

Extensor
pollicis
brevis

Extensor
pollicis
longus

C5
C6
C7
C8
T1

Radial n.
To: Extensor pollicis brevis
C7–C8
Extensor pollicis longus
C7–C8

FIGURE 4-195

DORSAL

FIGURES 4-193,194

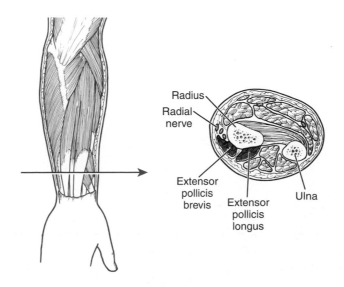

Radius
Radial
nerve

Extensor
pollicis
brevis

Extensor
pollicis
longus

Ulna

FIGURE 4-196

THUMB MP AND IP EXTENSION

(Extensor pollicis brevis and Extensor pollicis longus)

Range of Motion
MP extension: 50° to 0°
IP extension: 80° to 0°

Table 4-26 THUMB MP AND IP EXTENSION

I.D.	Muscle	Origin	Insertion
MP Extension			
168	Extensor pollicis brevis (Radiomedial wall of "anatomical snuffbox")	Radius (posterior surface) Adjacent interosseous membrane	Thumb (proximal phalanx, base, dorsolateral surface)
IP Extension			
167	Extensor pollicis longus (Ulnar wall of "anatomical snuffbox")	Ulna (shaft, middle 1/3 on posterior-lateral surface) Adjacent interosseous membrane	Thumb (base of distal phalanx)

The Extensor pollicis brevis is an inconstant muscle that often blends with the Extensor pollicis longus, in which event it is not possible to separate the brevis from the longus by clinical tests, and the test for the longus prevails.

THUMB MP EXTENSION TESTS

(Extensor pollicis brevis)

Grade 5 (Normal) to Grade 0 (Zero)

Position of Patient: Forearm in midposition and wrist in neutral; CMC and IP joints of the thumb are relaxed and in slight flexion. The MP joint of the thumb is in abduction and flexion.

Position of Therapist: Stabilize the first metacarpal firmly, allowing motion to occur only at the MP joint (Fig. 4–197). Resistance is provided with the other hand on the dorsal surface of the proximal phalanx in the direction of flexion. This normally is not a strong muscle.

Test: Patient extends the MP joint of the thumb while keeping the IP joint slightly flexed.

Instructions to Patient: "Bring your thumb up so it points toward the ceiling; don't move the end joint. Hold it. Don't let me push it down."

Grading

Grade 5 (Normal) and Grade 4 (Good): Only the experienced examiner can accurately distinguish between Grades 5 and 4. Resistance should be applied carefully and slowly because this usually is a weak muscle.

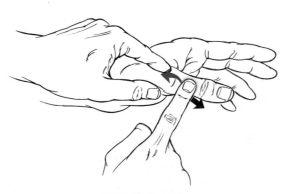

FIGURE 4–197

Grade 5 (Normal) to Grade 0 (Zero) Continued

Grade 3 (Fair): Patient moves proximal phalanx of the thumb through full range of extension with some resistance.

Grade 2 (Poor): Patient moves proximal phalanx through partial range of motion.

Grade 1 (Trace): The tendon of the Flexor pollicis brevis is palpated (Fig. 4–198) at the base of the 1st metacarpal where it lies between the tendons of the Abductor pollicis and the Extensor pollicis longus.

Grade 0 (Zero): No contractile activity.

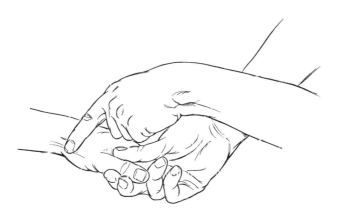

FIGURE 4–198

Substitution
Extension of the IP joint of the thumb with CMC adduction in addition to extension of the MP joint indicates substitution by the Extensor pollicis longus.

THUMB MP AND IP EXTENSION

(Extensor pollicis brevis and Extensor pollicis longus)

THUMB IP EXTENSION TESTS
(Extensor pollicis longus)

Grade 5 (Normal), Grade 4 (Good), and Grade 3 (Fair)

Position of Patient: Forearm in midposition, wrist in neutral with ulnar side of hand resting on the table. Thumb relaxed in a flexion posture.

Position of Therapist: Use the table to support the ulnar side of the hand and stabilize the proximal phalanx of the thumb (Fig. 4–199). Apply resistance over the dorsal surface of the distal phalanx of the thumb in the direction of flexion.

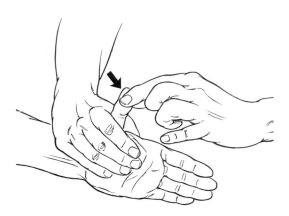

FIGURE 4–199

Test: Patient extends the IP joint of the thumb.

Instructions to Patient: "Straighten the end of your thumb. Hold it. Don't let me push it down."

Grading

Grade 5 (Normal) and Grade 4 (Good): Completes full range of motion. This is not a strong muscle, so resistance must be applied accordingly. The distinction between Grades 5 and 4 is based on comparison with the contralateral normal hand and, barring that, extensive experience in testing the hand.

Grade 3 (Fair): Completes full range of motion with no resistance.

Grade 2 (Poor), Grade 1 (Trace), and Grade 0 (Zero)

Position of Patient: Forearm in pronation with wrist in neutral and thumb in relaxed flexion posture to start.

Position of Therapist: Stabilize the wrist over its dorsal surface. Stabilize the fingers by gently placing the other hand across the fingers just below the MP joints (Fig. 4–200).

Test: Patient extends distal joint of the thumb (see Fig. 4–200).

Instructions to Patient: "Straighten the end of your thumb."

Grading

Grade 2 (Poor): Thumb completes range of motion.

Grade 1 (Trace): Palpate the tendon of the Extensor pollicis longus on the ulnar side of the "anatomical snuffbox" or, alternatively, on the dorsal surface of the proximal phalanx (Fig. 4–201).

Grade 0 (Zero): No contractile activity.

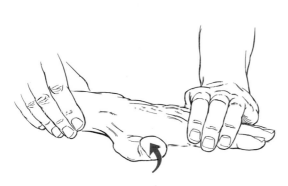

FIGURE 4–200

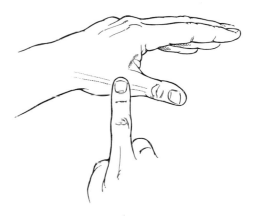

FIGURE 4–201

Substitution

The muscles of the thenar eminence (Abductor pollicis brevis, Flexor pollicis brevis, and Adductor pollicis) can extend the IP joint by flexing the CMC joint (an extensor tenodesis).

Helpful Hints

- Continued action by the Extensor pollicis longus will extend the MP and CMC joints.

- A quick way to assess the functional status of the long thumb extensor is to flick the distal phalanx into flexion; if the finger rebounds or snaps back, it is a useful muscle

THUMB ABDUCTION

(Abductor pollicis longus and Abductor pollicis brevis)

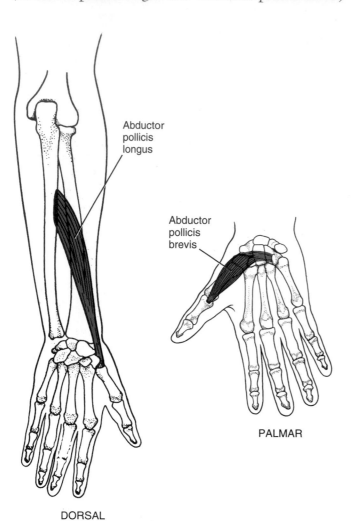

Abductor pollicis longus

Abductor pollicis brevis

DORSAL

PALMAR

FIGURES 4–202, 203

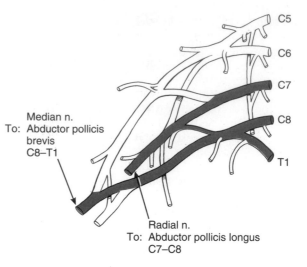

Median n.
To: Abductor pollicis brevis
C8–T1

Radial n.
To: Abductor pollicis longus
C7–C8

FIGURE 4–204

Range of Motion
0° to 70°

Table 4-27 THUMB ABDUCTION

I.D.	Muscle	Origin	Insertion
166	Abductor pollicis longus (Radiolateral wall of "anatomical snuffbox")	Ulna (posterior surface laterally) Radius (shaft, middle 1/3 of posterior aspect) Interosseous membrane	Thumb: 1st metacarpal (radial side of base) Trapezium bone
171	Abductor pollicis brevis	Flexor retinaculum Scaphoid bone (tubercle) Trapezium bone (tubercle) Tendon of Abductor pollicis longus	Medial fibers: Thumb (base of proximal phalanx, radial side) Lateral fibers: Extensor expansion of thumb

Others

152	Palmaris longus		
168	Extensor pollicis brevis		
172	Opponens pollicis		

ABDUCTOR POLLICIS LONGUS TEST

Grade 5 (Normal) to Grade 0 (Zero)

Position of Patient: Forearm supinated and wrist in neutral; thumb relaxed in adduction.

Position of Therapist: Stabilize the metacarpals of the four fingers and the wrist (Fig. 4–205). Resistance is given on the distal end of the 1st metacarpal in the direction of adduction.

Test: Patient abducts the thumb away from the hand in a plane parallel to the finger metacarpals.

Instructions to Patient: "Lift your thumb straight up." Demonstrate motion to the patient.

Grading

Grade 5 (Normal) and Grade 4 (Good): Completes full range of motion against resistance. Distinguishing Grades 5 and 4 may be difficult.

Grade 3 (Fair): Completes full range of motion with no resistance.

Grade 2 (Poor): Completes partial range of motion.

Grade 1 (Trace): Palpate tendon of the Abductor pollicis longus at the base of the 1st metacarpal on the radial side of the Extensor pollicis brevis (Fig. 4–206). It is the most lateral tendon at the wrist.

Grade 0 (Zero): No contractile activity.

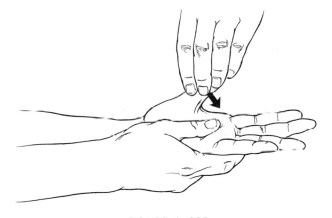

FIGURE 4–205

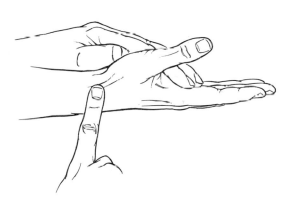

FIGURE 4–206

Substitution

The Extensor pollicis brevis can substitute for the Abductor pollicis longus. If the line of pull is toward the dorsal surface of the forearm (Extensor pollicis brevis), substitution is occurring.

Helpful Hints

• If the Abductor pollicis longus is stronger than the brevis, the thumb will deviate toward the radial side of the hand.

• If the Abductor pollicis brevis is stronger, deviation will be toward the ulnar side.

THUMB ABDUCTION

(Abductor pollicis longus and Abductor pollicis brevis)

ABDUCTOR POLLICIS BREVIS TEST

Grade 5 (Normal), Grade 4 (Good), and Grade 3 (Fair)

Position of Patient: Forearm in supination, wrist in neutral, and thumb relaxed in adduction.

Position of Therapist: Stabilize the metacarpals (Fig. 4–207) by placing the examiner's hand across the patient's palm with the thumb on the dorsal surface of the patient's hand (somewhat like a handshake but maintaining the patient's wrist in neutral). Apply resistance to the lateral aspect of the proximal phalanx of the thumb in the direction of adduction.

Test: Patient abducts the thumb in a plane perpendicular to the palm. Observe wrinkling of the skin over the thenar eminence and watch for the tendon of the Palmaris longus to "pop out."

Instructions to Patient: "Lift your thumb vertically until it points to the ceiling." Demonstrate motion to the patient.

Grading

Grade 5 (Normal): Completes full range of motion with maximal finger resistance.

Grade 4 (Good): Tolerates moderate resistance.

Grade 3 (Fair): Completes full range of motion with no resistance.

Grade 2 (Poor), Grade 1 (Trace), and Grade 0 (Zero)

Position of Patient: Forearm in midposition, wrist in neutral, and thumb relaxed in adduction.

Position of Therapist: Stabilize wrist in neutral.

Test: Patient abducts thumb in a plane perpendicular to the palm.

Instructions to Patient: "Try to lift your thumb so it points at the ceiling."

Grading

Grade 2 (Poor): Completes partial range of motion.

Grade 1 (Trace): Palpate the belly of the Abductor pollicis brevis in the center of the thenar eminence, medial to the Opponens pollicis (Fig. 4–208).

Grade 0 (Zero): No contractile activity.

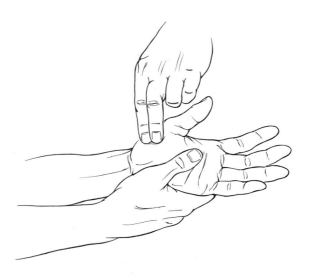

FIGURE 4–208

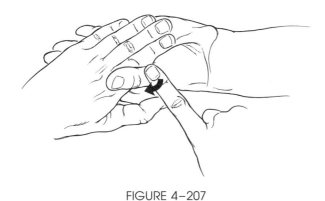

FIGURE 4–207

Substitution
If the plane of motion is not perpendicular, but toward the radial side of the hand, the substitution may be by the Abductor pollicis longus.

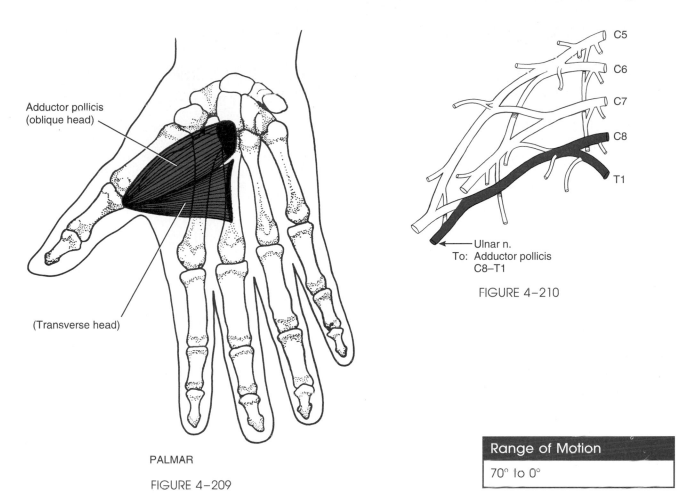

Adductor pollicis
(oblique head)

(Transverse head)

PALMAR

FIGURE 4-209

C5
C6
C7
C8
T1

Ulnar n.
To: Adductor pollicis
C8–T1

FIGURE 4-210

Range of Motion
70° to 0°

Table 4-28 THUMB ADDUCTION

I.D.	Muscle	Origin	Insertion
173	Adductor pollicis		Thumb (proximal phalanx, ulnar side of base)
	Oblique head	Capitate bone 2nd and 3rd metacarpals (bases) Palmar ligaments of carpal bones Sheath of tendon of Flexor carpi radialis	
	Transverse head	3rd metacarpal bone (palmar surface of distal 2/3)	
Other			
164	1st dorsal Interosseus		

THUMB ADDUCTION

(Adductor pollicis)

Grade 5 (Normal), Grade 4 (Good), and Grade 3 (Fair)

Position of Patient: Forearm in pronation, wrist in neutral, and thumb relaxed and hanging down in abduction.

Position of Therapist: Stabilize the metacarpals of the four fingers by grasping the patient's hand around the ulnar side (Fig. 4–211). Resistance is given on the medial side of the proximal phalanx of the thumb in the direction of abduction.

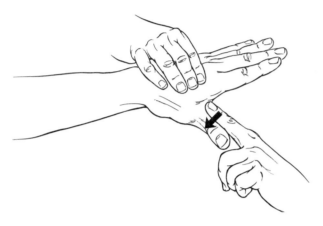

FIGURE 4–211

Test: Patient adducts the thumb by bringing the 1st metacarpal up to the 2nd metacarpal. Alternatively, place a sheet of paper between the thumb and the 2nd metacarpal (palmar pinch) and ask the patient to hold it while you try to pull the paper away.

Instructions to Patient: "Bring your thumb up to your index finger." Demonstrate motion to the patient.

Grading

Grade 5 (Normal) and Grade 4 (Good): Completes full range of motion and holds against maximal resistance. Patient can resist rigidly (Grade 5), or the muscle yields (Grade 4).

Grade 3 (Fair): Completes full range of motion with no resistance.

Grade 2 (Poor), Grade 1 (Trace), and Grade 0 (Zero)

Position of Patient: Forearm in midposition, wrist in neutral resting on table, and thumb in abduction.

Position of Therapist: Stabilize wrist on the table, and use a hand to stabilize the finger metacarpals (Fig. 4–212).

Test: Patient moves thumb horizontally in adduction. The end position is shown in Figure 4–212.

Instructions to Patient: "Return your thumb to its place next to your index finger." Demonstrate motion to patient.

Grading

Grade 2 (Poor): Completes full range of motion.

Grade 1 (Trace): Palpate the Adductor pollicis on the palmar side of the web space of the thumb by grasping the web between the index finger and thumb (Fig. 4–213). The Adductor lies between the 1st dorsal Interosseus and the 1st metacarpal bone. This muscle is difficult to palpate, and the therapist may have to ask the patient to perform a palmar pinch to assist in its location.

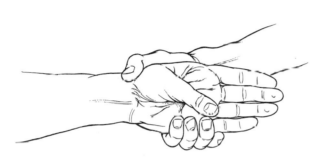

FIGURE 4–212

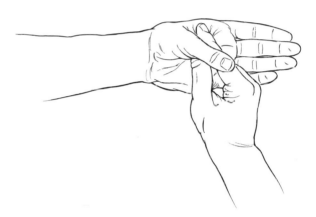

FIGURE 4–213

Substitution

- The Flexor pollicis longus and the Flexor pollicis brevis will flex the thumb, drawing it across the palm. These muscles should be kept inactive during the adduction test.
- The Extensor pollicis longus may attempt to substitute for the thumb adductor, in which case the CMC joint will extend.

OPPOSITION (THUMB TO LITTLE FINGER)

(Opponens pollicis and Opponens digiti minimi)

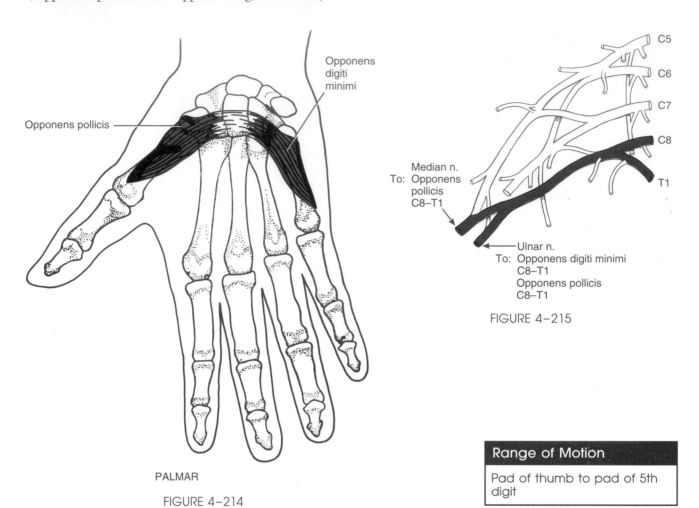

Opponens pollicis

Opponens digiti minimi

PALMAR

FIGURE 4–214

Median n.
To: Opponens pollicis
C8–T1

Ulnar n.
To: Opponens digiti minimi
C8–T1
Opponens pollicis
C8–T1

FIGURE 4–215

Range of Motion
Pad of thumb to pad of 5th digit

Table 4-29 OPPOSITION (THUMB TO LITTLE FINGER)

I.D.	Muscle	Origin	Insertion
172	Opponens pollicis	Trapezium bone (tubercle) Flexor retinaculum	1st metacarpal (entire length of lateral border and adjoining lateral half of palmar surface)
161	Opponens digiti minimi	Hamate (hook) Flexor retinaculum	5th metacarpal (whole length of ulnar margin and adjacent palmar surface)
Others			
171	Abductor pollicis brevis		
170	Flexor pollicis brevis		

(Opponens pollicis and Opponens digiti minimi)

This motion is a combination of abduction, flexion, and medial rotation of the thumb (Fig. 4–216).

The two muscles in thumb-to-5th digit opposition (Opponens pollicis and Opponens digiti minimi) should not be tested together and also should be graded separately.

Grade 5 (Normal) to Grade 0 (Zero)

Position of Patient: Forearm is supinated, wrist in neutral, and thumb in adduction with MP and IP flexion.

Position of Therapist: Stabilize the hand by holding the wrist on the dorsal surface. The examiner may prefer the hand to be stabilized on the table.

Opponens pollicis: Apply resistance for the Opponens pollicis at the head of the 1st metacarpal in the direction of lateral rotation, extension, and adduction (see Fig 4–216).

Opponens digiti minimi: Give resistance for the Opponens digiti minimi on the palmar surface of the 5th metacarpal in the direction of medial rotation (flattening the palm) (Fig. 4–217).

Test: Patient raises the thumb away from the palm and rotates it so that its distal phalanx opposes the distal phalanx of the little finger. Such apposition must be pad to pad and not tip to tip. Opposition also can be evaluated by asking the patient to hold an object between the thumb and little finger (in opposition), which the examiner tries to pull away.

Instructions to Patient: "Bring your thumb to your little finger and touch the two pads, forming the letter 'O' with your thumb and little finger." Demonstrate motion to the patient and require practice.

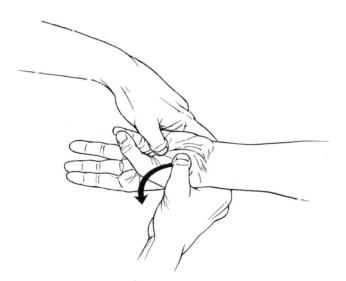

FIGURE 4–216

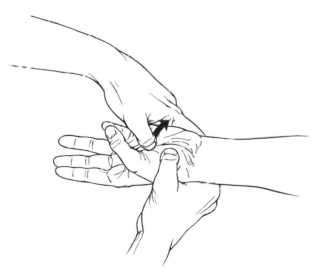

FIGURE 4–217

OPPOSITION (THUMB TO LITTLE FINGER)

(Opponens pollicis and Opponens digiti minimi)

Grade 5 (Normal) to Grade 0 (Zero) Continued

Grading

Grade 5 (Normal): Completes the full motion correctly against maximal thumb resistance.

Grade 4 (Good): Completes the range against moderate resistance.

Grade 3 (Fair): Moves thumb and 5th digit through full range of opposition with no resistance.

Grade 2 (Poor): Moves through range of opposition. (The two Opponens muscles are evaluated separately.)

Grade 1 (Trace): Palpate the Opponens pollicis along the radial shaft of the 1st metacarpal (Fig. 4–218). It lies lateral to the Abductor pollicis brevis. During Grade 5 and Grade 4 contractions the examiner will have difficulty in palpating the opponens pollicis because of nearby muscles. In Grade 3 muscles and below, the weaker contractions do not obscure palpation.

Palpate the Opponens digiti minimi on the hypothenar eminence on the radial side of the 5th metacarpal (Fig. 4–219). Be careful not to cover the muscle with the finger or thumb used for palpation lest any contractile activity be missed.

Grade 0 (Zero): No contractile activity.

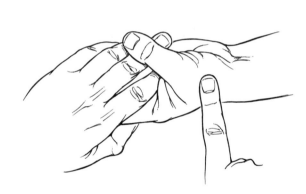

FIGURE 4–218

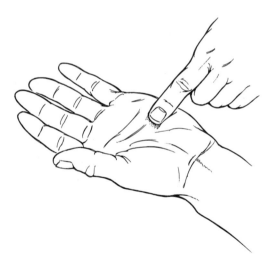

FIGURE 4–219

Substitutions

- The Flexor pollicis longus and the Flexor pollicis brevis can draw the thumb across the palm toward the little finger. If such motion occurs in the plane of the palm it is not opposition; contact will be at the tips, not the pads, of the digits.
- The Abductor pollicis brevis may substitute, but the rotation component of the motion will not be present.

References

Cited References

1. Kendall FP, McCreary EK, Provance PG. *Muscles: Testing and Function,* 4th ed. Baltimore: Williams & Wilkins, 1993.
2. Perry J. Shoulder function for the activities of daily living. In Matsen FA, Fu FH, Hawkins RJ. *The Shoulder: A Balance of Mobility and Stability.* Rosemont, IL: American Academy of Orthopedic Surgeons, 1993, Chap 10.

Other Readings

Bagg SD, Forrest WJ. Electromyographic study of scapular rotation during arm abduction in the scapular plane. Am J Phys Med 65:111–124, 1986.

Basmajian JV, Travill J. Electromyography of the pronator muscles in the forearm. Anat Rec 139:45–49, 1961.

Basmajian JV. *Muscles and Movements: A Basis for Human Kinesiology,* 2nd ed. New York: Kriger, 1977.

Basmajian JV, DeLuca, CJ. *Muscles Alive,* 5th ed. Baltimore: Williams & Wilkins, 1985.

Bearn JG. An electromyographic study of the trapezius, deltoid, pectoralis major, biceps and triceps muscles during static loading of the upper limb. Anat Rec 140:103–108, 1961.

Bharihoke VB, Gupta M. Muscular attachments along the medial border of the scapula. Surg Radiol Anat 8:1–13, 1986.

Catton WT, Gray JE. Electromyographic study of the action of the Serratus anterior in respiration. J Anat 85:412P, 1951.

Chang L, Blair WF. The origin and innervation of the Adductor pollicus muscle. J Anat 140:381–388, 1985.

Close JR, Kidd CC. The functions of the muscles of the thumb, the index and long fingers. J Bone Joint Surg 51-A:1601, 1969.

Greis PE, Kuhn JE, Schultheis J, et al. Validation of the lift-off test and analysis of subscapularis activity during maximal internal rotation. Am J Sports Med 24:589–593, 1996.

Inman VT, Saunders JB de CM, Abbott LC. Observations on the function of the shoulder joint. J Bone Joint Surg 26:1–30, 1944.

Jonsson B, Hagberg M. Effect of different working heights on the Deltoid muscle. Scand J Rehab Med Suppl 3:26–32, 1974.

Kasai T, Chiba S. True nature of the muscular arch of the axilla and its nerve supply. Kaibogaku Zasshi 25:657–669, 1977.

Lewis OJ. The comparative morphology of M. Flexor accessorius and the associated flexor tendons. J Anat 96:321–333, 1962.

Levy AS, Kelly BT, Lintner SA, et al. Function of the long head of the biceps at the shoulder: Electromyographic analysis. J Shoulder Elbow Surg 10:250–255, 2001.

Long C, Brown ME. Electromyographic kinesiology of the hand: Muscles moving the long finger. J Bone Joint Surg 46-A:1683–1706, 1964.

Long C. Intrinsic—extrinsic control of the fingers: Electromyographic studies. J Bone Joint Surg 50-A:973–984, 1968.

Testing the Muscles of the Lower Extremity

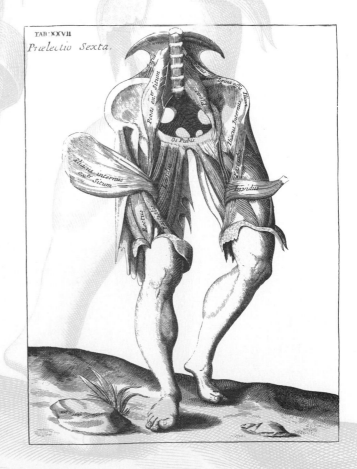

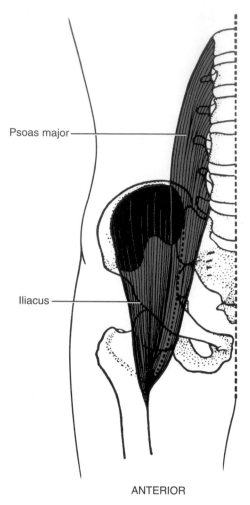

(Psoas major and Iliacus)

Psoas major
Iliacus
ANTERIOR

FIGURE 5-1

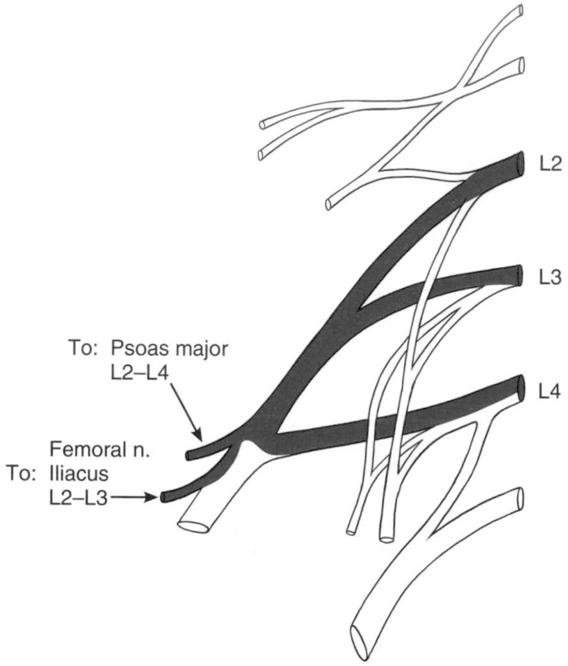

L2
L3
L4
To: Psoas major
L2–L4
Femoral n.
To: Iliacus
L2–L3

FIGURE 5-2

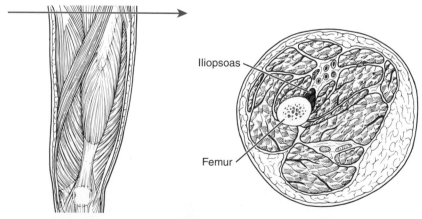

Iliopsoas
Femur

FIGURE 5-3

(Psoas major and Iliacus)

Range of Motion
0° to 120°

Table 5-1 HIP FLEXION

I.D.	Muscle	Origin	Insertion
174	Psoas major	L1–L5 vertebrae (transverse processes) T12–L5 vertebral bodies (sides) and their intervertebral discs	Femur (lesser trochanter)
176	Iliacus	Iliac fossa (upper 2/3) Iliac crest (inner lip) Sacroiliac and iliolumbar ligaments Sacrum (upper lateral surface)	Femur (lesser trochanter; joins tendon of Psoas major) Femoral shaft below lesser trochanter
Others			
196	Rectus femoris		
195	Sartorius		
185	Tensor fasciae latae		
177	Pectineus		
180	Adductor brevis		
179	Adductor longus		
181	Adductor magnus (superior fibers)		
183	Gluteus medius (anterior)		

(Psoas major and Iliacus)

Grade 5 (Normal), Grade 4 (Good), and Grade 3 (Fair)

Position of Patient: Short sitting with thighs fully supported on table and legs hanging over the edge. Patient may use arms to provide trunk stability by grasping table edge or with hands on table at each side (Fig. 5–4).

Position of Therapist: Standing next to limb to be tested. Contoured hand to give resistance over distal thigh just proximal to the knee joint (see Fig. 5–4).

Test: Patient flexes hip to end of range, clearing the table and maintaining neutral rotation, holding that position against the examiner's resistance, which is given in a downward direction toward the floor.

Instructions to Patient: "Lift your leg off the table and don't let me push it down."

For Grade 3: "Lift your leg straight up off the table."

Grading

Grade 5 (Normal): Thigh clears table. Patient tolerates maximal resistance.

Grade 4 (Good): Hip flexion holds against strong to moderate resistance. There may be some "give" at the end position.

Grade 3 (Fair): Patient completes test range and holds the position without resistance (Fig. 5–5).

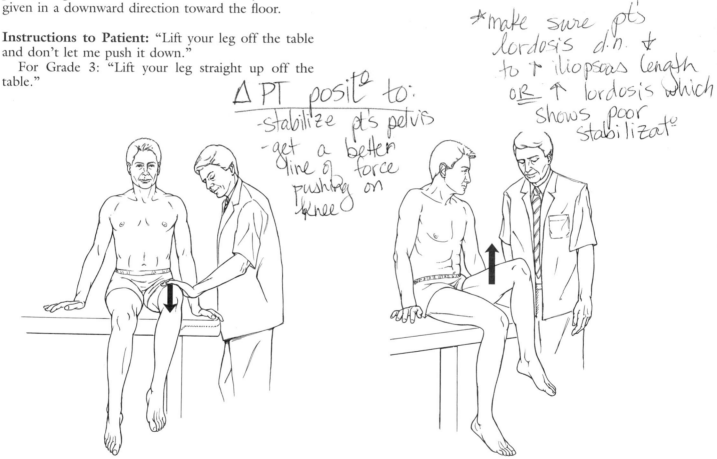

[handwritten annotations:]

Δ PT posit⁰ to:
- stabilize pt's pelvis
- get a better line of force pushing on knee

*make sure pt's lordosis d.n. ↑ to ↑ iliopsoas length OR ↑ lordosis which shows poor stabilizat⁰

FIGURE 5–4   FIGURE 5–5

Helpful Hints

Knowledge of the ranges of motion of the hip is imperative before manual tests of hip strength are conducted. If the examiner does not have a clear idea of hip joint ranges, especially tightness in the hip flexor muscles, test results will be contaminated. For example, in the presence of a hip flexion contracture, the patient must be standing and leaning over the edge of the table to test hip extension strength. This position (described on page 194) will decrease the influence of the flexion contracture and will allow the patient to move against gravity through the available range.

Grade 2 (Poor)

Position of Patient: Side-lying with limb to be tested uppermost and supported by examiner (Fig. 5–6). Trunk in neutral alignment. Lowermost limb may be flexed for stability.

Position of Therapist: Standing behind patient. Cradle test limb in one arm with hand support under the knee. Opposite hand maintains trunk alignment at hip (see Fig. 5–6).

Test: Patient flexes supported hip. Knee is permitted to flex to prevent hamstring tension.

Instructions to Patient: "Bring your knee up toward your chest."

Grading

Grade 2 (Poor): Patient completes the range of motion in side-lying position.

Grade 1 (Trace) and Grade 0 (Zero)

Position of Patient: Supine. Test limb supported by examiner under calf with hand behind knee (Fig. 5–7).

Position of Therapist: Standing at side of limb to be tested. Test limb is supported under calf with hand behind knee. Free hand palpates the muscle just distal to the inguinal ligament on the medial side of the Sartorius (see Fig. 5–7).

Test: Patient attempts to flex hip.

Instructions to Patient: "Try to bring your knee up to your nose."

Grading

Grade 1 (Trace): Palpable contraction but no visible movement.

Grade 0 (Zero): No palpable contraction of muscle.

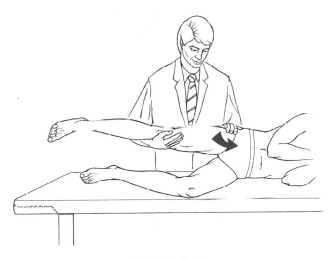

FIGURE 5–6

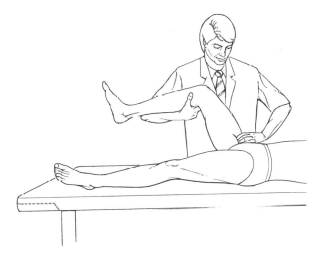

FIGURE 5–7

Substitutions

- Use of the Sartorius will result in external rotation and abduction of the hip. The Sartorius, because it is superficial, will be seen and can be palpated in most limbs (Fig. 5–8).
- If the Tensor fasciae latae substitutes for the hip flexors, internal rotation and abduction of the hip will result. If, however, the patient is tested in the supine position, gravity will cause the limb to externally rotate. The Tensor may be seen and palpated at its origin on the anterior superior iliac spine (ASIS).

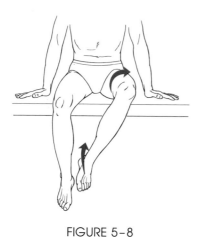

FIGURE 5–8

Helpful Hints

- When the trunk is weak the test will be more accurate from a supine position.
- Hip flexion is not a strong motion, so experience is necessary to appreciate what constitutes a normal level of resistance.

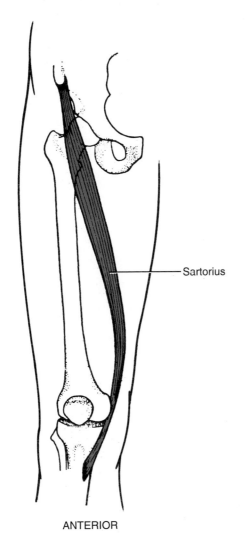

ANTERIOR

FIGURE 5-9

Sartorius

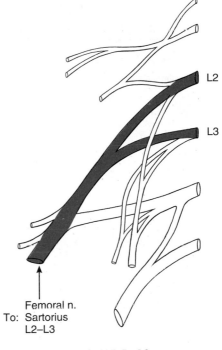

L2

L3

Femoral n.
To: Sartorius
L2–L3

FIGURE 5-10

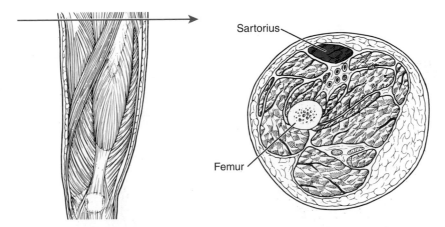

Sartorius

Femur

FIGURE 5-11

HIP FLEXION, ABDUCTION, AND EXTERNAL ROTATION WITH KNEE FLEXION

(Sartorius)

Range of Motion

Since this is a two-joint muscle, no specific range-of-motion value can be assigned solely to the Sartorius.

Table 5-2 HIP FLEXION, ABDUCTION, AND EXTERNAL ROTATION

I.D.	Muscle	Origin	Insertion
195	Sartorius	Ilium (anterior superior iliac spine (ASIS)) Iliac notch below ASIS	Tibia (shaft, proximal medial surface) Capsule of knee joint (via slip) Medial side fascia of leg

Others

Hip and knee flexors

Hip external rotators

Hip abductors

Grade 5 (Normal), Grade 4 (Good), and Grade 3 (Fair)

Position of Patient: Short sitting with thighs supported on table and legs hanging over side. Arms may be used for support.

Position of Therapist: Standing lateral to the leg to be tested. Place one hand on the lateral side of knee; the other hand grasps the medial-anterior surface of the distal leg (Fig. 5–12).

Hand at knee resists hip flexion and abduction (down and inward direction) in the Grade 5 and 4 tests. Hand at the ankle resists hip external rotation and knee flexion (up and outward) in Grade 5 and 4 tests. No resistance for Grade 3 test.

Test: Patient flexes, abducts, and externally rotates the hip and flexes the knee (Fig. 5–12).

Instructions to Patient: Therapist may demonstrate the required motion passively and then ask the patient to repeat the motion, or the therapist may place the limb in the desired end position.

"Hold it! Don't let me move your leg or straighten your knee."

Alternate instruction: "Slide your heel up the shin of your other leg."

Grading

Grade 5 (Normal): Holds end point against maximal resistance.

Grade 4 (Good): Tolerates moderate to heavy resistance.

Grade 3 (Fair): Completes movement and holds end position but takes no resistance (Fig. 5–13).

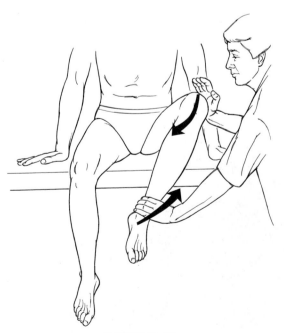

FIGURE 5-12

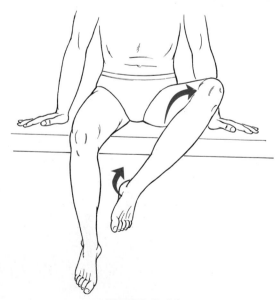

FIGURE 5-13

Grade 2 (Poor)

Position of Patient: Supine. Heel of limb to be tested is placed on contralateral shin (Fig. 5–14).

Position of Therapist: Standing at side of limb to be tested. Support limb as necessary to maintain alignment.

Test: Patient slides test heel upward along shin to knee.

Instructions to Patient: "Slide your heel up to your knee."

Grading

Grade 2 (Poor): Completes desired movement.

Grade 1 (Trace) and Grade 0 (Zero)

Position of Patient: Supine.

Position of Therapist: Standing on side to be tested. Cradle test limb under calf with hand supporting limb behind knee. Opposite hand palpates Sartorius on medial side of thigh where the muscle crosses the femur (Fig. 5–15). Examiner may prefer to palpate near the muscle origin just below the ASIS.

Test: Patient attempts to slide heel up shin toward knee.

Instructions to Patient: "Try to slide your heel up to your knee."

Grading

Grade 1 (Trace): Therapist can detect slight contraction of muscle; no visible movement.

Grade 0 (Zero): No palpable contraction.

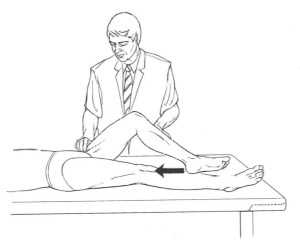

FIGURE 5–14

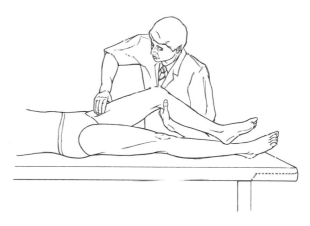

FIGURE 5–15

Substitution

Substitution by the Iliopsoas or the Rectus femoris results in pure hip flexion without abduction and external rotation.

Helpful Hints

- Therapist is reminded that failure of the patient to complete the full range of motion in the Grade 3 test is not an automatic Grade 2. Patient should be tested in the supine position to ascertain whether the correct grade is Grade 2 or less.

- Never grasp the belly of a muscle (the calf in this instance) during Poor and Trace tests.

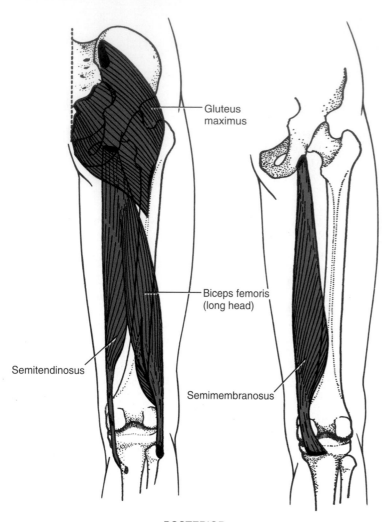

Gluteus maximus

Biceps femoris (long head)

Semitendinosus

Semimembranosus

POSTERIOR

FIGURE 5–16

FIGURE 5–17

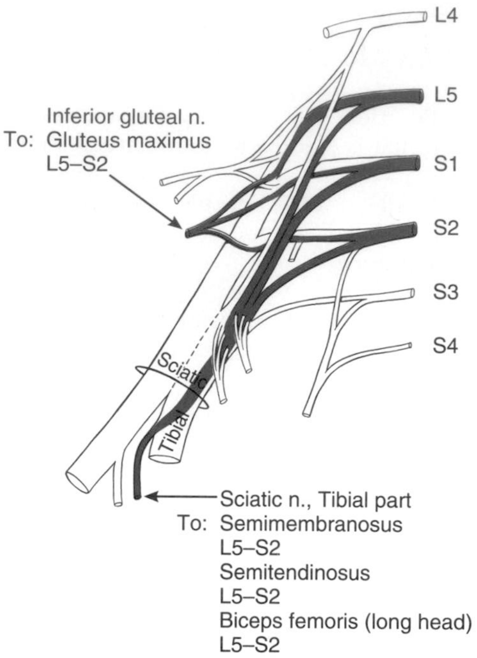

Inferior gluteal n.
To: Gluteus maximus
L5–S2

L4

L5

S1

S2

S3

S4

Sciatic

Tibial

Sciatic n., Tibial part
To: Semimembranosus
L5–S2
Semitendinosus
L5–S2
Biceps femoris (long head)
L5–S2

FIGURE 5–18

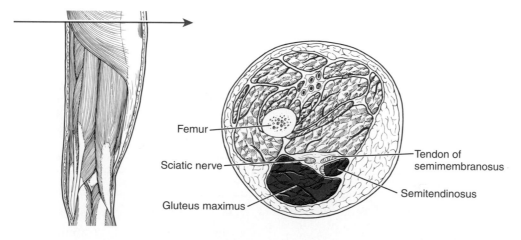

Femur

Sciatic nerve

Gluteus maximus

Tendon of semimembranosus

Semitendinosus

FIGURE 5–19

(Gluteus maximus and Hamstrings)

Range of Motion
0° to 20°
Some authors say as low as 0° to 5°.

Table 5-3 HIP EXTENSION

I.D.	Muscle	Origin	Insertion
182	Gluteus maximus	Ilium (posterior gluteal line) Iliac crest (posterior medial) Sacrum (dorsal surface of lower part) Coccyx (side) Sacrotuberous ligament Aponeurosis over Gluteus medius	Femur (gluteal tuberosity) Iliotibial tract of fascia lata
193	Semitendinosus	Ischial tuberosity (upper area, inferomedial impression via tendon shared with Biceps femoris) Aponeurosis (between the two muscles)	Tibia (proximal medial shaft) Pes anserina
194	Semimembranosus	Ischial tuberosity (superolateral impression)	Tibia (medial condyle, posterior aspect) Oblique popliteal ligament of knee joint Aponeurosis over distal muscle (variable)
192	Biceps femoris (long head)	Ischial tuberosity (inferomedial impression via tendon shared with Semitendinosus) Sacrotuberous ligament	Fibula (head) Tibia (lateral condyle)[37] Aponeurosis
Others			
181	Adductor magnus (inferior)		
183	Gluteus medius (posterior)		

(Gluteus maximus and Hamstrings)

Grade 5 (Normal), Grade 4 (Good), and Grade 3 (Fair) (Aggregate of All Hip Extensor Muscles)

Position of Patient: Prone. Arms may be overhead or abducted to hold sides of table. (Note: If there is a hip flexion contracture, immediately go to the test described for hip extension modified for hip flexion tightness [page 194]).

Position of Therapist: Standing at side of limb to be tested at level of pelvis. (Note: Fig. 5–20 shows examiner on opposite side to avoid obscuring activity.)

The hand providing resistance is placed on the posterior leg just above the ankle. The opposite hand may be used to stabilize or maintain pelvis alignment in the area of the posterior superior spine of the ilium (see Fig. 5–20). This is the most demanding test because the lever arm is longest.

Alternate Position: The hand that gives resistance is placed on the posterior thigh just above the knee (Fig. 5–21). This is a less demanding test.

Test: Patient extends hip through entire available range of motion. Resistance is given straight downward toward the floor. (No resistance is given in the Grade 3 test.)

Instructions to Patient: "Lift your leg off the table as high as you can without bending your knee."

Grading

Grade 5 (Normal): Patient completes available range and holds test position against maximal resistance.

Grade 4 (Good): Patient completes available range against strong to moderate resistance.

Grade 3 (Fair): Completes range and holds the position without resistance (Fig. 5–22).

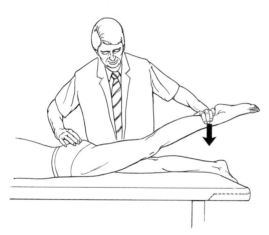

FIGURE 5–20

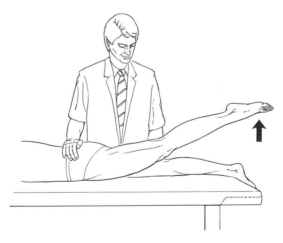

FIGURE 5–22

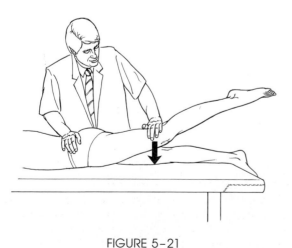

FIGURE 5–21

Grade 2 (Poor)

Position of Patient: Side-lying with test limb uppermost. Knee straight and supported by examiner. Lowermost limb is flexed for stability.

Position of Therapist: Standing behind patient at thigh level. Therapist supports test limb just below the knee, cradling the leg (Fig. 5–23). Opposite hand over the pelvic crest to maintain pelvic and hip alignment.

Test: Patient extends hip through full range of motion.

Instructions to Patient: "Bring your leg back toward me. Keep your knee straight."

Grading

Grade 2 (Poor): Completes range of extension motion in side-lying position.

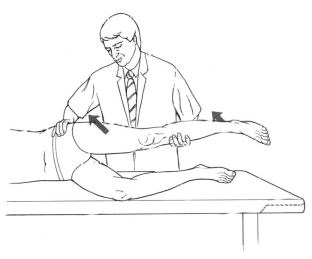

FIGURE 5–23

Grade 1 (Trace) and Grade 0 (Zero)

Position of Patient: Prone.

Position of Therapist: Standing on side to be tested at level of hips. Palpate hamstrings (deep into tissue with fingers) at the ischial tuberosity (Fig. 5–24). Palpate the Gluteus maximus with deep finger pressure over the center of the buttocks and also over the upper and lower fibers.

Test: Patient attempts to extend hip in prone position or tries to squeeze buttocks together.

Instructions to Patient: "Try to lift your leg from the table" OR "Squeeze your buttocks together."

Grading

Grade 1 (Trace): Palpable contraction of either hamstrings or Gluteus maximus but no visible joint movement. Contraction of Gluteus maximus will result in narrowing of the gluteal crease.

Grade 0 (Zero): No palpable contraction.

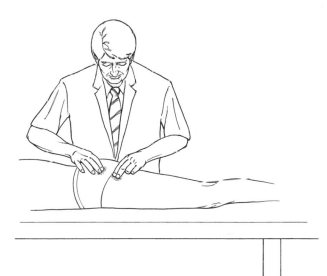

FIGURE 5–24

Helpful Hints

Therapist should be aware that the hip extensors are among the most powerful muscles in the body, and most therapists will not be able to "break" a Grade 5 hip extension. Care should be taken not to overgrade a Grade 4 muscle.

HIP EXTENSION

(Gluteus maximus and Hamstrings)

HIP EXTENSION TEST TO ISOLATE GLUTEUS MAXIMUS

Grade 5 (Normal), Grade 4 (Good), and Grade 3 (Fair)

Position of Patient: Prone with knee flexed to 90°. (Note: In the presence of a hip flexion contracture, do not use this test but refer to the test for hip extension modified for hip flexion tightness [see page 194].)

Position of Therapist: Standing at the side to be tested at the level of the pelvis. (Note: The therapist in the illustration is shown on the wrong side to avoid obscuring test positions.) Hand for resistance is contoured over the posterior thigh just above the knee. The opposite hand may stabilize or maintain the alignment of the pelvis (Fig. 5–25).

For the Grade 3 test the knee may need to be supported in flexion (by cradling at the ankle).

Test: Patient extends hip through available range, maintaining knee flexion. Resistance is given in a straight downward direction (toward floor).

Instructions to Patient: "Lift your foot to the ceiling" OR "Lift your leg keeping your knee bent."

Grading

Grade 5 (Normal): Completes available range of motion and holds end position against maximum resistance.

Grade 4 (Good): Limb position can be held against heavy to moderate resistance.

Grade 3 (Fair): Completes available range of motion and holds end position but takes no resistance (Fig. 5–26).

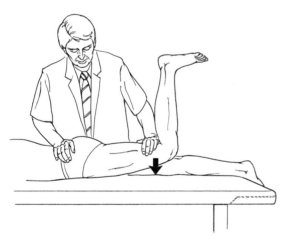

FIGURE 5–25

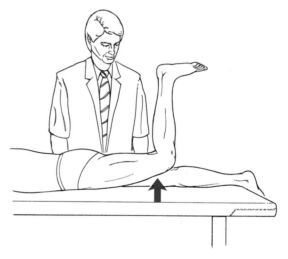

FIGURE 5–26

Grade 2 (Poor)

Position of Patient: Side-lying with test limb uppermost. Knee is flexed and supported by examiner. Lowermost hip and knee should be flexed for stability (Fig. 5–27).

Position of Therapist: Standing behind the patient at thigh level. Therapist cradles uppermost leg with forearm and hand under the flexed knee. Other hand is on pelvis to maintain postural alignment.

Test: Patient extends hip with supported knee flexed.

Instructions to Patient: "Move your leg back toward me."

Grading

Grade 2 (Poor): Completes available range of motion in side-lying position.

Grade 1 (Trace) and Grade 0 (Zero)

This test is identical to the Grade 1 and 0 tests for aggregate hip extension (see Fig. 5–24). The patient is prone and attempts to extend the hip or squeeze the buttocks together while the therapist palpates the Gluteus maximus.

Helpful Hints

Hip extension range is less when the knee is flexed because of tension in the Rectus femoris. A diminished range may be observed, therefore, in tests that isolate the Gluteus maximus.

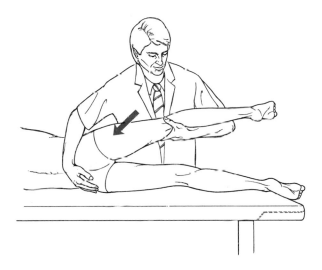

FIGURE 5–27

(Gluteus maximus and Hamstrings)

HIP EXTENSION TESTS MODIFIED FOR HIP FLEXION TIGHTNESS

Grade 5 (Normal), Grade 4 (Good), and Grade 3 (Fair)

Position of Patient: Patient stands with hips flexed and places torso prone on the table (Fig. 5–28). The arms are used to "hug" the table for support. The knee of the nontest limb should be flexed to allow test limb to rest on the floor at start of the test.

Position of Therapist: Standing at side of limb to be tested. (Note: Fig. 5–28 shows the examiner on the opposite side to avoid obscuring test positions.) The hand used to provide resistance is contoured over the posterior thigh just above the knee. The opposite hand stabilizes the pelvis laterally to maintain hip and pelvis posture (see Fig. 5–25).

Test: Patient extends hip through available range, but hip extension range is less when the knee is flexed (see page 193). Keeping the knee in extension will test all hip extensor muscles; with the knee flexed, the isolated Gluteus maximus will be evaluated.

Resistance is applied downward (toward floor) and forward.

Instructions to Patient: "Lift your foot off the floor as high as you can."

Grading

Grade 5 (Normal): Completes available range of hip extension. Holds end position against maximal resistance.

Grade 4 (Good): Completes available range of hip extension. (Note: Because of the intrinsic strength of these muscles, weakened extensor muscles frequently are overgraded.) Limb position can be held against heavy to moderate resistance.

Grade 3 (Fair): Completes available range and holds end position without resistance.

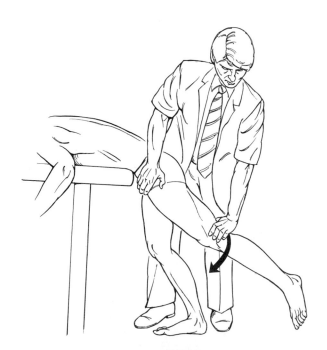

FIGURE 5–28

CROSS SECTIONS OF THE THIGH

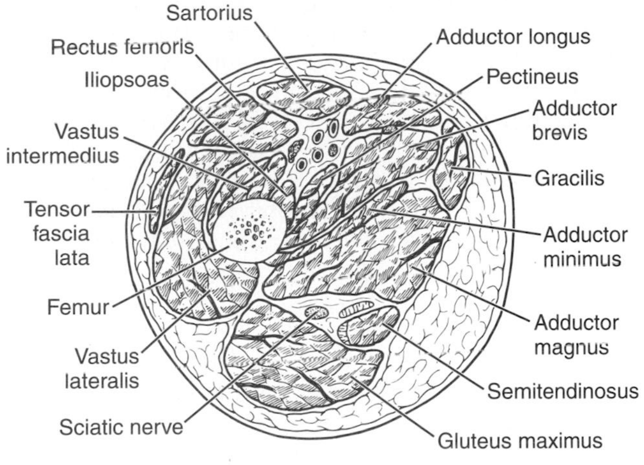

Sartorius
Rectus femoris
Iliopsoas
Vastus intermedius
Tensor fascia lata
Femur
Vastus lateralis
Sciatic nerve

Adductor longus
Pectineus
Adductor brevis
Gracilis
Adductor minimus
Adductor magnus
Semitendinosus
Gluteus maximus

HIGH
JUST BELOW LESSER
TROCHANTER

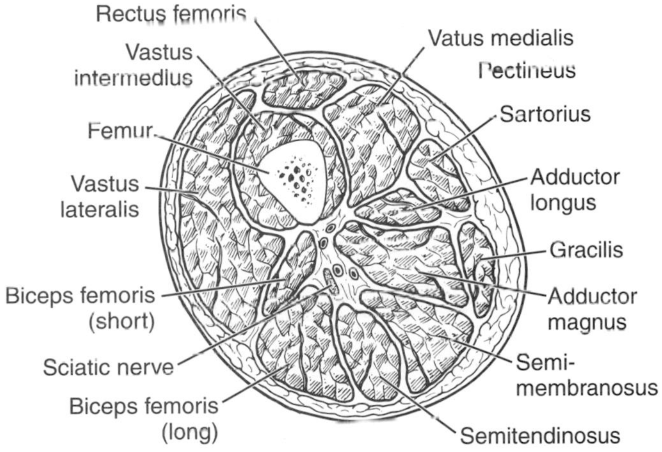

Rectus femoris
Vastus intermedius
Femur
Vastus lateralis
Biceps femoris (short)
Sciatic nerve
Biceps femoris (long)

Vatus medialis
Pectineus
Sartorius
Adductor longus
Gracilis
Adductor magnus
Semi-membranosus
Semitendinosus

MID
JUST ABOVE START OF TENDON
OF RECTUS FEMORIS (ABOUT
7–8" ABOVE CENTER OF KNEE)

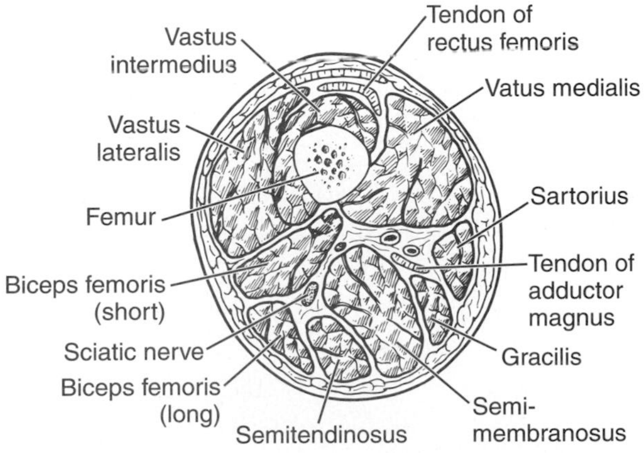

Vastus intermedius
Vastus lateralis
Femur
Biceps femoris (short)
Sciatic nerve
Biceps femoris (long)
Semitendinosus

Tendon of rectus femoris
Vatus medialis
Sartorius
Tendon of adductor magnus
Gracilis
Semi-membranosus

LOW
THROUGH TENDON OF
RECTUS FEMORIS (ABOUT 4"
ABOVE CENTER OF KNEE)

PLATE 6

(Gluteus maximus and Hamstrings)

Grade 2 (Poor), Grade 1 (Trace), and Grade 0 (Zero)

Do not test the patient with hip flexion contractures and weak extensors (less than Grade 3) in the standing position. Position the patient side-lying on the table. Conduct the test as described for the aggregate of extensor muscles (see page 190) or for the isolated Gluteus maximus (see page 192).

SUPINE HIP EXTENSION TEST

When for any reason a patient cannot lie prone and hip extension is expected to be above Grade 2 (Poor), use the supine hip extension test.[1] The test Grades 5, 4, 3, and 2 can be assigned. Although the traditional test for hip extension (Grade 2, Poor) is done with the patient side-lying, this supine hip extension test may be substituted to eliminate change of patient position. Grades 5, 4, 3, and 2 have been validated in this position (n = 44 subjects) by measuring maximum hip extension torques recorded via a strain gauge dynamometer.

Grade 5 (Normal), Grade 4 (Good), Grade 3 (Fair), and Grade 2 (Poor)

Position of Patient: Supine, heels off end of table. Arms folded across chest or abdomen. (Do not allow patient to push into table with upper extremities.)

Position of Therapist: Standing at end of table. Both hands are cupped under the heel (Fig. 5–29).

Test: Patient presses limb into table attempting to maintain full extension as the examiner raises the limb 24 to 26 inches from the table. (The opposite limb almost always rises involuntarily and should *not* be considered an aberrant test.)

Instruction to Patient: "Don't let me lift your leg from the table. Keep your hip locked tight and your whole body rigid as a board."

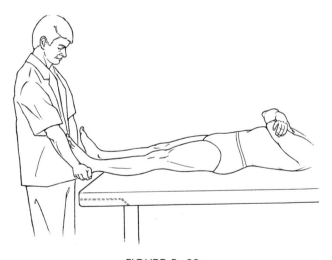

FIGURE 5–29

Grade 5 (Normal), Grade 4 (Good), Grade 3 (Fair), and Grade 2 (Poor) Continued

Grading

Grade 5 (Normal): Hip locks in neutral (full extension) throughout the test. Pelvis and back elevate as one locked unit as the examiner raises the limb (Fig. 5–30).

Grade 4 (Good): Hip flexes before pelvis and back elevate as the limb is raised by the examiner. Hip flexion should not exceed 30° (Fig. 5–31).

Grade 3 (Fair): Full elevation of the limb to the end of straight leg raising range with little or no elevation of the pelvis. Examiner feels strong resistance throughout the test (Fig. 5–32).

Grade 2 (Poor): Hip flexes fully with only minimal resistance felt (examiner should check to assure that the resistance felt exceeds weight of the limb) (see Fig. 5–32).

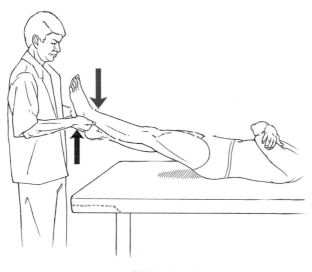

FIGURE 5–30

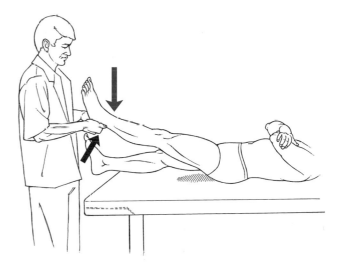

FIGURE 5–32

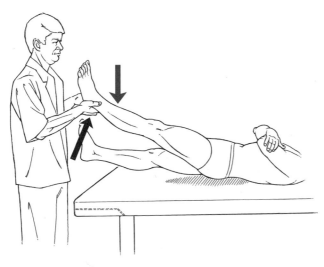

FIGURE 5–31

HIP ABDUCTION

(Gluteus medius and Gluteus minimus)

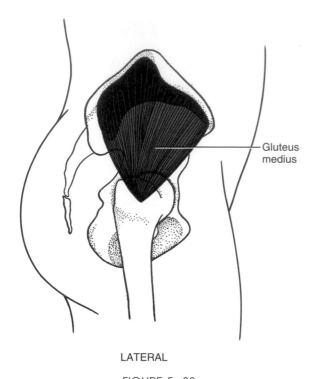

Gluteus medius

LATERAL

FIGURE 5-33

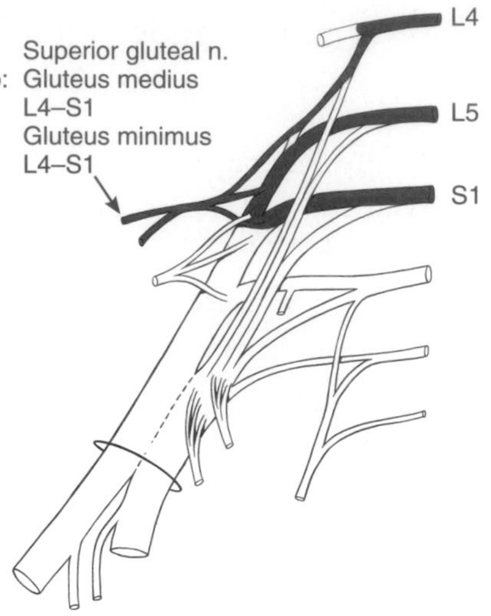

Superior gluteal n.
To: Gluteus medius
L4-S1
Gluteus minimus
L4-S1

L4

L5

S1

FIGURE 5-34

Range of Motion
0° to 45°

Table 5-4 HIP ABDUCTION

I.D.	Muscle	Origin	Insertion
183	Gluteus medius	Ilium (outer surface between crest and anterior and posterior gluteal lines) Fascia (over upper part)	Femur (greater trochanter, lateral aspect)
184	Gluteus minimus	Ilium (outer surface between anterior and inferior gluteal lines) Greater sciatic notch	Femur (greater trochanter, anterolateral ridge) Fibrous capsule of hip joint

Others

182	Gluteus maximus (upper fibers)		
185	Tensor fasciae latae		
187	Obturator internus (thigh flexed)		
189	Gemellus superior (thigh flexed)		
190	Gemellus inferior (thigh flexed)		
195	Sartorius		

(Gluteus medius and Gluteus minimus)

Grade 5 (Normal), Grade 4 (Good), and Grade 3 (Fair)

Position of Patient: Side-lying with test leg uppermost. Start test with the limb slightly extended beyond the midline and the pelvis rotated slightly forward. Lowermost leg is flexed for stability.

Position of Therapist: Standing behind patient. Hand used to give resistance is contoured across the lateral surface of the knee. The hand used to palpate the Gluteus medius is just proximal to the greater trochanter of the femur (Fig. 5–35). (No resistance is used in a Grade 3 test.)

Alternatively, resistance may be applied at the ankle, which gives a longer lever arm and requires greater strength on the part of the patient to achieve a grade of 5 or 4. Examiner is reminded always to use the same lever in a given test sequence and in subsequent comparison tests.

To distinguish a Grade 5 from a Grade 4 result, first apply resistance at the ankle and then at the knee.

Test: Patient abducts hip through the complete available range of motion without flexing the hip or rotating it in either direction. Resistance is given in a straight downward direction.

Instructions to Patient: "Lift your leg up in the air. Hold it. Don't let me push it down."

Grading

Grade 5 (Normal): Completes available range and holds end position against maximal resistance.

Grade 4 (Good): Completes available range and holds against heavy to moderate resistance.

Grade 3 (Fair): Completes range of motion and holds end position without resistance (Fig. 5–36).

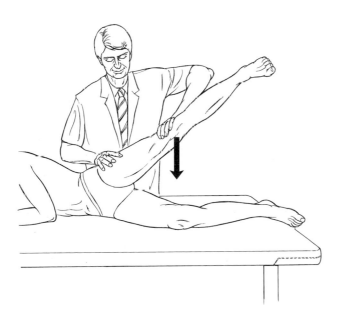

FIGURE 5–35

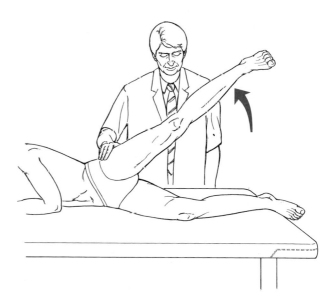

FIGURE 5–36

(Gluteus medius and Gluteus minimus)

Grade 2 (Poor)

Position of Patient: Supine.

Position of Therapist: Standing on side of limb being tested. One hand supports and lifts the limb by holding it under the ankle to raise limb just enough to decrease friction. This hand offers no resistance, nor should it be used to offer assistance to the movement. On some smooth surfaces such support may not be necessary (Fig. 5–37).

The other hand palpates the Gluteus medius just proximal to the greater trochanter of the femur.

Test: Patient abducts hip through available range.

Instructions to Patient: "Bring your leg out to the side. Keep your kneecap pointing to the ceiling."

Grading

Grade 2 (Poor): Completes range of motion supine with no resistance and minimal to zero friction.

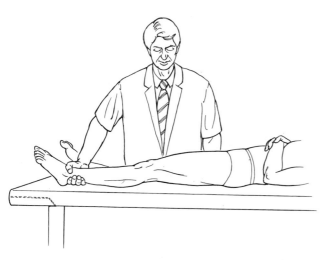

FIGURE 5–37

Grade 1 (Trace) and Grade 0 (Zero)

Position of Patient: Supine.

Position of Therapist: Standing at side of limb being tested at level of thigh. (Note: Fig. 5–38 shows therapist on opposite side to avoid obscuring test positions.) One hand supports the limb under the ankle just above the malleoli. The hand should provide neither resistance nor assistance to movement (Fig. 5–38). Palpate the Gluteus medius on the lateral aspect of the hip just above the greater trochanter.

Test: Patient attempts to abduct hip.

Instructions to Patient: "Try to bring your leg out to the side."

Grading

Grade 1 (Trace): Palpable contraction of Gluteus medius but no movement of the part.

Grade 0 (Zero): No palpable contraction.

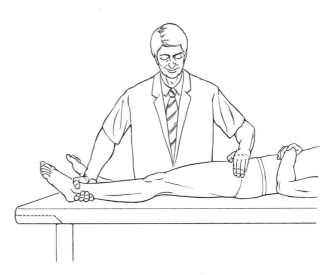

FIGURE 5–38

Substitutions

- Hip-hike substitution: Patient may "hike hip" by approximating pelvis to thorax using the lateral trunk muscles, which moves the limb through partial abduction range (Fig. 5–39). This movement may be detected by observing the lateral trunk and hip (move clothing aside) and palpating the Gluteus medius above the trochanter.

- External rotation and flexion substitution: The patient may try to externally rotate during the motion of abduction (Fig. 5–40). This could allow the oblique action of the hip flexors to substitute for the Gluteus medius.

- Tensor fasciae latae substitution: If the test is allowed to begin with active hip flexion or with the hip positioned in flexion, there is an opportunity for the Tensor fasciae latae to abduct the hip.

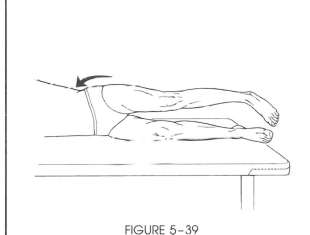

FIGURE 5–39

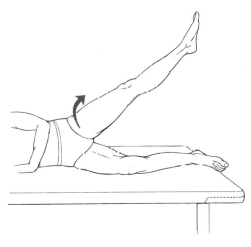

FIGURE 5–40

Helpful Hints

- The examiner should not be able to "break" a Grade 5 muscle and most therapists will not be able to "break" a Grade 4 muscle. A grade of 4 often masks significant weakness because of the intrinsic great strength of these muscles. Giving resistance at the ankle rather than at the knee assists in overcoming this problem.

- Do not attempt to palpate contractile activity of muscle through clothing. (This is one of the cardinal principles of manual muscle testing.)

- When the patient is supine, the weight of the opposite limb stabilizes the pelvis. It is not necessary, therefore, to use a hand to manually stabilize the contralateral limb.

(Tensor fasciae latae)

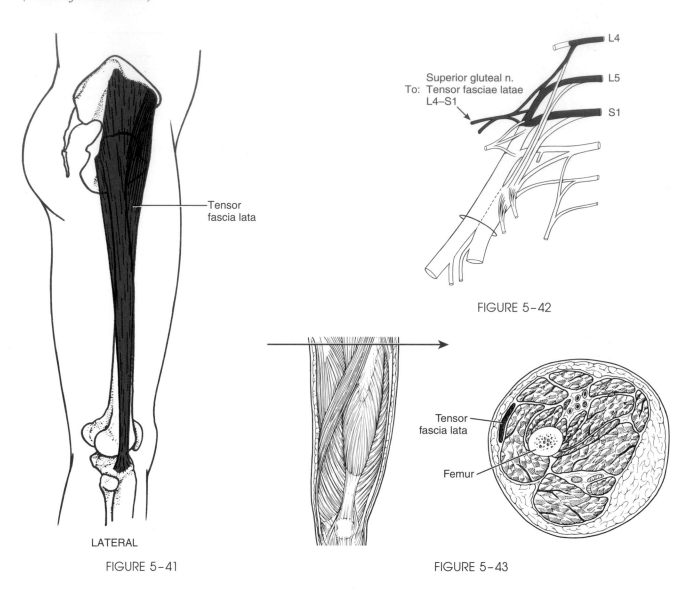

LATERAL

FIGURE 5-41

Superior gluteal n.
To: Tensor fasciae latae
L4–S1

L4

L5

S1

FIGURE 5-42

Tensor
fascia lata

Femur

FIGURE 5-43

Tensor
fascia lata

Range of Motion

Two-joint muscle. No specific range of motion can be assigned solely to the Tensor.

Table 5-5 HIP ABDUCTION FROM FLEXION

I.D.	Muscle	Origin	Insertion
185	Tensor fasciae latae	Iliac crest (outer lip) Fasciae latae (deep) Anterior superior iliac spine (lateral surface)	Iliotibial tract (between its two layers, ending 1/3 of the way down)
Others			
183	Gluteus medius		
184	Gluteus minimus		

(Tensor fasciae latae)

Grade 5 (Normal), Grade 4 (Good), and Grade 3 (Fair)

Position of Patient: Side-lying. Uppermost limb (test limb) is flexed to 45° and lies across the lowermost limb with the foot resting on the table (Fig. 5–44).

Position of Therapist: Standing behind patient at level of pelvis. Hand for resistance is placed on lateral surface of the thigh just above the knee. Hand providing stabilization is placed on the crest of the ilium (Fig. 5–45).

Test: Patient abducts hip through approximately 30° of motion. Resistance is given downward (toward floor) from the lateral surface of the distal femur. No resistance is given for the Grade 3 test.

Instructions to Patient: "Lift your leg and hold it. Don't let me push it down."

Grading

Grade 5 (Normal): Completes available range; holds end position against maximal resistance.

Grade 4 (Good): Completes available range and holds against strong to moderate resistance.

Grade 3 (Fair): Completes movement; holds end position but takes no resistance (Fig. 5–46).

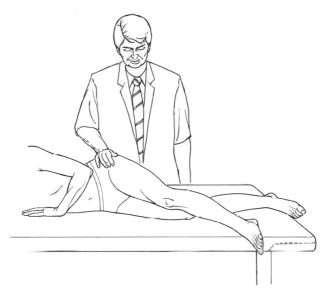

FIGURE 5–44

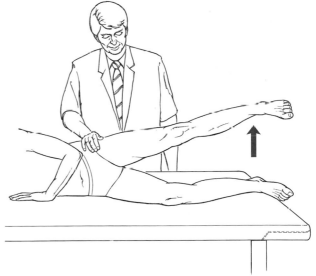

FIGURE 5–46

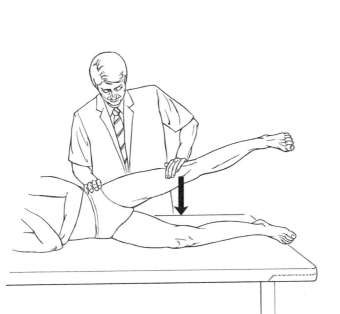

FIGURE 5–45

HIP ABDUCTION FROM FLEXED POSITION

(Tensor fasciae latae)

Grade 2 (Poor)

Position of Patient: Patient is in long-sitting position, supporting trunk with hands placed behind body on table. Trunk may lean backward up to 45° from vertical (Fig. 5–47).

Position of Therapist: Standing at side of limb to be tested. (Note: Fig. 5–47 deliberately shows therapist on wrong side to avoid obscuring test positions.) One hand supports the limb under the ankle; this hand will be used to reduce friction with the surface as the patient moves but should neither resist nor assist motion.

The other hand palpates the Tensor fasciae latae on the proximal anterolateral thigh where it inserts into the iliotibial band.

Test: Patient abducts hip through 30° of range.

Instructions to Patient: "Bring your leg out to the side."

Grading

Grade 2 (Poor): Completes hip abduction motion to 30°.

Grade 1 (Trace) and Grade 0 (Zero)

Position of Patient: Long sitting.

Position of Therapist: One hand palpates the insertion of the Tensor at the lateral aspect of the knee. The other hand palpates the Tensor on the anterolateral thigh (Fig. 5–48).

Test: Patient attempts to abduct hip.

Instructions to Patient: "Try to move your leg out to the side."

Grading

Grade 1 (Trace): Palpable contraction of Tensor fibers but no limb movement.

Grade 0 (Zero): No palpable contractile activity.

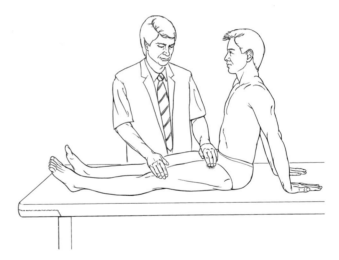

FIGURE 5–48

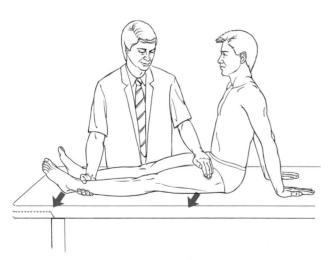

FIGURE 5–47

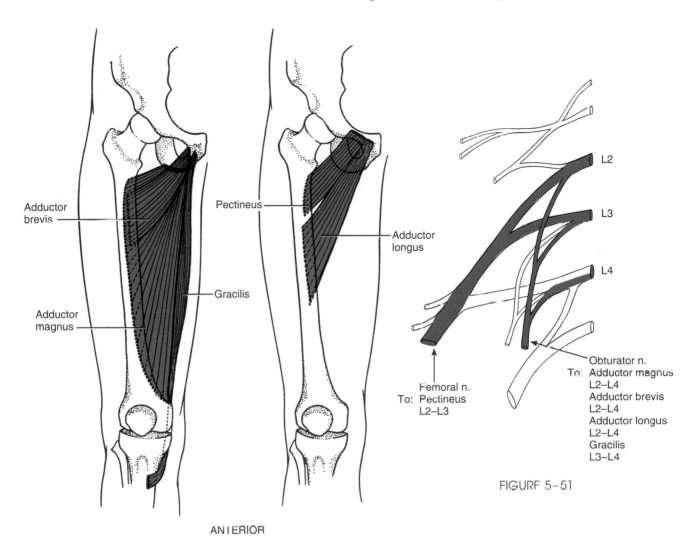

Adductor brevis

Pectineus

Adductor longus

Adductor magnus

Gracilis

Femoral n.
To: Pectineus
L2–L3

Obturator n.
To: Adductor magnus
L2–L4
Adductor brevis
L2–L4
Adductor longus
L2–L4
Gracilis
L3–L4

L2

L3

L4

ANTERIOR

FIGURE 5–49

FIGURE 5–50

FIGURF 5–51

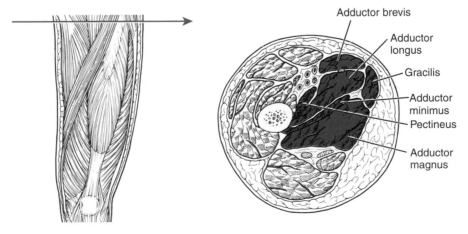

Adductor brevis

Adductor longus

Gracilis

Adductor minimus

Pectineus

Adductor magnus

FIGURE 5–52

HIP ADDUCTION

(Adductors magnus, brevis, and longus; Pectineus and Gracilis)

Table 5-6 HIP ADDUCTION

I.D.	Muscle	Origin	Insertion
181	Adductor magnus	Ischial tuberosity (inferolateral) Ischium (inferior ramus) Pubis (inferior ramus) Fibers from pubic ramus to femur (gluteal tuberosity), often named the *Adductor minimus*	Femur (linea aspera via aponeurosis; medial supracondylar line; and adductor tubercle on medial condyle)
180	Adductor brevis	Pubis (body and inferior ramus)	Femur (via aponeurosis to linea aspera)
179	Adductor longus	Pubis (anterior aspect between crest and symphysis)	Femur (linea aspera via aponeurosis)
177	Pectineus	Pubic pecten Fascia of Pectineus	Femur (on a line from lesser trochanter to linea aspera)
178	Gracilis	Pubis (body and inferior ramus) Ischial ramus	Tibia (medial shaft distal to condyle) Pes anserina Deep fascia of leg

Others

188	Obturator externus		
182	Gluteus maximus (lower)		

Grade 5 (Normal), Grade 4 (Good), and Grade 3 (Fair)

Position of Patient: Side-lying with test limb (lowermost) resting on the table. Uppermost limb (nontest limb) in 25° of abduction, supported by the examiner. The therapist cradles the leg with the forearm, the hand supporting the limb on the medial surface of the knee (Fig. 5–53).

Position of Therapist: Standing behind patient at knee level. The hand giving resistance to the test limb (lowermost limb) is placed on the medial surface of the distal femur, just proximal to the knee joint. Resistance is directed straight downward toward the table (Fig. 5–54).

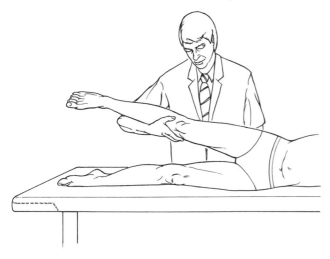

FIGURE 5–53

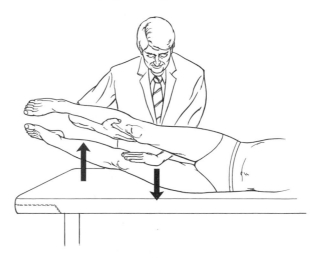

FIGURE 5–54

(Adductors magnus, brevis, and longus; Pectineus and Gracilis)

Grade 5 (Normal), Grade 4 (Good), and Grade 3 (Fair) Continued

Test: Patient adducts hip until the lower limb contacts the upper one.

Instructions to Patient: "Lift your bottom leg up to your top one. Hold it. Don't let me push it down."

For Grade 3: "Lift your bottom leg up to your top one. Don't let it drop!"

Grading

Grade 5 (Normal): Completes full range; holds end position against maximal resistance.

Grade 4 (Good): Completes full movement, but tolerates strong to moderate resistance.

Grade 3 (Fair): Completes full movement; holds end position but takes no resistance (Fig. 5–55).

Grade 2 (Poor)

Position of Patient: Supine. The nontest limb is positioned in some abduction to prevent interference with motion of the test limb.

Position of Therapist: Standing at side of test limb at knee level. One hand supports the ankle and elevates it slightly from the table surface to decrease friction as the limb moves across (Fig. 5–56). The examiner uses this hand neither to assist nor resist motion. The opposite hand palpates the adductor mass on the inner aspect of the proximal thigh.

Test: Patient adducts hip without rotation.

Instructions to Patient: "Bring your leg in toward the other one."

Grading

Grade 2 (Poor): Patient adducts limb through full range.

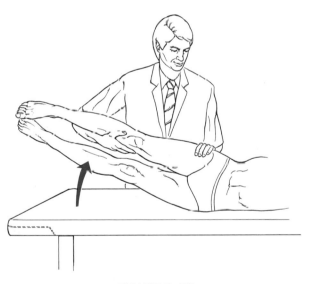

FIGURE 5–55

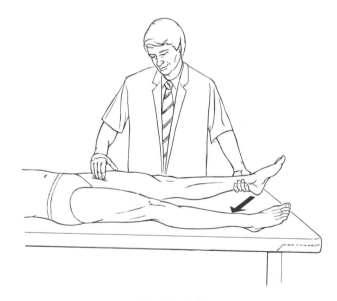

FIGURE 5–56

HIP ADDUCTION

(Adductors magnus, brevis, and longus; Pectineus and Gracilis)

Grade 1 (Trace) and Grade 0 (Zero)

Position of Patient: Supine.

Position of Therapist: Standing on side of test limb. One hand supports the limb under the ankle. The other hand palpates the adductor mass on the proximal medial thigh (Fig. 5–57).

Test: Patient attempts to adduct hip.

Instructions to Patient: "Try to bring your leg in."

Grading

Grade 1 (Trace): Palpable contraction, no limb movement.

Grade 0 (Zero): No palpable contraction.

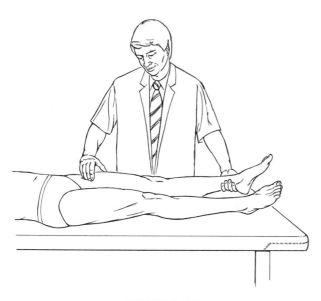

FIGURE 5–57

Substitutions

- Hip flexor substitution: The patient may attempt to substitute the hip flexors for the adductors by internally rotating the hip using a posterior pelvic tilt (Fig. 5–58). The patient will appear to be trying to turn supine from side-lying. Maintenance of true side-lying is necessary for an accurate test.

- Hamstring substitution: Patient may attempt to substitute the hamstrings for the adductors by externally rotating the test hip with an anterior pelvic tilt. Patient will appear to move toward prone. Again, true side-lying is important.

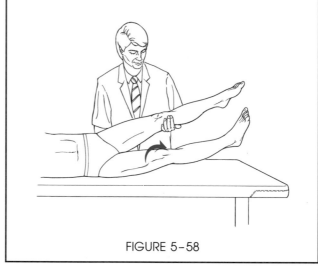

FIGURE 5–58

Helpful Hint

In the supine test position for Grades 2, 1, and 0, the weight of the opposite limb stabilizes the pelvis, so there is no need for manual stabilization of the nontest hip.

(Obturators internus and externus, Gemellae superior and inferior,
Piriformis, Quadratus femoris, Gluteus maximus [posterior])

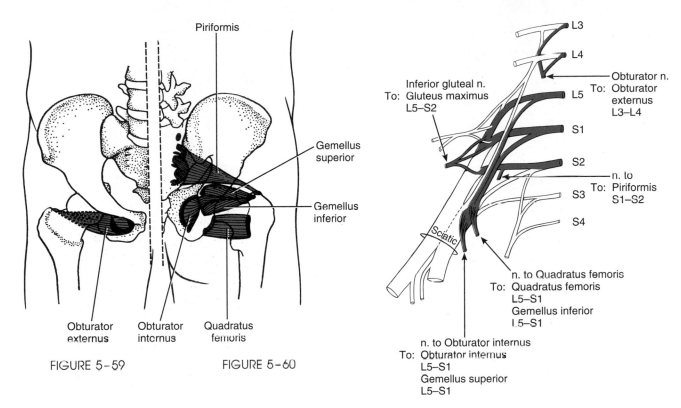

Piriformis

Gemellus
superior

Gemellus
inferior

Obturator
externus

Obturator
internus

Quadratus
femoris

FIGURE 5-59

FIGURE 5-60

L3

L4

Inferior gluteal n.
To: Gluteus maximus
L5–S2

Obturator n.
To: Obturator
externus
L3–L4

L5

S1

S2

n. to
To: Piriformis
S1–S2

S3

S4

Sciatic

n. to Quadratus femoris
To: Quadratus femoris
L5–S1
Gemellus inferior
L5–S1

n. to Obturator internus
To: Obturator internus
L5–S1
Gemellus superior
L5–S1

FIGURE 5-61

HIP EXTERNAL ROTATION

(Obturators internus and externus, Gemellae superior and inferior, Piriformis, Quadratus femoris, Gluteus maximus [posterior])

Range of Motion
0° to 45°

Table 5-7 HIP EXTERNAL ROTATION

I.D.	Muscle	Origin	Insertion
188	Obturator externus	Obturator membrane (external surface) Ischium (ramus) Pubis (inferior ramus) Pelvis (lesser pelvic cavity, inner surface)	Femur (trochanteric fossa)
187	Obturator internus	Pubis (inferior ramus) Ischium (ramus) Obturator fascia Obturator foramen (margin) Obturator membrane Upper brim of greater sciatic foramen	Femur (greater trochanter, medial) Tendon fuses with Gemelli
191	Quadratus femoris (may be absent)	Ischial tuberosity (external aspect)	Femur (quadrate tubercle on trochanteric crest)
186	Piriformis	Sacrum (anterior surface) Ilium (gluteal surface near posterior inferior iliac spine) Sacrotuberous ligament Capsule of sacroiliac joint	Femur (greater trochanter, medial side)
189	Gemellus superior (may be absent)	Ischium (spine, dorsal surface)	Femur (greater trochanter, medial surface) Blends with tendon of Obturator internus)
190	Gemellus inferior	Ischial tuberosity (upper part)	Femur (greater trochanter, medial surface) Blends with tendon of Obturator internus
182	Gluteus maximus	Ilium (posterior gluteal line and crest) Sacrum (dorsal and lower aspects) Coccyx (side) Sacrotuberous ligament Aponeurosis over Gluteus medius	Femur (gluteal tuberosity) Iliotibial tract of fascia lata

Others

195	Sartorius
192	Biceps femoris (long head)
183	Gluteus medius (posterior)
174	Psoas major
181	Adductor magnus (position-dependent)
179	Adductor longus
202	Popliteus (tibia fixed)

(Obturators internus and externus, Gemellae superior and inferior, Piriformis, Quadratus femoris, Gluteus maximus [posterior])

Grade 5 (Normal), Grade 4 (Good), and Grade 3 (Fair)

Position of Patient: Short sitting. (Trunk may be supported by placing hands flat or fisted at sides) (Fig. 5–62).

Position of Therapist: Sits on a low stool or kneels beside limb to be tested. The hand that gives resistance grasps the ankle just above the malleolus. Resistance is applied as a laterally directed force at the ankle (Fig. 5–62).

The other hand, which will offer counterpressure, is contoured over the lateral aspect of the distal thigh just above the knee. Resistance is given as a medially directed force at the knee. The two forces are applied in counterdirections for this rotary motion (Fig. 5–62).

Test: Patient externally rotates the hip. This is a test where it is preferable for the examiner to place the limb in the test end position rather than to ask the patient to perform the movement.

Instructions to Patient: "Don't let me turn your leg out."

Grading

Grade 5 (Normal): Holds at end of range against maximal resistance.

Grade 4 (Good): Holds at end of range against strong to moderate resistance.

Grade 3 (Fair): Holds end position but tolerates no resistance (Fig. 5–63).

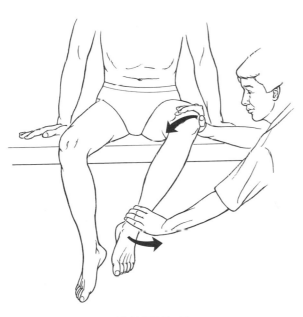

FIGURE 5–62

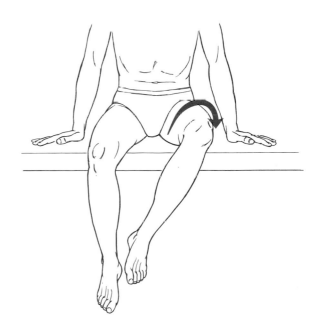

FIGURE 5–63

HIP EXTERNAL ROTATION

(Obturators internus and externus, Gemellae superior and inferior,
Piriformis, Quadratus femoris, Gluteus maximus [posterior])

Grade 2 (Poor)

Position of Patient: Supine. Test limb is in internal rotation.

Position of Therapist: Standing at side of limb to be tested.

Test: Patient externally rotates hip in available range of motion (Fig. 5–64). One hand may be used to maintain pelvic alignment at lateral hip.

Instructions to Patient: "Roll your leg out."

Grading

Grade 2 (Poor): Completes external rotation range of motion. As the hip rolls past the midline, minimal resistance can be offered to offset the assistance of gravity.

Alternate Test for Grade 2: With the patient short-sitting, the therapist places the test limb in maximal internal rotation. The patient then is instructed to return the limb actively to the midline (neutral) position against slight resistance. Care needs to be taken to ensure that gravity is not the predominant force. If this motion is performed satisfactorily, the test is assessed as a Grade 2.

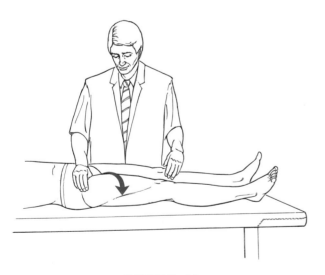

FIGURE 5–64

Grade 1 (Trace) and Grade 0 (Zero)

Position of Patient: Supine with test limb placed in internal rotation.

Position of Therapist: Standing at side of limb to be tested.

Test: Patient attempts to externally rotate hip.

Instructions to Patient: "Try to roll your leg out."

Grading

Grade 1 (Trace) and Grade 0 (Zero): The external rotator muscles, except for the Gluteus maximus, are not palpable. If there is any discernible movement (contractile activity), a grade of 1 should be given; otherwise, a grade of 0 is assigned on the principle that whenever uncertainty exists, the lesser grade should be awarded.

Helpful Hints

- There is wide variation in the amount of hip external rotation range of motion that can be considered normal. It is imperative, therefore, that a patient's accurate range (in each test position) be known before manual muscle testing takes place.

- There is greater range of rotation at the hip when the hip is flexed than when it is extended, probably secondary to laxity of joint structures.

- In short-sitting tests, the patient should not be allowed to use the following motions, lest they add visual distortion and contaminate the test results:
  a. lift the contralateral buttock off the table or lean in any direction to lift the pelvis;
  b. increase flexion of the test knee;
  c. abduct the test hip.

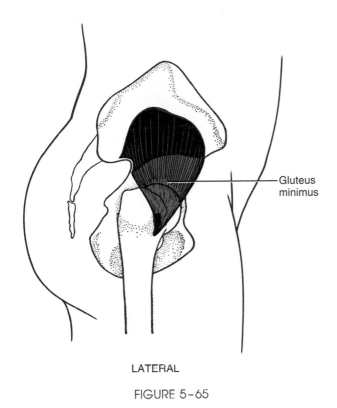

LATERAL

FIGURE 5-65

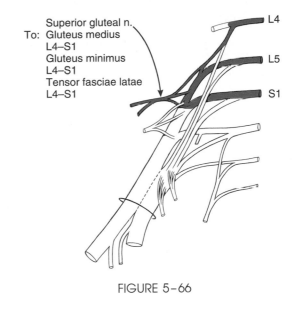

Superior gluteal n.

To: Gluteus medius
L4–S1
Gluteus minimus
L4–S1
Tensor fasciae latae
L4–S1

L4

L5

S1

FIGURE 5-66

Range of Motion
0° to 45°

Table 5-8 HIP INTERNAL ROTATION

I.D.	Muscle	Origin	Insertion
184	Gluteus minimus (anterior fibers)	Ilium (outer surface between anterior and inferior gluteal lines) Greater sciatic notch	Femur (greater trochanter, anterior aspect) Fibrous capsule of hip joint
185	Tensor fasciae latae	Iliac crest (outer lip) Fascia lata (deep) Anterior superior iliac spine (lateral surface)	Iliotibial tract (between its two layers ending 1/3 down femur)
183	Gluteus medius (anterior fibers)	Ilium (outer surface between crest and posterior gluteal line) Gluteal fascia	Femur (greater trochanter, lateral surface)

Others

193	Semitendinosus	
194	Semimembranosus	
181	Adductor magnus (position-dependent)	
179	Adductor longus (position-dependent)	

HIP INTERNAL ROTATION

(Glutei minimus and medius; Tensor fasciae latae)

Grade 5 (Normal), Grade 4 (Good), and Grade 3 (Fair)

Position of Patient: Short sitting. Arms may be used for trunk support at sides or may be crossed over chest.

Position of Therapist: Sitting or kneeling in front of patient. One hand grasps the lateral surface of the ankle just above the malleolus (Fig. 5–67). Resistance is given (Grades 5 and 4 only) as a medially directed force at the ankle.

The opposite hand, which offers counterpressure, is contoured over the medial surface of the distal thigh just above the knee. Resistance is applied as a laterally directed force at the knee. Note the counter-directions of the force applied.

Test: The limb should be placed in the end position of full internal rotation by the examiner for best test results (Fig. 5–67).

Grading

Grade 5 (Normal): Holds end position against maximal resistance.

Grade 4 (Good): Holds end position against strong to moderate resistance.

Grade 3 (Fair): Holds end position but takes no resistance (Fig. 5–68).

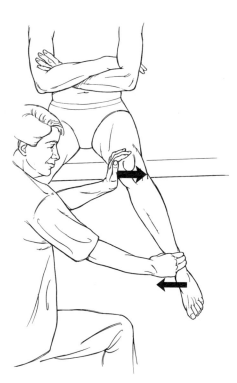

FIGURE 5–67

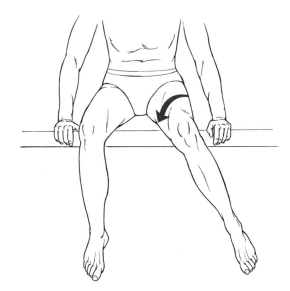

FIGURE 5–68

Grade 2 (Poor)

Position of Patient: Supine. Test limb in partial external rotation.

Position of Therapist: Standing next to test leg. Palpate the Gluteus medius proximal to the greater trochanter and the Tensor fasciae latae (Fig. 5–69) over the anterolateral hip below the ASIS.

Test: Patient internally rotates hip through available range.

Instructions to Patient: "Roll your leg in toward the other one."

Grading

Grade 2 (Poor): Completes the range of motion. As the hip rolls inward past the midline, minimal resistance can be offered to offset the assistance of gravity.

Alternate Test for Grade 2: With patient short sitting, the examiner places the test limb in maximal external rotation. The patient then is instructed to return the limb actively to the midline (neutral) position against slight resistance. Care needs to be taken to ensure that gravity is not the predominant force. If this motion is performed satisfactorily, the test may be assessed a Grade 2.

Grade 1 (Trace) and Grade 0 (Zero)

Position of Patient: Patient supine with test limb placed in external rotation.

Position of Therapist: Standing next to test leg.

Test: Patient attempts to internally rotate hip. One hand is used to palpate the Gluteus medius (over the posterolateral surface of the hip above the greater trochanter). The other hand is used to palpate the Tensor fasciae latae (on the anterolateral surface of the hip below the ASIS).

Instructions to Patient: "Try to roll your leg in."

Grading

Grade 1 (Trace): Palpable contractile activity in either or both muscles.

Grade 0 (Zero): No palpable contractile activity.

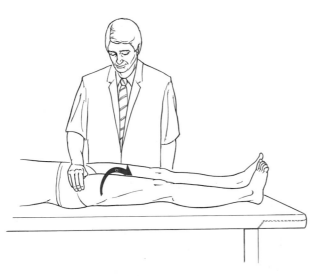

FIGURE 5–69

> ## Helpful Hints
>
> - In the short-sitting tests, do not allow the patient to assist internal rotation by lifting the pelvis on the side of the limb being tested.
> - Neither should the patient be allowed to extend the knee or adduct and extend the hip during performance of the test. These motions contaminate the test by offering visual distortion to the therapist.
> - For the external rotation test, the reader is referred to Helpful Hints 2 and 3 under External Rotation (page 212), which apply here as well.

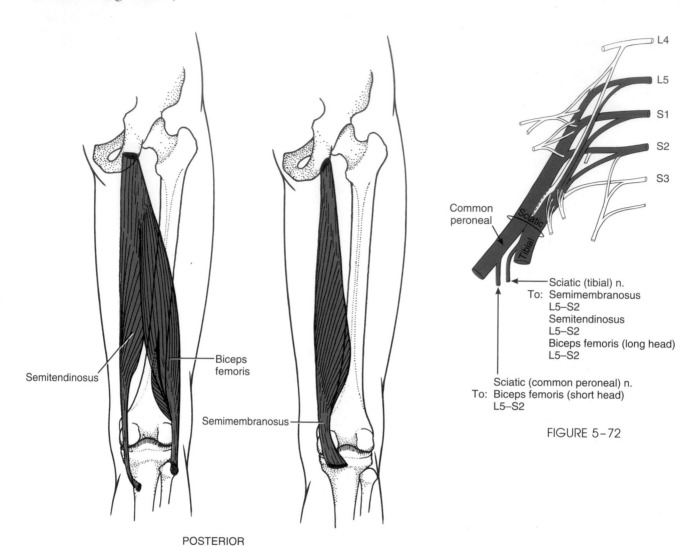

Semitendinosus

Biceps femoris

Semimembranosus

POSTERIOR

FIGURE 5-70

FIGURE 5-71

L4

L5

S1

S2

S3

Common peroneal

Sciatic

Tibial

Sciatic (tibial) n.
To: Semimembranosus
L5–S2
Semitendinosus
L5–S2
Biceps femoris (long head)
L5–S2

Sciatic (common peroneal) n.
To: Biceps femoris (short head)
L5–S2

FIGURE 5-72

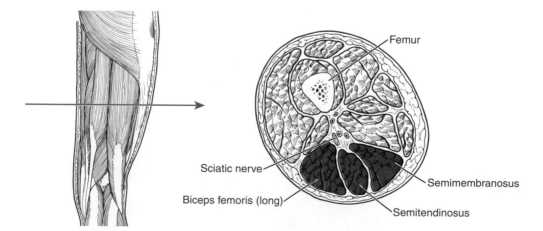

Femur

Sciatic nerve

Biceps femoris (long)

Semimembranosus

Semitendinosus

FIGURE 5-73

Range of Motion
0° to 135°

Table 5-9   KNEE FLEXION

I.D.	Muscle	Origin	Insertion
192	Biceps femoris		
	Long head	Ischium (tuberosity) Sacrotuberous ligament	Aponeurosis (posterior) Fibula (head, lateral aspect) Fibular collateral ligament
	Short head (may be absent)	Femur (linea aspera and lateral condylae) Lateral intermuscular septum	Tibia (lateral condyle)
193	Semitendinosus	Ischial tuberosity (inferior medial aspect) Tendon via aponeurosis shared with Biceps femoris (long)	Tibia (proximal shaft) Pes anserina Deep fascia of leg
194	Semimembranosus	Ischial tuberosity Sacrotuberous ligament	Distal aponeurosis Tibia (medial condyle) Oblique popliteal ligament of knee joint

Others

178	Gracilis
185	Tensor fasciae latae (knee flexed more than 30°)
195	Sartorius
202	Popliteus
205	Gastrocnemius
207	Plantaris

KNEE FLEXION

(All hamstring muscles)

Grade 5 (Normal), Grade 4 (Good), and Grade 3 (Fair)

There are three basic muscle tests for the hamstrings at Grades 5 and 4. The examiner should test first for the aggregate of the three hamstring muscles (with the foot in midline). Only if there is deviation (or asymmetry) in the movement or a question in the examiner's mind is there a need to test the medial and lateral hamstrings separately.

HAMSTRING MUSCLES IN AGGREGATE

Position of Patient: Prone with limbs straight and toes hanging over the edge of the table. Test may be started in about 45° of knee flexion.

Position of Therapist: Standing next to limb to be tested. (Illustration is deliberately incorrect to avoid obscuring test activity.) Hand giving resistance is contoured around the posterior surface of the leg just above the ankle (Fig. 5–74). Resistance is applied in the direction of knee extension for Grades 5 and 4.

The other hand is placed over the hamstring tendons on the posterior thigh (optional).

Test: Patient flexes knee while maintaining leg in neutral rotation.

Instructions to Patient: "Bend your knee. Hold it! Don't let me straighten it."

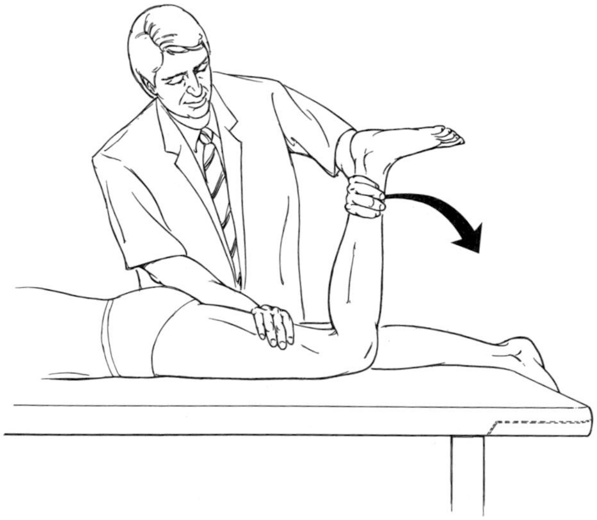

MEDIAL HAMSTRING TEST (SEMITENDINOSUS AND SEMIMEMBRANOSUS)

Position of Patient: Prone with knee flexed to less than 90°. Leg in internal rotation (toes pointing toward midline).

Position of Therapist: Hand giving resistance grasps the leg at the ankle. Resistance is applied in an oblique direction (down and out) toward knee extension (Fig. 5–75).

Test: Patient flexes knee, maintaining the leg in internal rotation (heel toward examiner, toes pointing toward midline).

FIGURE 5–74

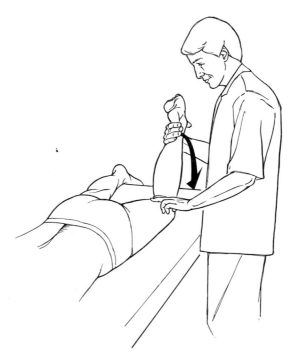

FIGURE 5–75

LATERAL HAMSTRING TEST (BICEPS FEMORIS)

Position of Patient: Prone with knee flexed to less than 90°. Leg is in external rotation (toes pointing laterally).

Position of Therapist: Therapist resists knee flexion at the ankle using a downward and inward force (Fig. 5–76).

Test: Patient flexes knee, maintaining leg in external rotation (heel away from examiner, toes pointing toward examiner) (Fig. 5–76).

Grading the Hamstring Muscles (Grades 5 to 3)

Grade 5 (Normal) for All Three Tests: Resistance will be maximal, and the end knee flexion position (approximately 90°) cannot be broken.

Grade 4 (Good) for All Three Tests: End knee flexion position is held against strong to moderate resistance.

Grade 3 (Fair) for All Three Tests: Holds end range position but tolerates no resistance (Fig. 5–77).

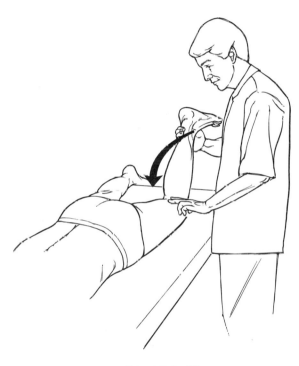

FIGURE 5–76

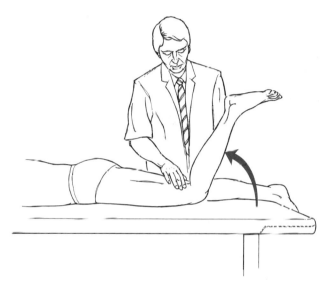

FIGURE 5–77

KNEE FLEXION

(All hamstring muscles)

Grade 2 (Poor)

Position of Patient: Side-lying with test limb (uppermost limb) supported by examiner. Lower limb flexed for stability.

Position of Therapist: Standing behind patient at knee level. One arm is used to cradle thigh, providing hand support at medial side of knee. Other hand supports the leg at the ankle just above the malleolus (Fig. 5–78).

Test: Patient flexes knee through available range of motion.

Instructions to Patient: "Bend your knee."

Grading

Grade 2 (Poor): Completes available range of motion in side-lying.

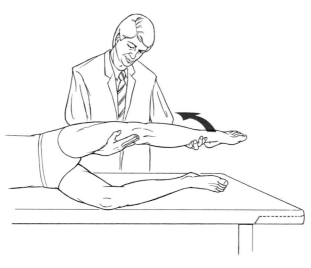

FIGURE 5–78

Grade 1 (Trace) and Grade 0 (Zero)

Position of Patient: Prone. Limbs are straight with toes extending over end of table. Knee is partially flexed and supported at ankle by examiner.

Position of Therapist: Standing next to test limb at knee level. One hand supports the flexed limb at the ankle (Fig. 5–79). The opposite hand palpates both the medial and lateral hamstring tendons just above the posterior knee.

Test: Patient attempts to flex knee.

Instructions to Patient: "Try to bend your knee."

Grading

Grade 1 (Trace): Tendons become prominent, but no visible movement occurs.

Grade 0 (Zero): No palpable contraction of the muscles, and tendons do not stand out.

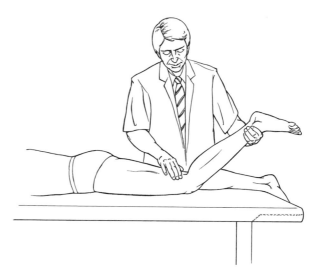

FIGURE 5–79

Substitutions

- Hip flexion substitution: The prone patient may flex the hip to start knee flexion. The buttock on the test side will rise as the hip flexes, and the patient may appear to roll slightly toward supine (Fig. 5–80).

- Sartorius substitution: The Sartorius may try to assist with knee flexion, but this also causes flexion and external rotation of the hip. Knee flexion when the hip is externally rotated is less difficult because the leg is not raised vertically against gravity.

- Gracilis substitution: Action of the Gracilis contributes a hip adduction motion.

- Gastrocnemius substitution: Do not permit the patient to strongly dorsiflex in an attempt to use the tenodesis effect of the Gastrocnemius.

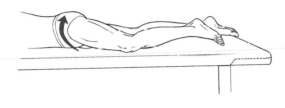

FIGURE 5-80

Helpful Hints

- If the Biceps femoris is stronger than the medial hamstrings, the leg will externally rotate during knee flexion. Similarly, if the Semitendinosus and Semimembranosus are the stronger components, the leg will internally rotate during knee flexion. This is the situation that, when observed, indicates asymmetry and the need to test the medial and lateral hamstrings separately.

- In tests for Grades 3 and 2, the knee may be placed in a 10° flexed position to start the test when Gastrocnemius weakness is present (the Gastrocnemius assists in knee flexion).

- If the hip flexes at the end of the knee flexion range of motion, check for a tight Rectus femoris muscle, because this tightness will limit the range of knee motion.

KNEE EXTENSION

(Quadriceps femoris)

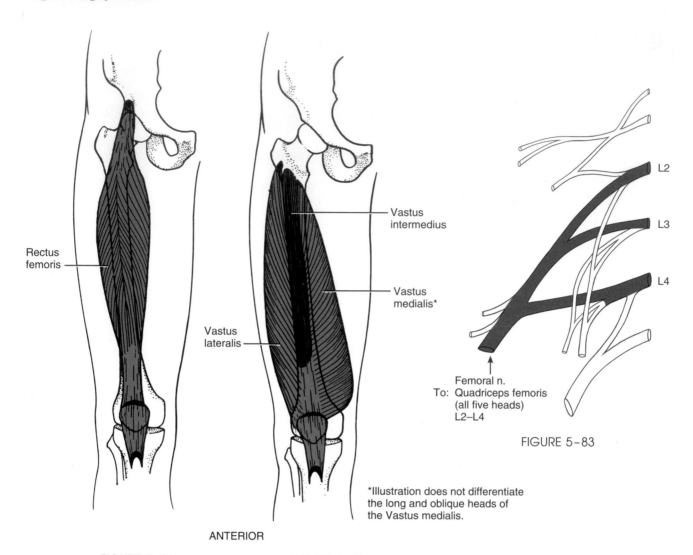

Rectus
femoris

Vastus
intermedius
Vastus
medialis*
Vastus
lateralis

ANTERIOR

FIGURE 5-81

FIGURE 5-82

*Illustration does not differentiate the long and oblique heads of the Vastus medialis.

L2
L3
L4
Femoral n.
To: Quadriceps femoris
(all five heads)
L2–L4

FIGURE 5-83

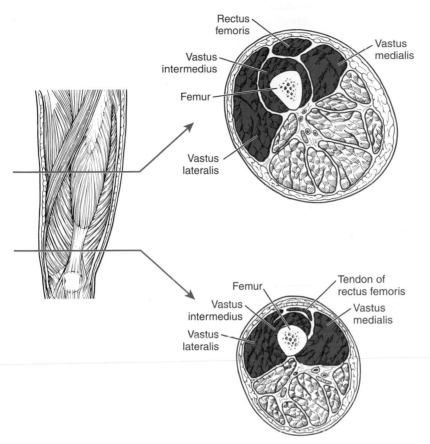

Rectus femoris

Vastus intermedius

Femur

Vastus lateralis

Vastus medialis

Femur

Vastus intermedius

Vastus lateralis

Tendon of rectus femoris

Vastus medialis

FIGURE 5–84

Range of Motion
135° to 0°
May extend 10° beyond 0° in those with hyperextension

Table 5-10 KNEE EXTENSION

I.D.	Muscle	Origin	Insertion
196	Rectus femoris	Ilium (anterior inferior iliac spine) Acetabulum (groove above) Capsule of hip joint Aponeurosis (anterior)	Aponeurosis (posterior) Patella (base via Quadriceps tendon) Tibial tuberosity via ligamentum patellae
198	Vastus intermedius	Femur (shaft, upper 2/3 lateral and anterior surfaces) Intermuscular septum (lateral)	Aponeurosis (anterior forming deep Quadriceps tendon) Patella (base, lateral aspect) Tibia (lateral condyle) Tibial tuberosity via ligamentum patellae

197	Vastus lateralis	Femur
		  Linea aspera (lateral lip)
		  Greater trochanter (inferior)
		  Intertrochanteric line (via aponeurosis)
		  Gluteal tuberosity (lateral lip)
		Lateral intermuscular septum
			Aponeurosis (deep surface, distal)
			Patella (base and lateral border via Quadriceps tendon)
			Lateral expansion to capsule of knee joint and iliotibial tract
			Tibial tuberosity via ligamentum patellae

199	Vastus medialis longus	Femur linea aspera, medial lip; intertrochanteric line Origin of Vastus medialis oblique Tendon of Adductor magnus Intermuscular septum (medial)	Aponeurosis (deep) Patella (medial border) Tibial tuberosity via ligamentum patellae
200	Vastus medialis oblique	Femur: linea aspera (distal); Supracondylar line Tendon of Adductor magnus Intermuscular septum	Aponeurosis to capsule of knee joint Patella (medial aspect) Quadriceps tendon (medial) Tibial tuberosity via ligamentum patellae
Other			
185	Tensor fasciae latae		

KNEE EXTENSION

(Quadriceps femoris)

The Quadriceps femoris muscles are tested together as a functional group. Any given head cannot be separated from any other by manual muscle testing. The Rectus femoris is isolated from the other Quadriceps during a hip flexion test.

Knowledge of the patient's hamstring range of motion is imperative before conducting tests for knee extension strength. Straight-leg raising (SLR) range dictates the optimal position for the knee extension test in the sitting position. In short sitting for Grades 5, 4, and 3, the less the range of SLR, the greater the backward trunk lean. Range of SLR also informs the examiner of the "available range" within the patient's comfort zone for side-lying tests.

Grade 5 (Normal), Grade 4 (Good), and Grade 3 (Fair)

Position of Patient: Short sitting. Place wedge or pad under the distal thigh to maintain the femur in the horizontal position. An experienced examiner may replace the padding under the thigh with his or her hand (Fig. 5–85). Hands rest on the table on either side of the body for stability, or may grasp the table edge. The patient should be allowed to lean backward to relieve hamstring muscle tension.

Do not allow the patient to hyperextend the knee because this may lock it into position.

Position of Therapist: Standing at side of limb to be tested. The hand giving resistance is contoured over the anterior surface of the distal leg just above the ankle. For Grades 5 and 4, resistance is applied in a downward direction (toward the floor) in the direction of knee flexion.

Test: Patient extends knee through available range of motion but not beyond 0°.

Instructions to Patient: "Straighten your knee. Hold it! Don't let me bend it."

Grading

Grade 5 (Normal): Holds end position against maximal resistance. Most physical therapists will not be able to break the Normal knee extensors.

Grade 4 (Good): Holds end position against strong to moderate resistance.

Grade 3 (Fair): Completes available range and holds the position without resistance (Fig. 5–86).

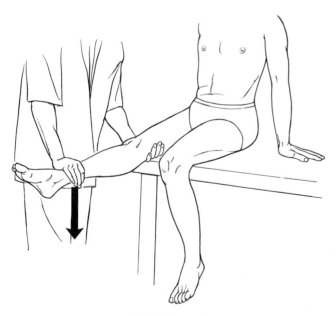

FIGURE 5–85

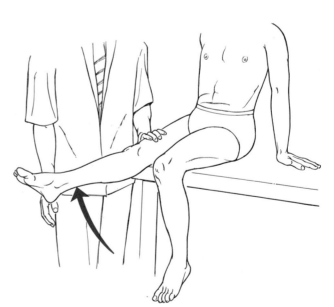

FIGURE 5–86

Grade 2 (Poor)

Position of Patient: Side-lying with test limb uppermost. Lowermost limb may be flexed for stability. Limb to be tested is held in about 90° of knee flexion. The hip should be in full extension.

Position of Therapist: Standing behind patient at knee level. One arm cradles the test limb around the thigh with the hand supporting the underside of the knee (Fig. 5–87). The other hand holds the leg just above the malleolus.

Test: Patient extends knee through the available range of motion. The therapist supporting the limb provides neither assistance nor resistance to the patient's voluntary movement. This is part of the art of muscle testing that must be acquired.

Be alert to activity by the internal rotators (see Substitution, below).

Instructions to Patient: "Straighten your knee."

Grading

Grade 2 (Poor): Completes available range of motion.

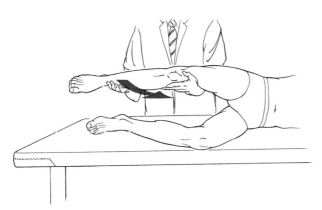

FIGURE 5–87

Grade 1 (Trace) and Grade 0 (Zero)

Position of Patient: Supine.

Position of Therapist: Standing next to limb to be tested at knee level. Hand used for palpation should be on the Quadriceps tendon just above the knee with the tendon "held" gently between the thumb and fingers. The examiner also may want to palpate the patellar tendon with two to four fingers just below the knee (Fig. 5–88).

Test: Patient attempts to extend knee.

As an alternate test, the therapist may place one hand under the slightly flexed knee; palpate either the Quadriceps or the patellar tendon while the patient tries to extend the knee.

Instructions to Patient: "Push the back of your knee down into the table" OR "Tighten your kneecap" (Quadriceps setting).

For Alternate Test: "Push the back of your knee down into my hand."

Grading

Grade 1 (Trace): Contractile activity can be palpated in muscle through the tendon. No joint movement occurs.

Grade 0 (Zero): No palpable contractile activity.

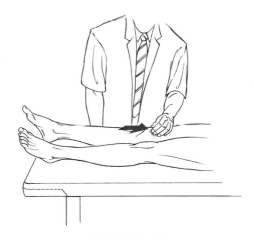

FIGURE 5–88

Substitution

When the patient is side-lying (as in the Grade 2 test), he or she may use the hip internal rotators to substitute for the Quadriceps, thereby allowing the knee to fall into extension.

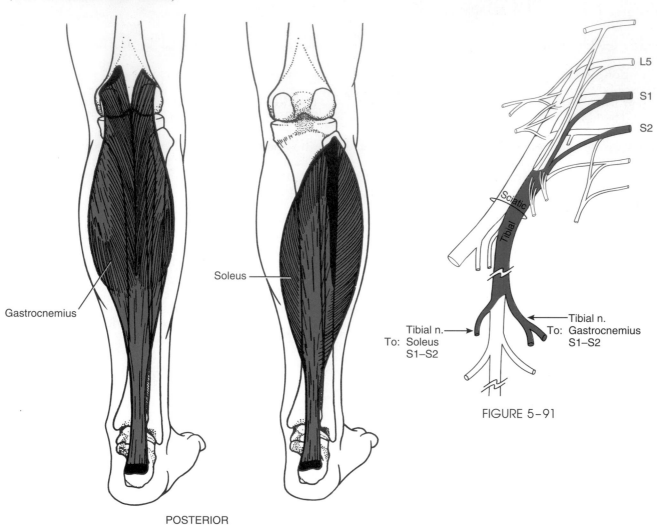

Gastrocnemius

Soleus

POSTERIOR

FIGURE 5-89

FIGURE 5-90

L5

S1

S2

Sciatic

Tibial

Tibial n.
To: Soleus
S1–S2

Tibial n.
To: Gastrocnemius
S1–S2

FIGURE 5-91

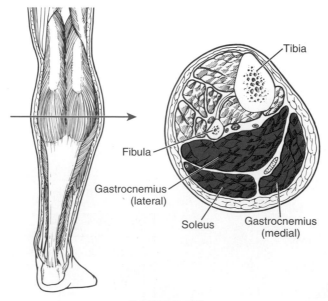

Tibia

Fibula

Gastrocnemius
(lateral)

Soleus

Gastrocnemius
(medial)

FIGURE 5-92

Range of Motion
0° to 45°

Table 5-11 PLANTAR FLEXION

I.D.	Muscle	Origin	Insertion
205	Gastrocnemius Medial head	Femur (medial condyle, popliteal surface) Capsule of knee joint	Anterior aponeurosis Tendo calcaneus (tendon of Achilles) formed when tendon of Gastrocnemius joins tendon of Soleus)
	Lateral head	Femur (lateral condyle, lateral surface, and supracondylar line) Capsule of knee joint Aponeurosis (posterior)	Calcaneus (posterior)
206	Soleus	Fibula (head, posterior aspect, and proximal 1/3 of shaft) Tibia (soleal line and middle 1/3 of medial shaft) Aponeurosis between tibia and fibula over popliteal vessels Aponeurosis (anterior)	Aponeurosis (posterior; tendinous raphe in midline of muscle) Tendo calcaneus when tendon of Soleus joins tendon of Gastrocnemius Calcaneus via Tendo calcaneus

Others

204	Tibialis posterior
207	Plantaris
208	Peroneus longus
209	Peroneus brevis
213	Flexor digitorum longus
222	Flexor hallucis longus

(Gastrocnemius and Soleus)

GASTROCNEMIUS AND SOLEUS TEST

Grade 5 (Normal), Grade 4 (Good), and Grade 3 (Fair)

Position of Patient: Patient stands on limb to be tested with knee extended. Patient is likely to need external support; no more than one or two fingers should be used on a table (or other surface) for balance assist only (Fig. 5–93).

Position of Therapist: Standing or sitting with a lateral view of test limb.

Test: Patient raises heel from floor consecutively through full range of plantar flexion.

Instructions to Patient: Therapist demonstrates correct heel rise to patient. "Stand on your right leg. Go up on your tiptoes. Now down. Repeat this 20 times." Repeat test for left limb.

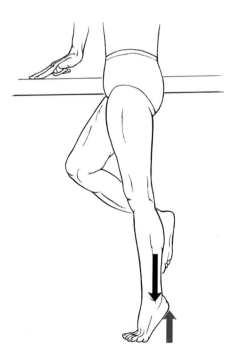

FIGURE 5–93

Grading

Grade 5 (Normal): Patient successfully completes a minimum of 20 heel rises through full range of motion without rest between rises and without fatigue.[2] (Twenty heel rises represent over 60 percent of maximum electromyographic activity of the plantar flexors.[2]) One study reported that a normal response required 25 complete heel rises.[3]

Grade 4 (Good): A Grade 4 is conferred when the patient completes any number of correct heel rises between 19 and 10 with no rest between repetitions and without fatigue. Grade 4 is conferred only if the patient uses correct form in all repetitions. Any failure to complete the full range in any given repetition automatically drops the grade to at least the next lower level.[2]

Grade 3 (Fair): Patient completes between nine and one heel rises correctly with no rest or fatigue.[2]

If the patient cannot complete at least one correct full-range heel rise in the standing position, the grade must be less than 3 (Fair). Regardless of any resistance in a nonstanding position for any reason, the patient must be given a grade of less than 3.[2]

Grade 2 (Poor)

STANDING TEST

Position of Patient: Standing on limb to be tested with knee extended, with a two-finger balance assist.

Position of Therapist: Standing or sitting with a clear lateral view of test limb.

Test: Patient attempts to raise heel from the floor through the full range of plantar flexion (Fig. 5–94).

Instructions to Patient: "Stand on your right leg. Try to go up on your tiptoes." Repeat test for left leg.

Grading

Grade 2+ (Poor+): The patient can just clear the heel from the floor and cannot get up on the toes for the end test position.

    Note: This is a rare exception for the use of a 2+ (Poor+) grade. There is no Grade 2 from the standing position.

PRONE TEST

Position of Patient: Prone with feet off end of table.

Position of Therapist: Standing at end of table in front of foot to be tested. One hand is contoured under and around the test leg just above the ankle (Fig. 5–95). Heel and palm of hand giving resistance are placed against the plantar surface at the level of the metatarsal heads.

Test: Patient plantar flexes ankle through the available range of motion. Manual resistance is down and forward toward dorsiflexion.

Grading

Grade 2+ (Poor+): Completes plantar flexion range and holds against maximal resistance.

Grade 2 (Poor): Patient completes plantar flexion range but tolerates no resistance.

Grade 2– (Poor–): Patient completes only a partial range of motion.

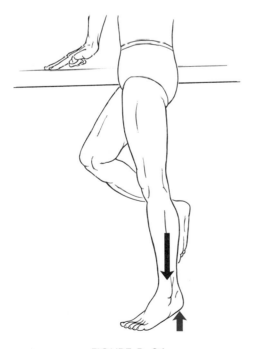

FIGURE 5–94

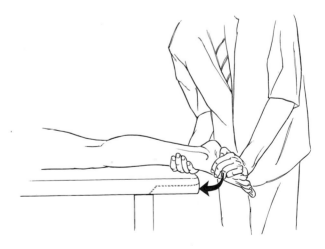

FIGURE 5–95

Grade 1 (Trace) and Grade 0 (Zero)

Position of Patient: Prone with feet off end of table.

Position of Therapist: Standing at end of table in front of foot to be tested. One hand palpates Gastrocnemius-Soleus activity by monitoring tension in the Achilles tendon just above the calcaneus (Fig. 5–96). The muscle bellies of the two muscles also may be palpated (not illustrated).

Test: Patient attempts to plantar flex the ankle.

Instructions to Patient: "Point your toes down, like a toe or ballet dancer."

Grading

Grade 1 (Trace): Tendon reflects some contractile activity in muscle, but no joint motion occurs. Contractile activity may be palpated in muscle bellies. The best location to palpate the Gastrocnemius is at midcalf with thumb and fingers on either side of the midline but above the Soleus. Palpation of the Soleus is best done on the posterolateral surface of the distal calf. In most people with calf strength of Grade 3 or better, the two muscles can be observed and differentiated during plantar flexion testing because their definition is clear.

Grade 0 (Zero): No palpable contraction.

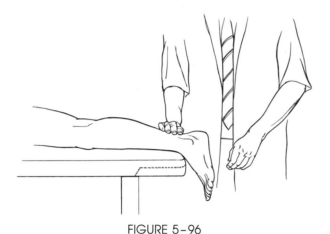

FIGURE 5–96

PLANTAR FLEXION, SOLEUS ONLY

All plantar flexor muscles are active in all positions of plantar flexion testing; therefore, no true isolation of the Soleus is possible. Testing during standing with the test leg flexed results in a 70 percent decrease in Gastrocnemius activity.[4] The test performed to "isolate" the Soleus should be interpreted with this caveat in mind. Thus, in the test to "isolate" the Soleus, the knee is placed in flexion to put slack on the Gastrocnemius, which crosses the knee joint.

Grade 5 (Normal), Grade 4 (Good), and Grade 3 (Fair)

Position of Patient: Standing on limb to be tested with knee slightly flexed (Fig. 5–97). Use one or two fingers for balance assist.

Position of Therapist: Standing or sitting with clear lateral view of test limb.

Test: Patient raises heel from floor through full range of plantar flexion, maintaining flexed position of knee (see Fig. 5–97). Twenty correct heel raises must be done consecutively without rest and without great fatigue.

Instructions to Patient: Therapist demonstrates test position and motion. "Stand on your right leg with your knee bent. Keep your knee bent and go up and down on your toes at least 20 times." Repeat test for left leg.

Grading

Grade 5 (Normal): Patient completes 20 consecutive heel rises to full range without rest or complaint of fatigue.[2]

Grade 4 (Good): Patient completes between 19 and 10 correct heel rises without rest.[2]

Grade 3 (Fair): Patient completes between nine and one correct heel rises with the knee flexed.

Note: If patient cannot complete all heel rises through a full range, the grade must be lower than 3. If the patient partially completes one heel rise, he or she may be given a grade of 2+. If the patient is unable to stand for the Grade 3 test for any reason, the grade awarded may not exceed a 2.

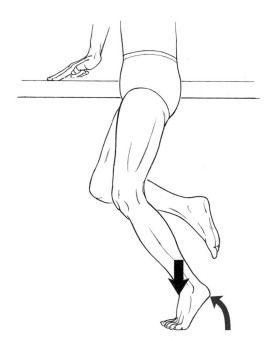

FIGURE 5–97

ANKLE PLANTAR FLEXION

(Gastrocnemius and Soleus)

Grade 2 (Poor), Grade 1 (Trace), and Grade 0 (Zero)

Position of Patient: Prone with knee flexed to 90°.

Position of Therapist: Standing next to patient. Resistance is given with the heel of the hand placed under plantar surface of forefoot in the direction of dorsiflexion.

Test: Patient attempts to plantar flex the ankle while the knee is maintained in flexion.

Instructions to Patient: "Point your toes toward the ceiling."

Grading

Grade 2+ (Poor+): Completes full plantar flexion range against maximal resistance.

Grade 2 (Poor): Completes full plantar flexion range with no resistance.

Grade 2− (Poor−): Completes only a partial range of motion with knee flexed.

Grades 1 and 0: Palpable contraction or Achilles tendon tightening is Grade 1. No contractile activity is Grade 0.

Substitutions

- By Flexor hallucis longus and Flexor digitorum longus: When substitution by the toe flexors occurs, their motions will be accompanied by plantar flexion of the forefoot and incomplete movement of the calcaneus (Fig. 5–98).

- By Peroneus longus and Peroneus brevis: These muscles substituting for the Gastrocnemius and Soleus will pull the foot into eversion.

- By Tibialis posterior: The foot will move into inversion during plantar flexion testing if the Tibialis posterior substitutes for the primary plantar flexors.

- By Tibialis posterior, Peroneus longus, and Peroneus brevis: Substitution by these three muscles will plantar flex the forefoot instead of the ankle.

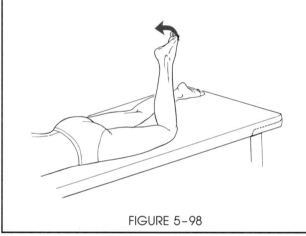

FIGURE 5–98

Helpful Hints

- If for any reason the patient cannot lie prone for Grades 2, 1, or 0, an alternative for the Grade 2, 1, or 0 test is to use the supine position for non–weight-bearing testing. The highest grade awarded in this case may not exceed a 2+.

- If the patient is unable to perform a standing plantar flexion test but has a stable forefoot, a different application of resistance may be used with the patient supine. The resistance is applied against the sole of the foot with the forearm while the heel is cupped with the hand of the same arm and the ankle is forced into dorsiflexion. The highest grade that may be awarded in this case is a 2+.

- During standing plantar flexion tests, the Tibialis posterior and the Peroneus longus and brevis muscles must be Grade 5 or 4 to stabilize the forefoot to attain and hold the tiptoe position.

- During standing heel rise testing, it is important to be sure that the patient maintains a fully erect posture. If the subject leans forward, such posture can bring the heel off the ground, creating a testing artifact.

CROSS SECTIONS OF THE LEG

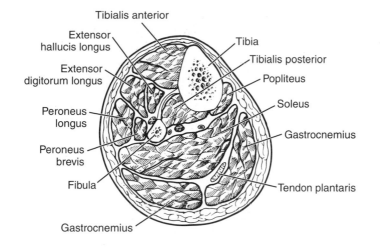

Tibialis anterior

Extensor hallucis longus

Extensor digitorum longus

Peroneus longus

Peroneus brevis

Fibula

Gastrocnemius

Tibia

Tibialis posterior

Popliteus

Soleus

Gastrocnemius

Tendon plantaris

MID LEG
AT UPPER PORTION OF
GASTROCNEMIUS AND
SOLEUS AT LARGEST
CIRCUMFERENCE OF CALF

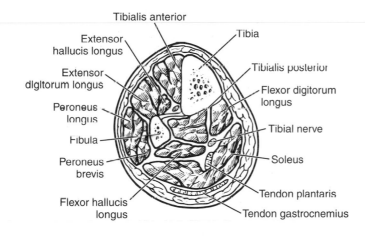

Tibialis anterior

Extensor hallucis longus

Extensor digitorum longus

Peroneus longus

Fibula

Peroneus brevis

Flexor hallucis longus

Tibia

Tibialis posterior

Flexor digitorum longus

Tibial nerve

Soleus

Tendon plantaris

Tendon gastrocnemius

LOWER LEG
NEAR END OF MUSCULAR
PORTIONS OF TRICEPS
SURAE. GASTROCNEMIUS
IS ALL TENDINOUS.

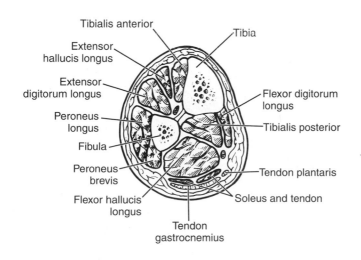

Tibialis anterior

Extensor hallucis longus

Extensor digitorum longus

Peroneus longus

Fibula

Peroneus brevis

Flexor hallucis longus

Tendon gastrocnemius

Tibia

Flexor digitorum longus

Tibialis posterior

Tendon plantaris

Soleus and tendon

HIGH ANKLE
LOWER LEG WHERE
GASTROCNEMIUS,
SOLEUS, AND PLANTARIS
ARE TENDINOUS

PLATE 7

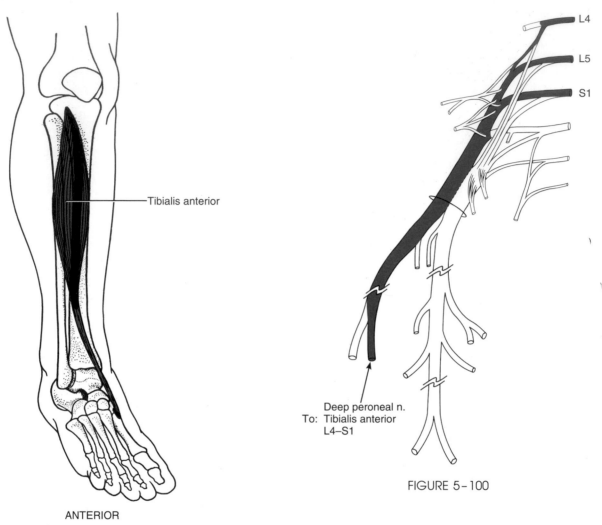

Tibialis anterior

ANTERIOR

FIGURE 5–99

L4

L5

S1

Deep peroneal n.
To: Tibialis anterior
L4–S1

FIGURE 5–100

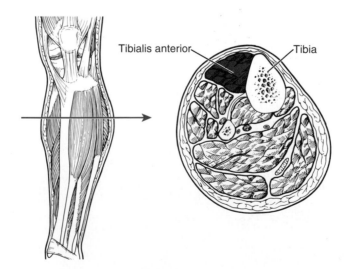

Tibialis anterior

Tibia

FIGURE 5–101

(Tibialis anterior)

Range of Motion
0° to 20°

Table 5-12 FOOT DORSIFLEXION AND INVERSION

I.D.	Muscle	Origin	Insertion
203	Tibialis anterior	Tibia (lateral condyle and proximal 2/3 of lateral shaft) Interosseous membrane Fascia cruris (deep) Intermuscular septum	1st (medial) cuneiform (on medial and plantar surfaces) 1st metatarsal (base)

Others

210	Peroneus tertius		
211	Extensor digitorum longus		
221	Extensor hallucis longus		

Grades 5 (Normal) to 0 (Zero)

Position of Patient: Short sitting. Alternatively, patient may be supine.

Position of Therapist: Sitting on stool in front of patient with patient's heel resting on thigh. One hand is contoured around the posterior leg just above the malleoli for Grades 5 and 4 (Fig. 5-102). The hand providing resistance for the same grades is cupped over the dorsomedial aspect of the foot (see Fig. 5-102).

Test: Patient dorsiflexes ankle and inverts foot, keeping toes relaxed.

Instructions to Patient: "Bring your foot up and in. Hold it! Don't let me push it down.

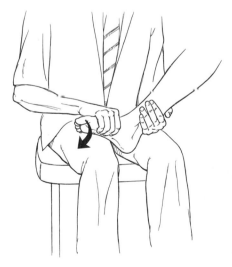

FIGURE 5-102

Grades 5 (Normal) to 0 (Zero) Continued

Grading

Grade 5 (Normal): Completes full range and holds against maximal resistance.

Grade 4 (Good): Completes available range against strong to moderate resistance.

Grade 3 (Fair): Completes available range of motion and holds end position without resistance (Fig. 5–103).

Grade 2 (Poor): Completes only a partial range of motion.

Grade 1 (Trace): Therapist will be able to detect some contractile activity in the muscle, or the tendon will "stand out." There is no joint movement.

Palpate the tendon of the Tibialis anterior on the anteromedial aspect of the ankle at about the level of the malleoli (Fig. 5–104, lower hand). Palpate the muscle for contractile activity over its belly just lateral to the "shin" (Fig. 5–104, upper hand)

Grade 0 (Zero): No palpable contraction.

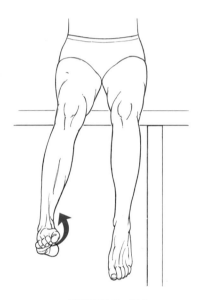

FIGURE 5–103

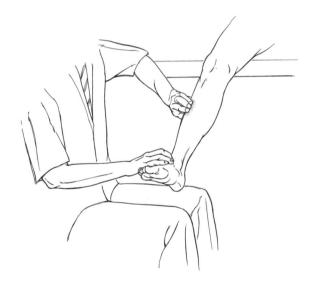

FIGURE 5–104

Substitution

Substitution by the Extensor digitorum longus and the Extensor hallucis longus muscles results also in toe extension. Instruct the patient, therefore, to keep the toes relaxed so that they are not part of the test movement.

Helpful Hints

- In the sitting and supine positions, make sure the knee is flexed to put the Gastrocnemius on slack. If the knee is extended and there is Gastrocnemius tightness, the patient will not be able to achieve full dorsiflexion range.

- If the supine position is used in lieu of the short-sitting position for the Grade 3 test, the therapist should add a degree of difficulty to the test to compensate for the lack of gravity. For example, give mild resistance in the supine position but award no more than a Grade 3.

- In the supine position, to earn a Grade 2 the patient must complete a full range of motion.

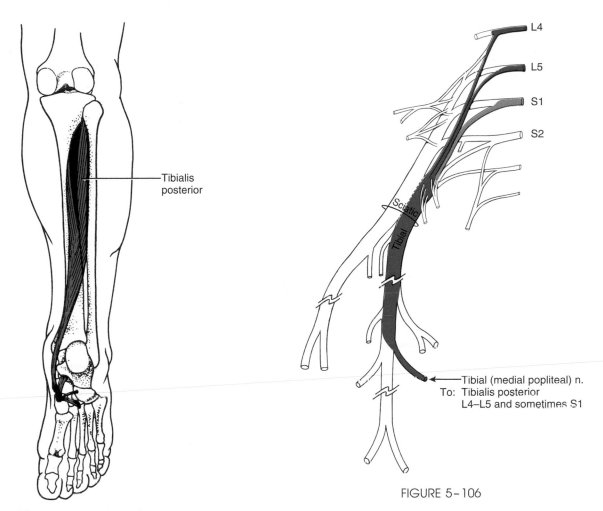

Tibialis posterior

POSTERIOR VIEW OF LEG
PLANTAR VIEW OF FOOT

FIGURE 5–105

L4

L5

S1

S2

Sciatic

Tibial

Tibial (medial popliteal) n.
To: Tibialis posterior
L4–L5 and sometimes S1

FIGURE 5–106

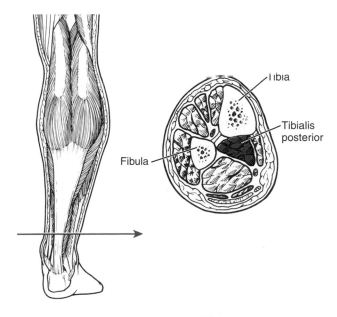

Tibia

Tibialis
posterior

Fibula

FIGURE 5–107

FOOT INVERSION
(Tibialis posterior)

Table 5-13 FOOT INVERSION

I.D.	Muscle	Origin	Insertion
204	Tibialis posterior	Tibia (proximal 2/3 of posterior lateral shaft below soleal line) Interosseous membrane (posterior) Fibula (shaft, proximal posterior medial 2/3) Deep transverse fascia Intermuscular septa	Navicular bone (tuberosity) Cuneiform bones Sustentaculum tali (distal) Metatarsals 2–4 (via tendinous band)

Others

203	Tibialis anterior		
213	Flexor digitorum longus		
222	Flexor hallucis longus		
206	Soleus		
221	Extensor hallucis longus		

Grades 5 (Normal) to 2 (Poor)

Position of Patient: Short sitting with ankle in slight plantar flexion.

Position of Therapist: Sitting on low stool in front of patient or on side of test limb. One hand is used to stabilize the ankle just above the malleoli (Fig. 5–108). Hand providing resistance is contoured over the dorsum and medial side of the foot at the level of the metatarsal heads. Resistance is directed toward eversion and slight dorsiflexion.

Test: Patient inverts foot through available range of motion.

Instructions to Patient: Therapist may need to demonstrate motion. "Turn your foot down and in. Hold it."

Grading

Grade 5 (Normal): The patient completes the full range and holds against maximal resistance.

Grade 4 (Good): The patient completes available range against strong to moderate resistance.

Grade 3 (Fair): The patient will be able to invert the foot through the full available range of motion (Fig. 5–109).

Grade 2 (Poor): The patient will be able to complete only a partial range of motion.

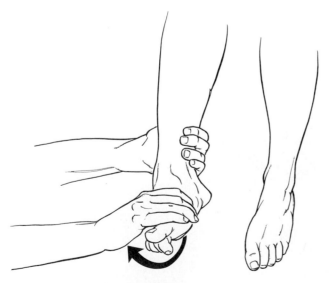

FIGURE 5-108

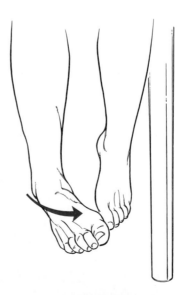

FIGURE 5-109

Grade 1 (Trace) and Grade 0 (Zero)

Position of Patient: Short-sitting or supine.

Position of Therapist: Sitting on low stool or standing in front of patient. Palpate tendon of the Tibialis posterior between the medial malleolus and the navicular bone (Fig. 5–110). Alternatively, palpate tendon above the malleolus.

Test: Patient attempts to invert foot.

Instructions to Patient: "Try to turn your foot down and in."

Grading

Grade 1 (Trace): The tendon will stand out if there is contractile activity in the muscle. If palpable activity occurs in the absence of movement, the grade is 1.

Grade 0 (Zero): No palpable contraction.

Substitution

Flexors of the toes should remain relaxed to prevent substitution by the Flexor digitorum longus and Flexor hallucis longus.

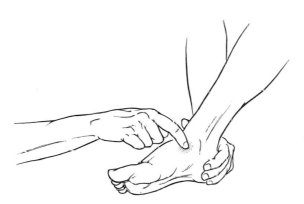

FIGURE 5–110

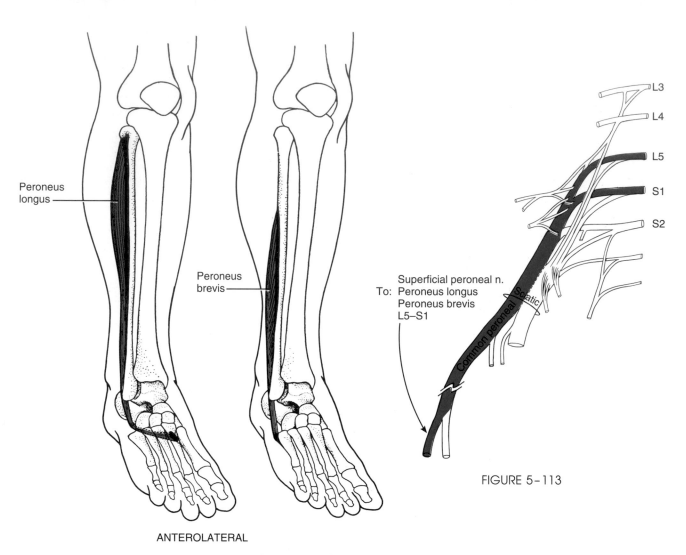

Peroneus
longus

Peroneus
brevis

ANTEROLATERAL

FIGURE 5–111

FIGURE 5–112

Superficial peroneal n.
To: Peroneus longus
Peroneus brevis
L5–S1

Common peroneal

Sciatic

L3
L4
L5
S1
S2

FIGURE 5–113

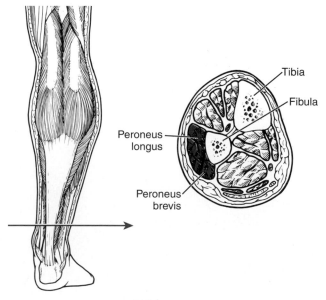

Tibia

Fibula

Peroneus
longus

Peroneus
brevis

FIGURE 5–114

(Peroneus longus and Peroneus brevis)

Range of Motion
0° to 25°

Table 5-14   FOOT EVERSION

I.D.	Muscle	Origin	Insertion
With Plantar Flexion			
208	Peroneus longus	Fibula (head and proximal 2/3 of shaft, lateral aspect) Tibia (lateral condyle) (occasionally) Fascia cruris Intermuscular septa	1st metatarsal (base and lateral aspect) Medial cuneiform (base and lateral aspect) Other metatarsals occasionally
209	Peroneus brevis	Fibula (distal and lateral 2/3 of shaft) Crural intermuscular septum	5th metatarsal (tuberosity at base, lateral aspect)
With Dorsiflexion			
211	Extensor digitorum longus		
210	Peroneus tertius		
Other			
205	Gastrocnemius		

Grade 5 (Normal) to Grade 2 (Poor)

Position of Patient: Short sitting with ankle in neutral position (midway between dorsiflexion and plantar flexion) (Fig. 5–115). Test also may be performed with patient supine.

Position of Therapist: Sitting on low stool in front of patient or standing at end of table if patient is supine.

One hand grips the ankle just above the malleoli for stabilization. Hand giving resistance is contoured around the dorsum and lateral border of the forefoot (Fig. 5–115). Resistance is directed toward inversion and slight dorsiflexion.

Test: Patient everts foot with depression of first metatarsal head and some plantar flexion.

Instructions to Patient: "Turn your foot down and out. Hold it! Don't let me move it in."

Grading

Grade 5 (Normal): Patient completes full range and holds end position against maximal resistance.

Grade 4 (Good): Patient completes available range of motion against strong to moderate resistance.

Grade 3 (Fair): Patient completes available range of eversion but tolerates no resistance (Fig. 5–116).

Grade 2 (Poor): The patient will be able to complete only a partial range of eversion motion.

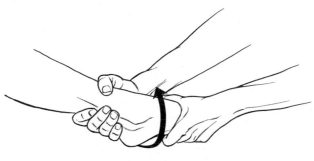

FIGURE 5–115

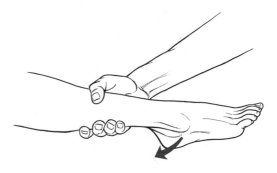

FIGURE 5–116

(Peroneus longus and Peroneus brevis)

Grade 1 (Trace) and Grade 0 (Zero)

Position of Patient: Short sitting or supine.

Position of Therapist: Sitting on low stool or standing at end of table. To palpate the Peroneus longus, place fingers on the lateral leg over the upper one-third just below the head of the fibula. The tendon of the muscle can be felt posterior to the lateral malleolus but behind the tendon of the Peroneus brevis.

To palpate the tendon of the Peroneus brevis, place index finger over the tendon as it comes forward from behind the lateral malleolus, proximal to the base of the 5th metatarsal (Fig. 5–117). The belly of the Peroneus brevis can be palpated on the lateral surface of the distal leg over the fibula.

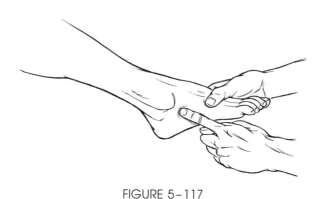

FIGURE 5–117

Grading

Grade 1 (Trace): Palpation will reveal contractile activity in either or both muscles, which may cause the tendon to stand out. No motion occurs.

Grade 0 (Zero): No palpable contractile activity.

Isolation of Peroneus Longus

Give resistance against the plantar surface of the head of the 1st metatarsal in a direction toward inversion and dorsiflexion.

Foot Eversion with Dorsiflexion

If the Peroneus tertius is present, it can be tested by asking the patient to evert and dorsiflex the foot. In this motion, however, the Extensor digitorum longus participates.

The tendon of the Peroneus tertius can be palpated on the lateral aspect of the dorsum of the foot, where it lies lateral to the tendon of the Extensor digitorum longus slip to the little toe.

Helpful Hints

- Foot eversion is accompanied by either dorsiflexion or plantar flexion. The toe extensors are the primary dorsiflexors accompanying eversion because the Peroneus tertius is an inconstant muscle.

- The primary motion of eversion with plantar flexion is accomplished by the Peroneus brevis because the Peroneus longus is primarily a depressor of the 1st metatarsal head rather than an evertor.

- The Peroneus brevis cannot be isolated if both peronei are innervated and active.

- If there is a difference in strength between the Peroneus longus and the Peroneus brevis, the stronger of the two can be ascertained by the relative amount of resistance taken in eversion versus the resistance taken at the 1st metatarsal head. If greater resistance is taken at the 1st metatarsal head, the Peroneus longus is the stronger muscle.

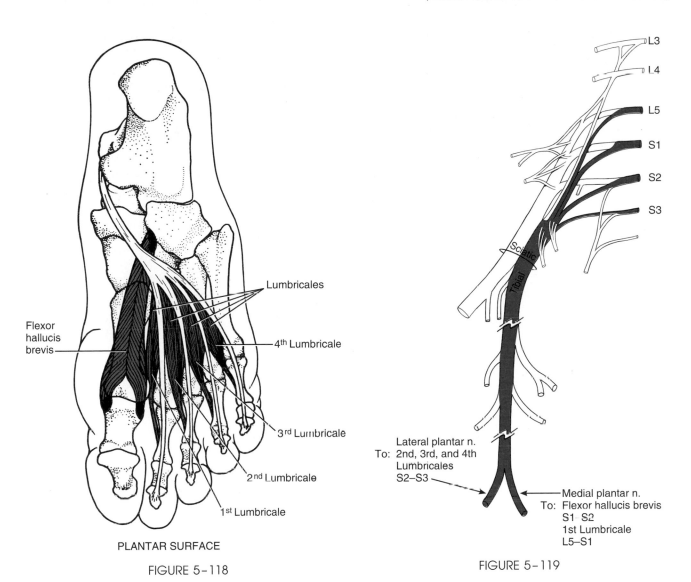

Lumbricales

4th Lumbricale

3rd Lumbricale

2nd Lumbricale

1st Lumbricale

Flexor
hallucis
brevis

PLANTAR SURFACE

FIGURE 5–118

L3
L4
L5
S1
S2
S3

Sciatic

Tibial

Lateral plantar n.
To: 2nd, 3rd, and 4th
Lumbricales
S2–S3

Medial plantar n.
To: Flexor hallucis brevis
S1 S2
1st Lumbricale
L5–S1

FIGURE 5–119

(Lumbricales and Flexor hallucis brevis)

Range of Motion	
Great toe, 0° to 45°	
Lateral four toes, 0° to 40°	

Table 5–15 FLEXION OF MP JOINTS OF TOES AND HALLUX

I.D.	Muscle	Origin	Insertion
Toes			
218	Lumbricales	Tendons of Flexor digitorum longus near angles of separation 1st Lumbricale (by a single head, tendon of Flexor digitorum longus bound for toe 2) 2nd–4th Lumbricales (arise by dual heads from adjacent sides of tendons of Flexor digitorum longus bound for toes 3–5)	All: Toes 2–5 (proximal phalanges and dorsal expansions of the tendons of Extensor digitorum longus)
Hallux			
223	Flexor hallucis brevis (rises by 2 heads)		
	Lateral head	Cuboid bone (plantar surface) Lateral cuneiform bone	Hallux (proximal phalanx on both sides of base) Blends with Adductor hallucis
	Medial head	Medial intermuscular septum Tibialis posterior (tendon)	Hallux (proximal phalanx on both sides of base) Blends with Abductor hallucis
Others			
219, 220	Interossei, dorsal and plantar		
216	Flexor digiti minimi brevis		
213	Flexor digitorum longus		
214	Flexor digitorum brevis		
222	Flexor hallucis longus		
224	Abductor hallucis		
225	Adductor hallucis		

HALLUX MP FLEXION *(Flexor hallucis brevis)*

Grades 5 (Normal) to 0 (Zero)

Position of Patient: Short sitting (alternate position: supine) with legs hanging over edge of table. Ankle is in neutral position (midway between dorsiflexion and plantar flexion).

Position of Therapist: Sitting on low stool in front of patient. Alternate position: standing at side of table near patient's foot.

Test foot rests on examiner's lap. One hand is contoured over the dorsum of the foot just below the ankle for stabilization (Fig. 5–120). The index finger of the other hand is placed beneath the proximal phalanx of the great toe. Alternatively, the tip of the finger (with very short fingernails) is placed up under the proximal phalanx.

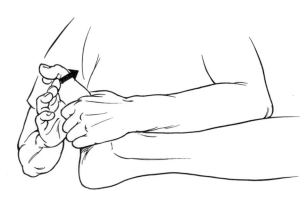

FIGURE 5–120

Grades 5 (Normal) to 0 (Zero) Continued

Test: Patient flexes great toe.

Instructions to Patient: "Bend your big toe over my finger. Hold it. Don't let me straighten it."

Grading

Grade 5 (Normal): Patient completes available range and tolerates strong resistance.

Grade 4 (Good): Patient completes available range and tolerates moderate to mild resistance.

Grade 3 (Fair): Patient completes available range of metatarsophalangeal (MP) flexion of the great toe but is unable to hold against any resistance.

Grade 2 (Poor): Patient completes only partial range of motion.

Grade 1 (Trace): Therapist may note contractile activity but no toe motion.

Grade 0 (Zero): No contractile activity.

Helpful Hints

- The muscle and tendon of the Flexor hallucis brevis cannot be palpated.

- When the Flexor hallucis longus is not functional, the Flexor hallucis brevis will flex the MP joint but with no flexion of the interphalangeal (IP) joint. In the opposite condition, when the Flexor hallucis brevis is not functional, the IP joint flexes and the MP joint may hyperextend. (When this condition is chronic, the posture is called hammer toe.)

TOE MP FLEXION

(Lumbricales)

Grades 5 (Normal) to 0 (Zero)

Position of Patient: Short sitting with foot on examiner's lap. Alternate position: supine. Ankle is in neutral (midway between dorsiflexion and plantar flexion).

Position of Therapist: Sitting on low stool in front of patient. Alternate position: standing next to table beside test foot.

One hand grasps the dorsum of the foot just below the ankle to provide stabilization (as in test for flexion of the hallux) (Fig. 5–121). The index finger of the other hand is placed under the MP joints of the four lateral toes to provide resistance to flexion.

Test: Patient flexes lateral four toes at the MP joints, keeping the IP joints neutral.

Instructions to Patient: "Bend your toes over my finger."

Grading

Grading is the same as that used for the great toe.

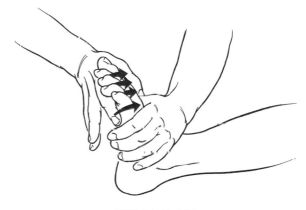

FIGURE 5–121

Helpful Hints

- In actual practice, the great toe and the lateral toes are rarely tested independently. Many patients cannot separate hallux motion from motion of the lateral toes, nor can they separate MP and IP motions.

- The examiner could test each toe separately because the Lumbricales are notoriously uneven in strength. This may not, however, be practicable.

HALLUX AND TOE DIP AND PIP FLEXION

(Flexor digitorum longus, Flexor digitorum brevis, Flexor hallucis longus)

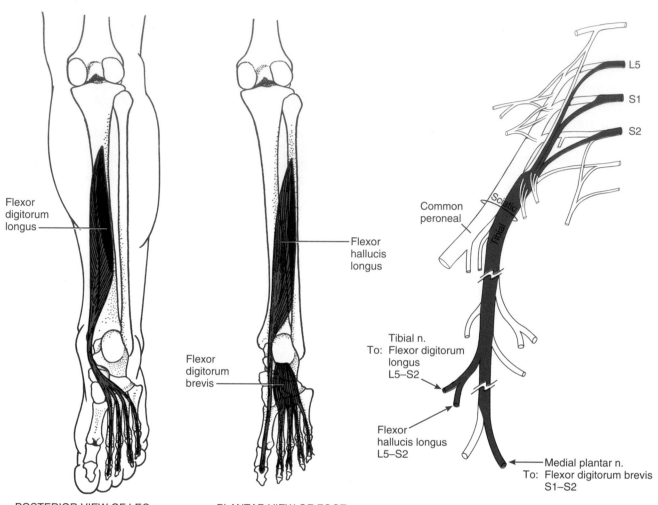

Flexor digitorum longus

POSTERIOR VIEW OF LEG

FIGURE 5-122

Flexor hallucis longus

Flexor digitorum brevis

PLANTAR VIEW OF FOOT

FIGURE 5-123

L5

S1

S2

Common peroneal

Sciatic

Tibial

Tibial n.
To: Flexor digitorum longus
L5–S2

Flexor hallucis longus
L5–S2

Medial plantar n.
To: Flexor digitorum brevis
S1–S2

FIGURE 5-124

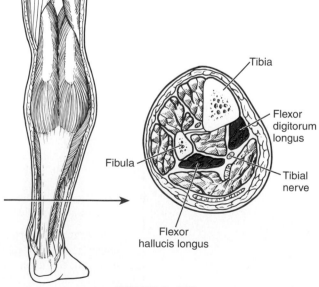

Tibia

Flexor digitorum longus

Fibula

Tibial nerve

Flexor hallucis longus

FIGURE 5-125

(Flexor digitorum longus, Flexor digitorum brevis, Flexor hallucis longus)

Range of Motion
PIP flexion, four lateral toes: 0° to 35°
DIP flexion, four lateral toes: 0° to 60°
IP flexion of hallux: 0° to 90°

Table 5-16 FLEXION OF IP JOINTS OF HALLUX AND TOES

I.D.	Muscle	Origin	Insertion
DIP, Toes			
213	Flexor digitorum longus	Tibia (shaft, posterior aspect of middle 2/3) Fascia over Tibialis posterior	Toes 2–5 (distal phalanges, plantar surfaces and base)
PIP, Toes			
214	Flexor digitorum brevis	Calcaneus (tuberosity, medial process) Plantar aponeurosis Intermuscular septum	Toes 2–5 (by four tendons to middle phalanges, both sides)
IP, Hallux			
222	Flexor hallucis longus	Fibula (shaft, 2/3 of posterior aspect) Interosseous membrane Intermuscular septum (posterior crural) Fascia over Tibialis posterior	Slip of tendon to Flexor digitorum longus Hallux (distal phalanx, base, plantar aspect)
Others			
DIP, Toes			
217	Quadratus plantae		
PIP, Toes			
213	Flexor digitorum longus		

(Flexor digitorum longus, Flexor digitorum brevis, Flexor hallucis longus)

Grades 5 (Normal) to 0 (Zero)

Position of Patient: Short sitting with foot on examiner's lap, or supine.

Position of Therapist: Sitting on short stool in front of patient or standing at side of table near patient's foot.

One hand grasps the anterior foot with the fingers placed across the dorsum of the foot and the thumb under the proximal phalanges (PIP) or distal phalanges (DIP) or under the IP of the hallux for stabilization (Figs. 5–126, 5–127, and 5–128).

The other hand applies resistance using the examiner's four fingers or thumb under the middle pha-

langes (for the IP test) (Fig. 5–126); under the distal phalanges for the DIP test (Fig. 5–127); and with the index finger under the distal phalanx of the hallux (Fig. 5–128).

Test: Patient flexes the toes or hallux.

Instructions to Patient: "Curl your toes; hold it. Curl your big toe and hold it."

Grading

Grades 5 (Normal) and 4 (Good): Patient completes range of motion of toes and then hallux; resistance in both tests may be minimal.

Grades 3 (Fair) and 2 (Poor): Patient completes range of motion with no resistance (Grade 3) or completes only a partial range (Grade 2).

Grades 1 (Trace) and 0 (Zero): Minimal to no palpable contractile activity occurs. Tendon of the Flexor hallucis longus may be palpated on the plantar surface of the proximal phalanx of the great toe.

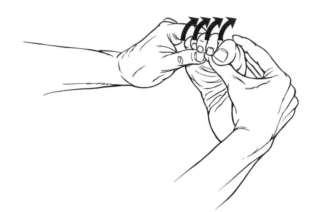

FIGURE 5–126

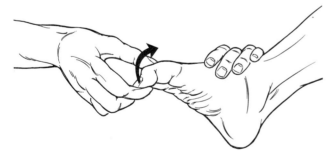

FIGURE 5–127

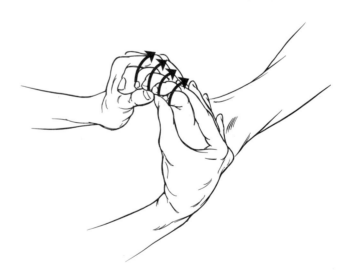

FIGURE 5–128

Helpful Hints

- As with all toe motions, the patient may not be able to move one toe separately from another or separate MP from IP activity among individual toes.

- Some persons can separate hallux activity from toe motions, but fewer can separate MP from IP hallux activity.

- Many people can "pinch" with their great toe (Adductor hallucis), but this is not a common clinical test.

- The Abductor hallucis is not commonly tested because it is only rarely isolated. Its activity can be observed by resisting adduction of the forefoot, which will bring the great toe into abduction, but the lateral toes commonly extend at the same time.

(Extensor digitorum longus and brevis, Extensor hallucis longus)

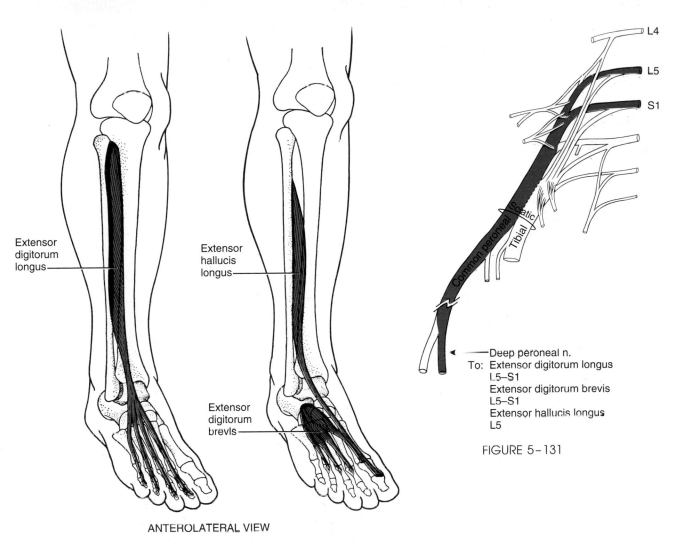

Extensor digitorum longus

Extensor hallucis longus

Extensor digitorum brevis

ANTEROLATERAL VIEW

FIGURE 5-129

FIGURE 5-130

Deep peroneal n.
To: Extensor digitorum longus
L5–S1
Extensor digitorum brevis
L5–S1
Extensor hallucis longus
L5

FIGURE 5-131

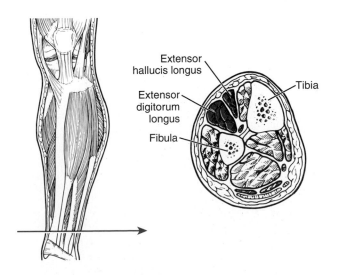

Extensor hallucis longus

Extensor digitorum longus

Fibula

Tibia

FIGURE 5-132

Chapter 5 / Testing the Muscles of the Lower Extremity **249**

(Extensor digitorum longus and brevis, Extensor hallucis longus)

Range of Motion °
Hallux: 0° to 75°–80°
Digits 2–5: 0° to 40°

Table 5-17 EXTENSION OF MP JOINTS OF TOES AND IP JOINT OF HALLUX

I.D.	Muscle	Origin	Insertion
211	Extensor digitorum longus	Tibia (lateral condyle) Fibula (shaft, proximal 3/4 of medial surface) Fascia cruris (deep) Interosseous membrane (anterior) Intermuscular septum	Toes 2–5 (to each middle and each distal phalanx, dorsal surface)
212	Extensor digitorum brevis	Calcaneus (anterior superolateral surface) Lateral talocalcaneal ligament Extensor retinaculum (inferior)	Ends in four tendons: Hallux (proximal phalanx, dorsal surface) (may be named *Extensor hallucis brevis*)) Toes 2–4: join tendons of Extensor digitorum longus (lateral sides)
221	Extensor hallucis longus	Fibula (shaft, middle 1/2 of medial aspect) Interosseous membrane	Hallux (distal phalanx, dorsal aspect of base) Expansion to proximal phalanx

Grades 5 (Normal) to 0 (Zero)

Position of Patient: Short sitting with foot on examiner's lap. Alternate position: supine. Ankle in neutral (midway between plantar flexion and dorsiflexion).

Position of Therapist: Sitting on low stool in front of patient, or standing beside table near the patient's foot.

Lateral Toes: One hand stabilizes the metatarsals with the fingers on the plantar surface and the thumb on the dorsum of the foot (Fig. 5–133). The other hand is used to give resistance with the thumb placed over the dorsal surface of the proximal phalanges of the toes.

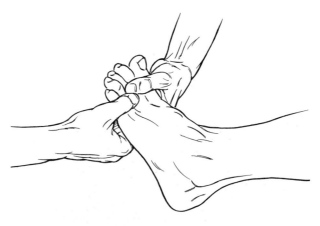

FIGURE 5–133

Grades 5 (Normal) to 0 (Zero) Continued

Hallux: Stabilize the metatarsal area by contouring the hand around the plantar surface of the foot with the thumb curving around to the base of the hallux (Fig. 5–134). The other hand stabilizes the foot at the heel. For resistance, place thumb over the MP joint (Fig. 5–134) or over the IP joint (Fig. 5–135).

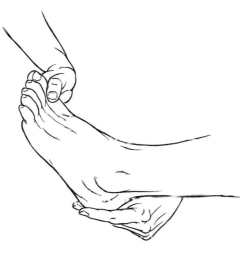

FIGURE 5–134

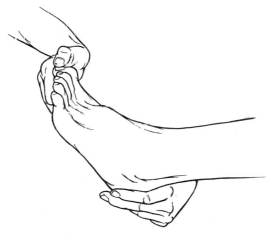

FIGURE 5–135

Test: Patient extends lateral four toes or extends hallux.

Instructions to Patient: "Straighten your big toe. Hold it." "Straighten your toes and hold it."

Grading

Grades 5 (Normal) and 4 (Good): Patient can extend the toes fully against variable resistance (which may be small).

Grades 3 (Fair) and 2 (Poor): Patient can complete range of motion with no resistance (Grade 3) or can complete a partial range of motion (Grade 2).

Grades 1 (Trace) and 0 (Zero): Tendons of the Extensor digitorum longus can be palpated or observed over dorsum of metatarsals. Tendon of the Extensor digitorum brevis often can be palpated on the lateral side of the dorsum of the foot just in front of the malleolus.

Palpable contractile activity is a Grade 1; no contractile activity is a Grade 0.

Helpful Hints

- Many (if not most) patients cannot separate great toe extension from extension of the four lateral toes. Nor can most separate MP from IP activity.

- The test is used not so much to ascertain strength as to determine whether the toe muscles are active.

References

Cited References

1. Perry J, Weiss W, Gronley J. The Supine Hip Extension Test. Manuscript in preparation, January, 2001.
2. Mulroy S. Functions of the triceps surae during strength testing and gait. PhD Dissertation, Department of Biokinesiology and Physical Therapy, University of Southern California, Los Angeles, 1994.
3. Lunsford BR, Perry J. The standing heel-rise test for ankle plantar flexion: Criterion for normal. Phys Ther 75:694–698, 1995.
4. Perry J, Easterday CS, Antonelli DJ. Surface versus intramuscular electrodes for electromyography for superficial and deep muscles. Phys Ther 61:6–15, 1981.

Other Readings

Cummins EJ, Anson BJ, Carr BW, Wright RR. Structure of the calcaneal tendon (of Achilles) in relation to orthopedic surgery (with additional observations on the Plantaris muscle). Surg Gynecol Obstet 3:107–116, 1046.

DeSousa OM, Vitti M. Estudio electromigrafico de los musculos adductores largo y mayor. Arch Mex Anat 7:52–53, 1966.

Johnson CE, Basmajian JV, Dasher W. Electromyography of Sartorius muscle. Anat Rec 173:127–130, 1972.

Jonsson B, Olofsson BM, Steffner LCH. Function of the teres major, latissimus dorsi, and pectoralis major muscles. Acta Neerl Scand 9:275, 1972.

Jonsson B, Steen B. Function of the hip and thigh muscles in Romberg's test and "standing at ease." Acta Morphol Neerl Scand 5:267–276, 1962.

Joseph J, Williams PL. Electromyography of certain hip muscles. J Anat 91:286–294, 1957.

Kaplan EB. The iliotibial tract. Clinical and morphological significance. J Bone Joint Surg 40[A]:817–831, 1958.

Keagy RD, Brumlik J, Bergen JL. Direct electromyography of the Psoas major muscle in man. J Bone Joint Surg 48[A]:1377–1382, 1966.

Markee JE, Logue JT Jr, Williams M, et al. Two joint muscles of the thigh. J Bone Joint Surg 37A:125–142. 1955.

Pare EB, Stern JT, Schwartz JM. Functional differentiation within the Tensor fasciae latae. J Bone Joint Surg 63[A]:1457–1471, 1981.

Perry J. Gait Analysis: Normal and Pathological Function. Thorofare, NJ, Slack, Inc., 1992.

Sneath RS. The insertion of the Biceps femoris. J Anat 89:550–553, 1955.

CHAPTER 6

Testing of Infants, Toddlers, and Preschool Children

Jack E. Turman, Jr., P.T., Ph.D., and
Teresa Van Vranken, D.P.T.

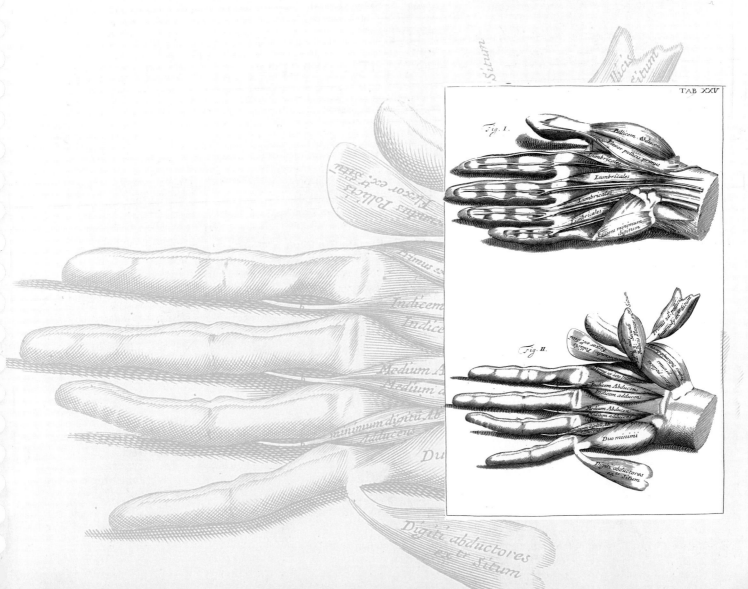

Manual muscle testing of infants and children traditionally has posed problems to pediatric practitioners because of validity issues. These problems stem from the child's inability to understand the evaluator's instructions as well as potential confounding of the results via evaluator handling. Trends in early intervention and pediatric rehabilitation focus on evaluating and treating infants and children in their natural environments (e.g., home, classroom, playground, preschool).[1,2] This focus encourages therapists to rely on their observation skills and their ability to engage infants and children in age-appropriate behaviors, thereby refraining from excessive handling of the infant or toddler in the evaluation process.[3] It requires that therapists possess a mature understanding of developmental milestones, as these milestones provide a framework for understanding the behaviors of infants and children. This chapter was designed to provide clinicians with a means to analyze muscle function associated with the classic gross and fine motor developmental milestones observed during infancy and early childhood. In using this approach, physical therapists will be able to provide other members of pediatric care teams with functionally relevant data. These data will form the basis for establishing developmental treatment goals and outcomes desired by clinicians and educators alike.

This chapter is designed to be compatible with developmental assessments commonly used in a wide range of pediatric clinics (Alberta Infant Motor Scale[3]; Revised Gessell and Amatruda Developmental Neurological Examination[4]; Bayley Scales of Infant Development II[5]; Peabody Developmental Motor Scales[6]). Chapter contents will assist physical therapists who work with children to analyze their clients' muscle function in the context of those clients' developmental assessment. It provides clinicians with a checklist of the major muscle groups associated with each particular posture or movement. These movements are complex, and the analysis of muscle function associated with each posture or movement is not exhaustive. By using the information provided, however, clinicians will be able to detect when aberrant muscle function is a contributory factor to the infant or child's atypical posture or movement, and may be altering an appropriate developmental progression.

Each posture or movement analyzed in the chapter is observed commonly in the pediatric population. The age range presented for each posture and movement is based on chronological age (age since the individual's birth date). Therapists are reminded to calculate a corrected age when evaluating an infant or toddler born prematurely. Infants born prior to 37 weeks' gestation are considered premature.[7] A corrected age is calculated by subtracting the number of weeks of gestation from 40 and then subtracting this number from the chronological age. We recommend calculating a corrected age until the chronological age of 24 months. The age range presented with each posture or movement in the infant section was adapted from Piper and Darrah.[4] With each movement, a normal muscle activity pattern is listed. An analysis of functional activities associated with each movement is provided to relate both evaluation and interventions to functional outcomes. Also provided is a brief discourse on the spectrum of muscle activity associated with each posture and movement to address the transitional processes that infants and children may use in progressing to the next milestone. These last two sections were included to help in establishing goals and treatment planning.

We recognize that the approach taken in this chapter is not the traditional one used in evaluating strength in children. Therefore, we have provided three case studies as examples using the information presented in this chapter. These cases exemplify a physical therapy evaluation occurring in a natural setting for each child. In each case a grading scale has been used to measure the child's functional performance on particular milestones. The grading system is used to illustrate that while aberrant muscle function may be present, functional participation in the child's natural environment is possible. It also must be noted that while a child may be able to perform all developmental milestones up to his or her highest ability level, it is not necessary to facilitate or observe each milestone. Many muscle synergies are demonstrated at several levels of performance. The child or the child-parent dyad must determine the direction of the assessment with appropriate suggestions and minimal manual facilitation by the therapist to determine the child's highest performance level. During assessment of the child, the therapist should note the movements being observed and document the presence or absence of individual muscle activity. We do not suggest providing resistance until later in childhood, when traditional manual muscle testing can be employed. After observing the child in a number of developmentally appropriate movements, the therapist will analyze the results of muscle activity and determine a pattern of muscle strengths and weaknesses that can be used to develop specific interventions.

This chapter is designed to produce material that is useful to experienced and novice pediatric physical therapists, and to students interested in working with infants and children. We hope it helps physical therapists become more proficient in analyzing muscle activity patterns of infants and children, and that by using this type of muscle assessment, make valuable contributions to pediatric teams caring for children with disabilities.

Note to Reader: Throughout this chapter, the term "movement" is used to refer generally to both *posture* and *movement*, unless one term or the other is specifically indicated. Likewise, unless a specific age group is indicated, the word "child" is used to refer to infants, toddlers, and children alike.

The necessity to write reports in a client's chart and to compare results over different periods of time has led to a grading scale described below.

Description	Grade[1-7]
Functional (F)	Normal for age or only slight impairment or delay
Weak functional (WF)	Moderate impairment or delay that affects activity pattern, base of support, or control against gravity, or decreases functional exploration
Nonfunctional (NF)	Severe impairment or delay; activity pattern has only elements of correct muscular activity
No function (0)	Cannot do activity

POSITION: *PRONE*

Activity: *"Swimming"* (19–32 weeks)

Base of Support

Weight bearing on abdomen.

Muscle Activity Pattern

> Concentric contraction of head and neck extensors
> Concentric contraction of rhomboids
> Concentric contraction of back extensors
> Concentric contraction of gluteals
> Concentric contraction of hamstrings

Functional Activity

Elevation of visual perspective. Preparation for higher levels of antigravity mobility.

Spectrum of Muscle Function

In this position the child is using all extensor musculature against gravity. The head and upper chest are elevated; scapulae are retracted (Fig. 6–1). Elevating the lower extremities may activate the gluteal muscles. The child may rock back and forth, but there is no forward motion.

Activity: *Rolling Prone to Supine with Rotation* (28–36 weeks)

Base of Support

Weight bearing on one side of body (Fig. 6–2).

Muscle Activity Pattern

> Active rotation against gravity of head, shoulder, or pelvis
> Concentric contraction of neck rotators
> Concentric contraction of ipsilateral rhomboids (those participating in initiating the rolling activity)
> Concentric contraction of ipsilateral obliques (those participating in initiating the rolling activity)
> Concentric contraction of hip flexors and abductors (those participating in initiating the rolling activity)

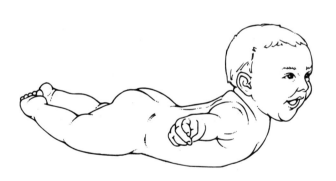

FIGURE 6–1

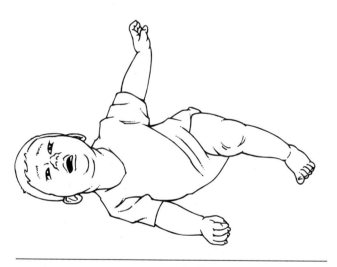

FIGURE 6–2

In Figure 6–2 the child is rolling to the left; therefore a concentric contraction of the left rhomboids, obliques, hip flexors, and abductors would be observed.

Functional Activity

Transitional skill with selective muscle control against gravity. Environmental exploration involving change in perspective. Coupled with supine to prone, this transitional skill provides for infant mobility.

Spectrum of Muscle Activity

The child's head, shoulder, or pelvis may initiate movement. One observes a dissociation of the head, trunk, and pelvis. Generally, the hip is flexed prior to abduction.

Activity: *Reciprocal Crawling* (30–37 weeks)

Base of Support

Elbow, forearm, and opposite leg. Fingers extended, palms on the ground. Abdomen resting on the ground (Fig. 6–3).

Muscle Activity Pattern

Shoulder flexion and internal rotation moving into extension
Hip flexion and external rotation
Knee flexion moving into extension and adduction
Trunk rotation away from lead arm

Functional Activity

Initial form of quadruped mobility. Increased efficient access to the environment. The movement is generally object- or activity-directed.

Spectrum of Muscle Activity

Head and neck extension maintained efficiently against gravity. Movement is seen in all four limbs in opposite, alternating fashion. Weight shifting to the weight-bearing arm allows reach of the opposite arm for objects.

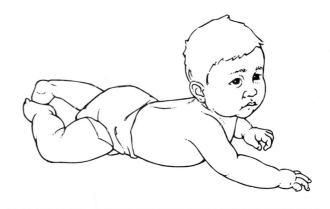

FIGURE 6–3

Activity: *Modified Four-Point Kneeling* (34–46 weeks)

Base of Support

Weight bearing on hands, one foot, and opposite knee (Fig. 6–4). Base of support is widened from quadruped.

Muscle Activity Pattern

Head neutral or concentric contraction of neck extensors for increased upward gaze

Shoulders flexed, scapulae protracted

Arms extended, palms on floor

Hip flexed at or past 90° with concordant knee flexion

Opposite hip flexed at or past 90° with external rotation, 90° or less of knee flexion, foot on the floor. Foot may be slightly plantar-flexed for greater stability

Functional Activity

Modified quadruped position affords the child increased opportunities for exploration via a widened base of support to obtain or manipulate objects. Figure 6–4 demonstrates three-point kneeling in which the child has weight-shifted laterally and posteriorly to obtain a toy. This is an example of increased ability to manage the center of gravity, against the force of gravity, over the base of support while in an elevated position.

Spectrum of Muscle Activity

With the placement of one foot on the floor, the pelvis is rotated toward the opposite side for greater stability, thus allowing the child to visualize or obtain an object.

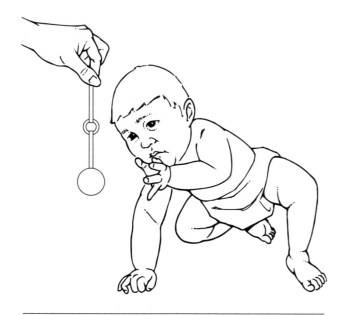

FIGURE 6–4

Activity: *Reciprocal Creeping* (34–44 weeks)

Base of Support

Alternating weight bearing of opposite hand and knee. Abdomen is raised from the surface.

Muscle Activity Pattern

Concentric contraction of neck extensors
Isometric shoulder protraction during weight-bearing phases
Alternating concentric contractions of shoulder flexors and extensors
Alternating isometric and concentric contractions of triceps
Hips and knees alternating between concentric flexion and extension
Feet plantar-flexed

Functional Activity

Increased mobility in the quadruped position. Affords the child the ability to obtain an object with increased speed and efficiency versus crawling.

Spectrum of Muscle Activity

Mature representation of creeping is presented with a neutral spine and limb placement directly underneath the respective girdles, narrowing the base of support. Child's management of body mass against gravity is much improved. Immature presentation shows increased lumbar lordosis and abduction of the limbs, lowering the center of gravity and widening the base of support (Fig. 6–5).

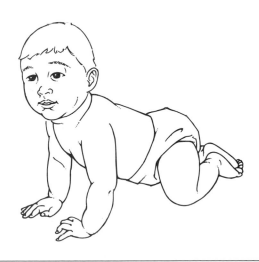

FIGURE 6–5

POSITION: *SUPINE*

Activity: *Hands to Feet* (18–24 weeks)

Base of Support

Weight bearing on the back and posterior aspect of the head.

Muscle Activity Pattern

Concentric contraction of shoulder flexors
Isometric contraction of pectorals
Concentric contraction of abdominals
Concentric contraction of hip flexors

Functional Activity

Regard and exploration of body parts via hands and eyes.

Spectrum of Muscle Activity

Initially, child may only approximate feet and hands. With increased strength the child may bring the feet to the mouth with either muscular contraction of the hip flexors against gravity or use of hands (Fig. 6–6). The pelvis may tilt posterior, indicating increased abdominal strength. The head also may be raised toward the feet.

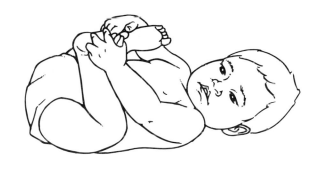

FIGURE 6–6

Activity: *Rolling Supine to Prone with Rotation* (25–36 weeks)

Base of Support

Weight bearing on one side of body (Fig. 6–7A and B).

Muscle Activity Pattern

Concentric contraction of neck flexors
Concentric contraction of neck rotators toward the roll
Concentric contraction of pectorals as non–weight-bearing arm is horizontally adducted
Concentric contraction of obliques
Pelvic rotation
Concentric contraction of non–weight-bearing hip flexors
Concentric contraction of non–weight-bearing adductors

Functional Activity

Transitional skill for change in perspective, object regard, or acquisition.

Spectrum of Muscle Activity

Selective muscle control as seen with dissociation of the trunk and hips. The child may lead with head, arm, and shoulder, or leg and pelvis (Fig. 6–7B).

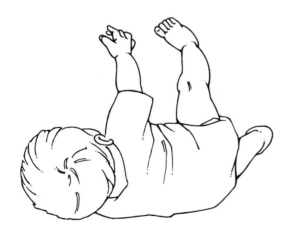

FIGURE 6–7A

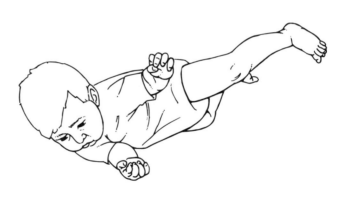

FIGURE 6–7B

POSITION: *SITTING*

Activity: *Pull to Sit* (13–27 weeks)

Base of Support

Weight bearing on buttocks and lumbar spine (Fig. 6–8).

Muscle Activity Pattern

Concentric contraction of head and neck flexors
Shoulder stabilization
Concentric contraction of elbow flexors
Concentric contraction of abdominals
Concentric contraction of hip flexors

Spectrum of Muscle Activity

Immature presentation may show increased head lag and decreased hip flexion. As child's muscle control and strength increase, the head will be maintained in line with the body against gravity as the upright position is achieved.

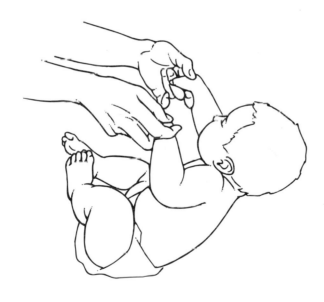

FIGURE 6-8

Activity: *Sitting with Propped Arms* (10–25 weeks)

Base of Support

Weight bearing on buttocks, legs, and hands.

Muscle Activity Pattern

Head erect
Isometric contraction of shoulder flexors
Concentric contraction of pectorals
Shoulder stabilization during support phase
Concentric contraction of back extensors

Functional Activity

This posture allows for perception of the environment at an elevated perspective, object acquisition, and play.

Spectrum of Muscle Activity

Spine generally kyphotic, indicating lack of general back extensor strength. Hips flexed and externally rotated to widen base of support. Knees flexed with the feet between buttocks and hands for additional support (Fig. 6–9). As muscular strength increases, the child is able to maintain spine erect against gravity, with the assistance of upper extremities, and he or she may move outside of base of support to reach for objects.

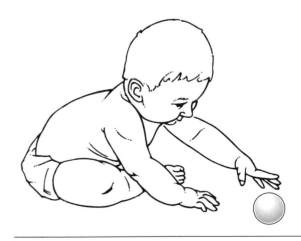

FIGURE 6-9

Activity: *Sitting Without Arm Support: Unsustained* (21–27 weeks)

Base of Support

Weight bearing on buttocks and legs.

Muscle Activity Pattern

Head erect
Alternating concentric contractions of back extensors and abdominals

Functional Activity

Initial independent sitting with arms free to manipulate objects.

Spectrum of Muscle Activity

Initially, the child will make adjustments as he or she tries to maintain the center of gravity over the base of support. This results because the child has yet to achieve mature muscle control patterns. Legs are abducted and externally rotated for widened base of support. Increased maturity is seen via decreased kyphosis of the spine, the child's willingness to move arms within the base of support, as well as decreasing the width of the base of support (Fig. 6–10).

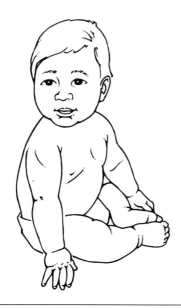

FIGURE 6–10

Case Study #1

Taylor is a 9-month-old boy diagnosed with hypotonia and was referred by his early intervention teacher for positioning techniques. He is the product of a 31-week pregnancy, delivered via cesarean section secondary to perceived fetal distress. He has no medical precautions and is not taking medication. Hearing and vision are reported as normal. Mother reports concerns regarding independent sitting.

Observed Behaviors

While supported against his mother Taylor was able to maintain his head at midline in the upright position with minimal difficulty. When placed at his mother's right shoulder he appeared to brace himself with his hands against her body. In this position he was able to turn his head to the right to observe a key ring the therapist was jingling. Taylor demonstrated visual tracking 180°.

When the keys were placed within arm's length, he reached out with his left hand and acquired them, grasping and holding, as well as resisting, when the therapist pulled gently. He brought them to midline, manipulated them briefly with both hands, and brought them to his mouth.

When placed in the prone position, Taylor was able to lift his head, with minimal difficulty, at midline to 90° (see Fig. 6–3). His hands were flat on the floor, his arms flexed at the shoulder and elbow, supporting his upper body weight. His legs were abducted and flexed, bilaterally, at both the hip and the knee. He was able to follow the path of his favorite toy with his eyes a full 180°. When the toy was brought beyond 180°, he weight-shifted to his left side, right elbow extended, flexing and abducting the right leg minimally and maintaining visual contact. He did not reach for the toy, but his mother reported that at times he will reach out for a toy. When the toy was moved to his far left, he weight-shifted to the right side, as previously described, and reached out his left hand to grasp the toy. Once the toy was acquired he rolled from prone to supine (see Fig. 6–2) with minimal dissociation of the trunk and hips (shoulder leading hips) and utilized both hands to bring the toy to his mouth. His mother reported that he rolls supine to and from the prone position from either side (see Fig. 6–7A and B.)

In the supine position, his legs remained abducted with flexion at the hip and knee bilaterally. Some slight adduction (lacking midline) and hip flexion (<90°) was seen intermittently as he was playing with a toy held above him. His mother reported that he currently does not bring his legs up and does not play with his feet (see Fig. 6–6). His mother reported that he does not move to a sitting position by himself.

When pulled to a sitting position, he showed a slight head lag (see Fig. 6–8). Once seated upright with the therapist holding his hands, he was able to move his head to midline and the upright position. His legs were abducted and externally rotated with his knees just slightly off the ground. He was unable to sit without therapist support (see Fig. 6–10). When his hands were placed on the ground (right arm within circle of legs, left arm lateral to left leg at the knee) he was able to maintain a propped position for approximately 3 minutes, arms fully extended (see Fig. 6–9). He presented with capital extension, cervical flexion, increased thoracic kyphosis, decreased lumbar lordosis, and posterior pelvic tilt. He maintained his head in the upright position with minimal difficulty and was able to turn his head 45° to either side. He did not attempt to reach for objects in this position and weight shifting was not observed.

Analysis

Milestone	Figure	Grade
Prone to supine	6–2	WF
Supine to prone	6–7A and B	WF
Hands to feet	6–6	NF
Pull to sit	6–8	WF
Sitting without arm support: unsustained	6–10	NF
Sitting with propped arms	6–9	WF

Taylor presented with a physical developmental age of approximately 4 to 6 months. He was able to perform the basic tasks of upright "regard" in the prone position, rolling, and maintaining a propped sitting position. He did not possess the overall strength to overcome the effects of global hypotonia in an upright position against gravity. This was seen in the head lag as he was pulled to sit and in the difficulty he had in maintaining an upright head position without utilizing his arms against a support surface (i.e., his mother's body or the floor).

When in both prone and supine positions or sitting, he demonstrated decreased strength of the pelvic and leg musculature. This was most marked in the supine and sitting positions. The posture of his legs was abducted and flexed at both hip and knee. This provided him with a larger base of support but restricted his mobility as he was unable to decrease the base of support to explore alternative positions. When rolling he led slightly with his shoulders, as opposed to his hips and legs, further indicating decreased strength of abdominals, hip flexors, and abductors.

In sitting he was restricted to the most basic effort of head and trunk support. Head, neck, and upper trunk musculature were decreased in strength and endurance. His arms remained in an extended position, shoulders abducted, and protracted hands flat on the floor. His inability to maintain sitting while performing a weight shift decreased his ability to explore the environment with his hands. Decreased back extensor strength was seen in the persistent rounded posture of the spine and posterior pelvic tilt.

Activity: *Dynamic Sitting Without Arm Support: Sustained* (25–32 weeks)

Base of Support

Weight bearing on buttocks and legs.

Muscle Activity Pattern

Head erect
Isometric contractions of back extensors and abdominals to maintain position
Concentric contraction of back extensors or abdominals as child moves outside of base of support

Functional Activity

Erect sitting with balance and stability to obtain and manipulate objects. Attention to the task of sitting is decreased, affording the child the ability to give increased attention to the environment outside of his immediate surroundings.

Spectrum of Muscle Activity

Increased maturity is seen via (a) decreased base of support as one or both legs may be extended with continued maintenance of erect posture against gravity; (b) increased movement of the arms and legs both in and outside of the base of support; and (c) rotation of the trunk while reaching. The child is able to lean forward outside the base of support and manage the center of gravity as the arms are lifted to obtain a toy (Fig. 6–11).

POSITION: *STANDING*

Activity: *Supported Standing* (18–30 weeks)

Base of Support

Weight bearing on both feet. Adult support at chest level.

Muscle Activity Pattern

Head erect
Concentric co-contraction of back extensors and abdominals
Concentric co-contraction of lower limb flexors and extensors

Functional Activity

This is a preindependent standing activity that develops strength and balance and provides the child with the experience of standing.

Spectrum of Muscle Activity

Initially the child will require support at chest level while bearing weight (Fig. 6–12). The child may bounce up and down with active control and flexion/extension of the trunk. As the child becomes more experienced, he or she will be able to utilize support surface while maintaining standing position.

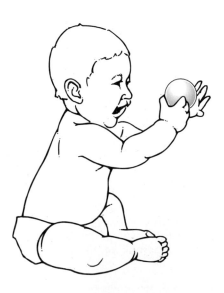

FIGURE 6–11

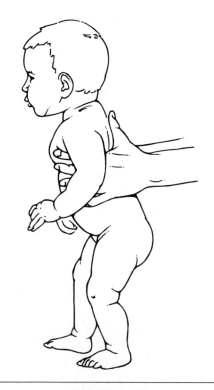

FIGURE 6–12

Activity: *Pulls to Stand, Stands with Support* (32-40 weeks)

Base of Support

Weight bearing through feet. Balance and stability with hands on the support surface or adult assistance (Fig. 6-13A).

Muscle Activity Pattern

Head erect
Concentric contraction of shoulder flexors (reaching for support surface)
Concentric contraction of shoulder extensors (pulling to stand)
Shoulder stabilization while moving to stand
Concentric contraction of transition limb hip flexor
Isometric contraction of contralateral hip abductor
Concentric contraction of bilateral quadriceps as full stand is achieved

Functional Activity

This skill allows for the acquisition of objects and environmental exploration higher than floor level. This provides the initial experience of transitioning from floor to stand.

Spectrum of Muscle Activity

Initially, the child may require assistance when moving to the standing position. The adult is able to control the child's inability to manage the increased number of degrees of freedom during the transition to stand. As the child matures, he or she is able to control the center of gravity over the base of support, against gravity, and use the support surface to move to stand. Once stance is acquired, the base of support is generally widened with the legs externally rotated (Fig. 6-13B).

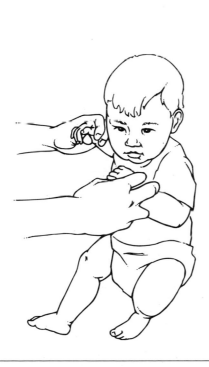

FIGURE 6-13A

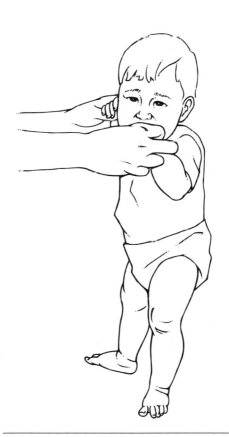

FIGURE 6-13B

Activity: *Side-Step Cruising* (36–56 weeks)

Base of Support

Weight bearing through alternating double- and single-limb support with weight shifting. Some weight bearing is seen through the arms on the support surface (Fig. 6–14).

Muscle Activity Pattern

Isometric contraction of shoulder extensors during single-limb support

Trunk co-contraction and stabilization

Concentric contraction of swing limb abductors

Eccentric contraction of stance limb adductors

Isometric co-contraction of weight-bearing limb flexors and extensors

Concentric contraction of plantar flexors of the foot for stability as weight is transferred

Functional Activity

One of the first attempts at erect independent mobility. The child can acquire objects or move to desired places or people using support surfaces throughout the environment.

Spectrum of Muscle Activity

Initially, the child may rest the abdomen on the support surface as he or she manipulates objects and cruises sideways. Hips are abducted and externally rotated to increase the base of support. As competence increases, the child will rely less on the support surface.

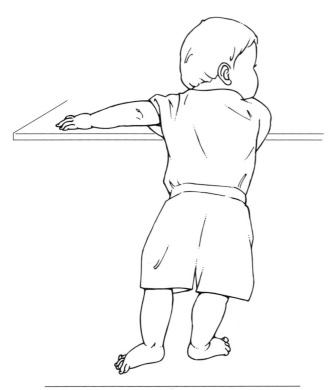

FIGURE 6-14

Activity: Controlled Lowering with Support (36–45 weeks)

Base of Support

Weight bearing on both feet with single upper extremity using support surface.

Muscle Activity Pattern

Eccentric contraction of abductors and flexors of the support arm
Eccentric gluteal activity
Eccentric quadriceps activity
Eccentric contraction of plantar flexors

Functional Activity

Utilization of a support surface affords the child the ability to transition from an upright position to the floor safely. This also provides the opportunity for the child to reach and acquire objects on the floor for manipulation or to transfer them to the surface of the support at which he or she is standing.

Spectrum of Muscle Activity

As the child moves downward, he may move to a half-kneel position for increased stability as he or she addresses or manipulates objects that are on the floor (Fig. 6–15). This transition is the first in which the child must manage his or her entire mass in the direction of gravity with eccentric control.

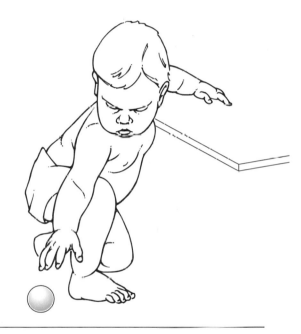

FIGURE 6–15

Activity: *Stand Without Support* (42–56 weeks)

Base of Support

Weight bearing on feet. Hips are abducted and externally rotated for increased base of support.

Muscle Activity Pattern

Abdominal and back extensor co-contraction for erect posture

Concentric contraction of gluteals

Isometric co-contraction of hip flexors and extensors

Isometric co-contraction of abductors and adductors

Functional Activity

Preparation for independent walking. Support surface not required; thus, the environment has a decreased impact on the child's mobility.

Spectrum of Muscle Activity

Child initially is generally hyperlordotic; arms may be at high or medium guard during initial stages. As the child becomes more stable, arms and hands will lower and may be used to manipulate objects; base of support narrows; legs become less externally rotated (Fig. 6–16).

Activity: *Stand from Modified Squat* (46–60 weeks)

Base of Support

Weight bearing on feet.

Muscle Activity Pattern

Concentric contraction of back extensors

Concentric contraction of gluteals

Concentric contraction of Quadriceps

Concentric contraction of ankle plantar flexors

Functional Activity

Child has the ability to reach for objects on the ground and transfer them to an alternative location without using a support surface; thus, environmental restrictions have less impact (Fig. 6–17).

Spectrum of Muscle Activity

Initially, the child may present with increased lumbar lordosis; the base of support is widened with external rotation of the hips. As the child moves to a standing position the increased lumbar lordosis may result in plantar flexion in an attempt to manage the center of gravity over the base of support.

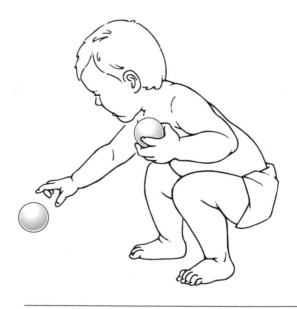

FIGURE 6–17

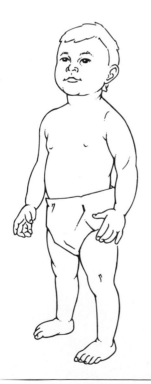

FIGURE 6–16

Activity: *Walks Alone* (46–57 weeks)

Base of Support

Weight bearing on feet.

Muscle Activity Pattern

Concentric co-contraction of abdominal and back extensors for stabilization

Alternating concentric hip and knee flexion and extension

Eccentric contraction of hamstrings during swing phase

Concentric contraction of stance limb abductors

Functional Activity

Independent physical access to the environment increases the child's ability to explore and obtain objects from the surrounding environment.

Spectrum of Muscle Activity

Initially, the child has a widened base of support. External rotation at the hip. Arms at high guard for increased balance and protective readiness. As child becomes more efficient, the base of support will narrow; external rotation of the legs will decrease; the arms will move down from high guard, affording the child the ability to acquire objects in the environment (Fig. 6–18).

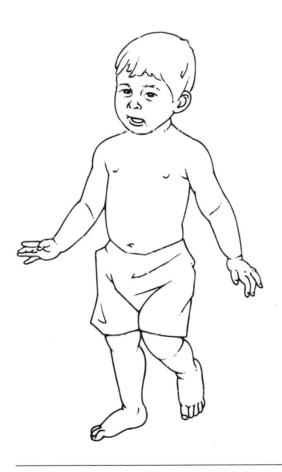

FIGURE 6–18

Activity: *Squatting* (52–59 weeks)

Base of Support

Weight bearing on feet. Base of support is widened.

Muscle Activity Pattern

Concentric co-contraction of abdominals and back extensors for stabilization

Isometric contraction of Quadriceps and gluteal muscles

Concentric co-contraction of anterior and posterior lower leg muscles for posture maintenance

Isometric contraction of abductors

Functional Activity

Child is able to move easily from a standing position to obtain objects from the floor and stand again without using a support surface (Fig. 6–19).

Spectrum of Muscle Activity

As the child becomes more competent, the base of support will narrow, external rotation of legs will decrease, and the child will be able to reach farther outside the base of support during play.

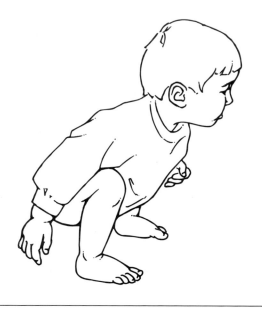

FIGURE 6–19

Case Study #2

Maya is a 23-month-old girl referred for falling and difficulties walking. She is the product of a full-term pregnancy with vaginal delivery and an unremarkable birth history. She was seen at home with her mother and father present, seated in her mother's lap. Her mother reported that Maya had no current medical diagnosis. She sat alone at 9 months (delayed; see Figs. 6–9 and 6–10) and began walking independently at 18 months (delayed; see Fig. 6–18). She continues to fall without external challenges. A previous appointment with an orthopedic surgeon revealed no significant abnormalities of her spine or legs.

Observed Behaviors

A doll was placed on the floor slightly in front of the therapist as a history was elicited from Maya's parents. Maya used the following immature gait pattern: wide base of support and decreased step length and flat-footed contact. She was flexed at the hip and knee, in a crouched position, and her center of mass moved in the frontal plane toward the weight-bearing limb with little dissociation of trunk and legs. Arms were held at medium guard. She intermittently lost her balance, and rocked in the anteroposterior direction over her ankles (see Fig. 6–18).

In attempting to squat, Maya reached for the therapist's leg with her right hand but stopped as the support was removed. She moved directly over the doll and squatted. She bent at the knee and ankle before increasing her hip flexion and lowering her trunk (see Fig. 6–19). She lost her balance anteriorly, adjusted, and grasped the doll's head. When transitioning from squat to stand, the movement was initiated with extension of her head and neck, retraction and depression of the left shoulder, and slight back extension. She completed the movement by bringing her left hand to her left knee and pushing upward (see Fig. 6–17). She regained a standing position, but remained crouched, flexed at the hip, knee, and ankle (see Fig. 6–16).

Maya was asked to remove a truck from her toy box. The truck was in the farthest corner of the box and she could not reach it while standing. She lowered her hands to the edge of the box and squatted as previously described. She braced herself on the edge of the box and lowered first the right knee, then the left, to the ground (see Fig. 6–15). She continued to support herself with one hand while reaching for the toy, set it outside the box, and re-erected as previously described, using a support surface (see Figs. 6–13A and B).

Once erect, she reached for the truck with her right hand, squatting and re-erecting as previously described. She turned slowly to the right, holding the truck close to her body. She stepped forward on her right foot, but she undercompensated for the truck's weight. Her center of mass moved posteriorly over her left foot and she fell on her bottom to the floor. She rolled backward on her right ischial tuberosity, maintaining support on her right elbow. She shifted her weight to the left and pushed upward into a three-point position (see Fig. 6–4) from which she played with the truck, weight-bearing arm fully extended. (This movement was initiated with head and neck extension.)

When encouraged to stand, Maya moved onto her hands and knees and pushed up to a bear crawl position. Her center of mass moved back and forth between her hands and feet. She walked her feet slightly forward and managed to push herself upward, walking her hands up her thighs (Gowers' sign) until she was erect.

Analysis

Milestone	Figure	Grade
Walks alone	6–18	WF
Squatting	6–19	WF
Squat to stand	6–17	WF
Controlled lowering with support	6–15	WF
Pulls to stand	6–13A and B	WF
Modified four-point kneeling	6–4	WF
Stands alone	6–16	WF

Maya responded appropriately to her name and to environmental stimuli and followed directions. She has no medical diagnosis, but her parents are concerned because she has difficulty walking and often falls. She has a physical developmental age of 8 to 13 1/2 months. She demonstrates no overt indications of cognitive impairment. As the child is currently walking, an analysis of the more basic milestones (such as rolling or moving to sit) was not necessary. The motor requirements for such activities may be analyzed as the child demonstrates higher-level skills.

During both independent standing and ambulation, she presented a wide base of support. She demonstrated an immature gait pattern. Her immature stance and gait pattern revealed moderate to severe weakness of the extensor muscles. This weakness was also demonstrated in her transition to a squatting position. If a support surface was present, she used it to lower herself to the ground. Without the presence of a support surface, her nonreaching arm was placed in protective extension and her center of mass was directly above the toy she picked up. She initiated the movement with dorsiflexion and knee flexion at 45° to 50° before increasing hip flexion and lowering the trunk. This strategy allowed her to lower to the floor without having to maintain her center of mass outside of her base of support for an extended period of time.

When moving from a squat to stand she used a support surface if one was available. Her base of support continued to be widened. She compensated for lack of back extensor strength by moving her head, neck, and shoulder-arm complex posterior to her center of mass, thus decreasing the demand. During the movement she displayed a positive Gowers' sign.

When side-lying, the demand on the back extensors was not as great and Maya was able to achieve a modified four-point position by initiating movement with minimal head and neck extension. Using an atypical strategy for

Case Study #2 (Continued)

her age, however, both upper extremities remained weight-bearing until her center of mass was appropriately positioned, prior to moving the toy with her left arm. A more typical presentation would show a transfer of the demand caudally, to the lower extremities, with the trunk supported by back extensors. Her mobility was further restricted by the need to maintain her weight-bearing arm in an extended position during contralateral play.

From a modified four-point position without a support surface, Maya moved to a standing position via a bear crawl. Her base of support was widened and management of center of mass was difficult, requiring adjustments in foot position until the foot was centered between her base of support. Moving to a stand required the use of both arms, fully extended, on the lower extremities, indicating back extensor weakness. Head and neck were extended and bilateral shoulder retraction was seen as she achieved an upright posture. This is a typical presentation of Gowers' sign. It is generally seen in children with muscle disease.

Activity: *Low Kneel to High Kneel* (15 months–2 years)

Base of Support

Dorsal aspect of both feet (Fig. 6–20A). Anterior aspect of lower legs (Fig. 6–20B).

Muscle Activity Pattern

Trunk stabilization
Concentric gluteal contraction
Concentric quadriceps contraction

Functional Activity

Reaching for an object from floor to alternative level. Preparation to move to a standing position.

Spectrum of Muscle Activity

Child may initially use a support surface or place hands on the floor to stabilize trunk and compensate for inadequate strength of gluteals and Quadriceps. In the low-kneel position the child's legs may initially be abducted and internally rotated with the feet lateral to the knees. With growth and increased strength, the child is able to move the body mass against gravity and maintain position without a surface support and then can transition through the spectrum from low kneel to high kneel and finally to half kneel.

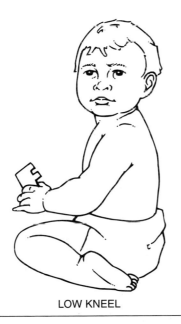

LOW KNEEL

FIGURE 6–20A

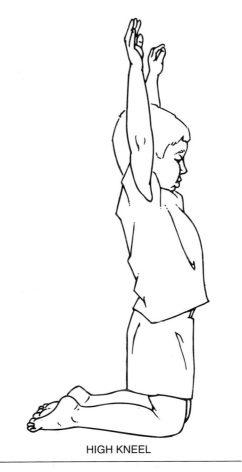

HIGH KNEEL

FIGURE 6–20B

Activity: *High Kneel to Half-Kneel* (18–27 months)

Base of Support

Anterior aspect of the leg and dorsum of one foot. Plantar surface of contralateral foot.

Muscle Activity Pattern

Concentric co-contraction of abdominals and back extensors
Concentric contraction of stable limb abductors
Isometric contraction of gluteals
Concentric contraction of moving limb hip flexors

Functional Activity

Preparation for moving to a standing position from the floor. Head is maintained in the frontal plane.

Spectrum of Muscle Activity

The child may initially lean to the contralateral side of the moving limb and place a hand on the floor for support, or may reach for a support surface as the moving leg is brought into position. The moving limb may also be abducted and the medial surface of the foot may remain in contact with the floor as it is swung through (Fig. 6–20C). Mature representation reflects maintenance of a level pelvis in the transverse plane. The moving limb is maintained in a fairly consistent sagittal plane.

Children move through the spectrum from low kneel to high kneel to half kneel as they mature.

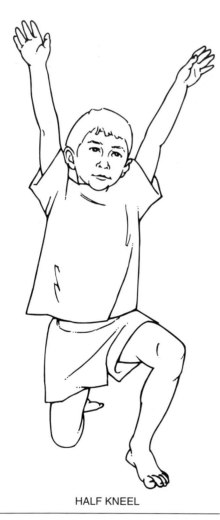

HALF KNEEL

FIGURE 6–20C

Activity: *Side Step* (18–30 months)

Base of Support

Weight bearing on both feet with intermittent bouts of single-limb support. Center of gravity maintenance over base of support in the frontal plane (Fig. 6–21).

Muscle Activity Pattern

Co-contraction of back extensors and abdominals for maintenance of erect trunk

Co-contraction of stance limb hip flexors and extensors

Isometric contraction of gluteals

Isometric contraction of stance limb abductors to maintain level pelvis

Concentric contraction of swing limb abductors

Eccentric contraction of stance limb adductors

Weight shift and weight acceptance onto swing limb

Isometric contraction of abductors of new stance limb

Concentric contraction of new swing limb adductors

Concentric contraction of ankle plantar flexors

Functional Activity

Increases child's maneuverability around and through obstacles in the environment. Increased single-limb stance period.

Spectrum of Muscle Activity

As the child becomes more proficient, side-step length will increase and will progress from frontal plane movement to associated diagonal planes. Figure 6–21 depicts a child demonstrating a mature representation of a side step.

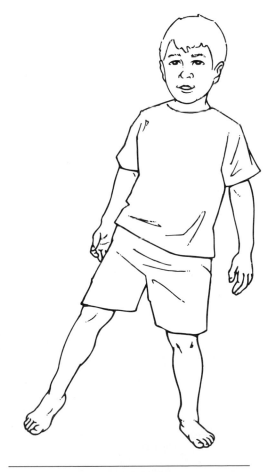

FIGURE 6–21

Activity: *Standing on One Foot* (2 1/2–3 1/2 years)

Base of Support

Weight bearing on a single foot.

Muscle Activity Pattern

Co-contraction of back extensors and abdominals for maintenance of erect trunk

Isometric contraction of Quadriceps to maintain locked knee

Isometric contraction of stance limb abductors

To account for anterior-posterior sway, transitions between concentric and isometric co-contractions of anterior and posterior compartment muscles are observed

To account for sagittal sway, transitions between concentric and isometric co-contractions of the foot invertors and evertors are observed

Concentric contraction of hamstrings in non–weight-bearing limb to lift foot

To maintain posture, a transition between concentric and isometric contractions of non–weight-bearing limb abductors is observed

Functional Activity

Development and increase of static and dynamic balance skills for higher-level play activities.

Spectrum of Muscle Activity

As seen in Figure 6–22A, a toddler may initiate brief periods of single-limb stance. Initially, the child may wrap the non–weight-bearing limb around the stance limb. The arms may be held out from the body for balance. The pelvis may tilt to the non–weight-bearing side secondary to decreased strength of abductors and movement of the center of gravity closer to the support limb. The toddler will present with increased sway. As the child becomes older and more proficient, arms will be maintained at sides of the body and pelvis symmetry is maintained (Fig. 6–22B).

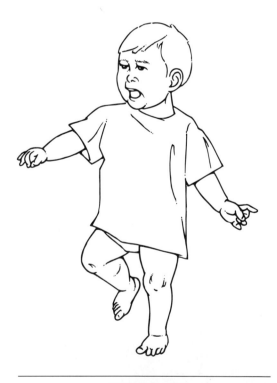

FIGURE 6-22A

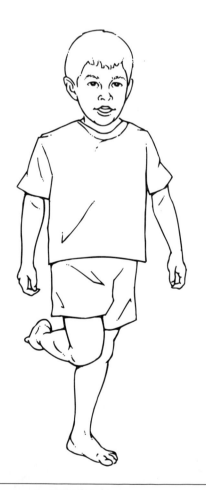

FIGURE 6-22B

Activity: *Jumping from Two Feet* (3–4 years)

Base of Support

Weight bearing on both feet.

Muscle Activity Pattern

Preparation Phase (Fig. 6–23A)
Trunk stabilization
Concentric hip and knee flexion
Eccentric contraction of hip extensors and ankle plantar flexors

Action Phase (Fig. 6–23B)
Concentric gluteal contraction
Concentric hip and knee extension
Concentric plantar flexion

Functional Activity

This activity allows for a rehearsal of higher level of gross motor play skills and an increased management of center of gravity.

Spectrum of Muscle Activity

As the child becomes more proficient, greater hip and knee flexion and ankle dorsiflexion are observed secondary to a desire for increased force production. As the child matures, an increased proficiency at managing the center of gravity over the base of support facilitates an increase in force production.

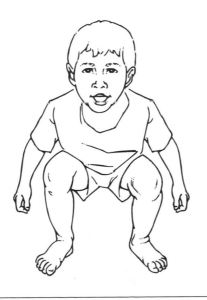

FIGURE 6–23A

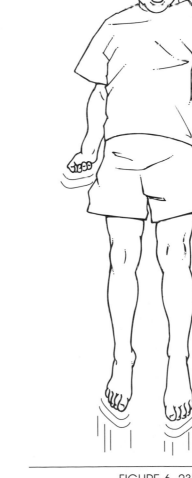

FIGURE 6–23B

Activity: *Jumping off a Step* (3–4 years)

Base of Support

Weight bearing on both feet.

Muscle Activity Pattern

Preparation Phase
Trunk stabilization
Concentric hip and knee flexion
Eccentric contraction of hip extensors and ankle
    plantar flexors

Action Phase (Fig. 6–24A)
Concentric hip and knee extension
Concentric contraction of back extensors
Concentric gluteal contraction
Concentric plantar flexion with a forward compo-
    nent

Landing Phase (Fig. 6–24B)
Trunk stabilization
Eccentric contraction of hip extensors
Eccentric contraction of knee extensors
Eccentric contraction of ankle plantar flexion

Functional Activity

This allows for a rehearsal of higher level of gross
motor play skills and an increased management of
center of gravity.

Spectrum of Muscle Activity

As the child becomes more proficient, greater hip
and knee flexion and ankle dorsiflexion are observed
secondary to desire for increased force production
(Fig. 6–24B).

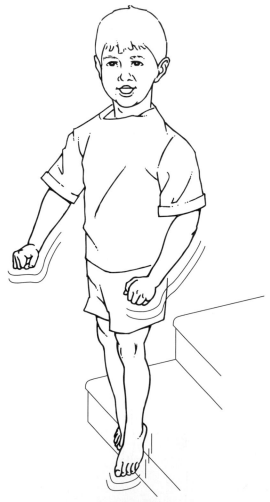

ACTION PHASE
FIGURE 6-24A

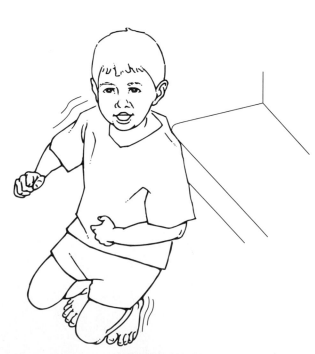

LANDING PHASE
FIGURE 6-24B

Activity: *Toe-Walking* (3–4 years)

Base of Support

Metatarsophalangeal (MTP) joints and digits.

Muscle Activity Pattern (Fig. 6–25)

> Trunk stabilization for erect posture
> Concentric contraction of hip flexors
> Isometric contraction of gluteals
> Isometric contraction of Quadriceps
> Concentric contraction of plantar flexors

Functional Activity

This allows for a rehearsal of higher level of gross motor play skills and an increased management of center of gravity.

Spectrum of Muscle Activity

Initially, the child may hold arms out to sides for balance. There also may be a drop in the heel as weight is accepted. As the child's strength develops, the center of gravity is maintained over the metatarsophalangeal joints, step length may increase, and the medial and lateral muscles of the lower limb will play an increasing role in stabilization.

Activity: *Heel-Walking* (4–5 years)

Base of Support

Bilateral calcanei.

Muscle Activity Pattern

> Trunk stabilization
> Concentric contraction of hip flexors
> Isometric contraction of Quadriceps
> Isometric contraction of gluteals
> Concentric contraction of dorsiflexors

Functional Activity

This allows for a rehearsal of higher level of gross motor play skills and an increased management of center of gravity.

Spectrum of Muscle Activity

Initially the toes may be raised only slightly from the floor; the base of support will be wide with increased trunk flexion and utilization of arms as balance. As the child's strength increases, toes are lifted and maintained a maximal distance from the floor (Fig. 6–26).

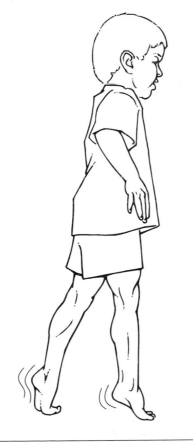

FIGURE 6–25

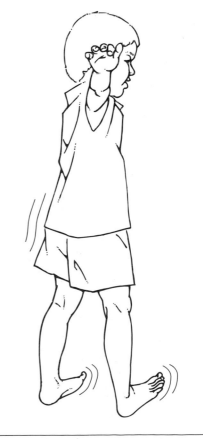

FIGURE 6–26

Activity: *Tandem-Walking* (5+ years)

Base of Support

Plantar aspects of bilateral feet.

Muscle Activity Pattern

Trunk stabilization

Stance Limb
Concentric co-contraction of hip flexors and extensors
Concentric contraction of abductors

Swing Limb
Concentric contraction of hip flexors
Concentric contraction of adductors
Concentric contraction of quadriceps
Concentric contraction of hip extensors as weight
 is transferred

Functional Activity

This allows for a rehearsal of higher level of gross motor play skills and an increased management of center of gravity.

Spectrum of Muscle Activity

The child may initially place the swing foot slightly in front of the stance foot (Fig. 6–27), moving it posteriorly into the appropriate position only after stance has been initiated. Increased trunk sway for balance maintenance is seen, as well as arms positioned away from body.

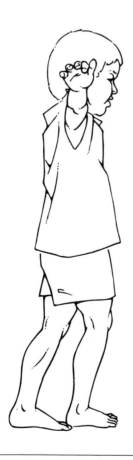

FIGURE 6–27

Activity: *Stair-Walking: Upstairs* (24–29 months)

Base of Support

Bilateral plantar aspects of feet. Alternating periods of single-limb stance.

Muscle Activity Pattern

Concentric contraction of abdominals
Isometric stabilization of back extensors
Concentric contraction of swing limb hip flexors
Concentric contraction of swing foot dorsiflexors
Isometric stabilization of stance limb abductors
Isometric contraction of stance limb gluteals
Concentric contraction of swing limb Quadriceps as weight is accepted
Concentric contraction of stance limb ankle plantar flexors
Concentric contraction of swing limb gluteals as increased weight is transferred

Functional Activity

Transitioning between ground and higher levels: for use in homes, apartments, and schools, and with playground equipment.

Spectrum of Muscle Activity

Initially, the child may use the rail or adult support. As the leg is brought to the upper step, a lateral trunk lean to the opposite side may be seen. As the child matures, weight will be maintained over the stance limb with forward trunk lean as ascension begins (Fig. 6–28).

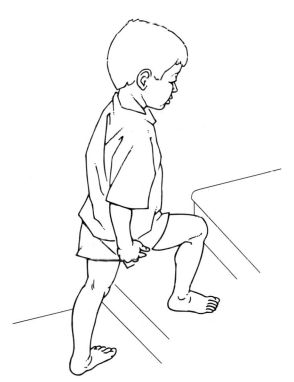

FIGURE 6-28

Activity: *Stair-Walking: Downstairs* (36–41 months)

Base of Support

Bilateral plantar aspects of feet. Alternating periods of single limb stance.

Muscle Activity Pattern

Trunk stabilization
Isometric contraction of gluteals
Concentric contraction of swing limb hip flexors
Concentric contraction of swing limb abductors
Eccentric contraction of stance limb Quadriceps
Isometric contraction of stance limb abductors
Eccentric contraction of swing limb plantar flexors
  as weight is accepted
Concentric contraction of swing limb abductors as
  full weight is accepted

Functional Activity

Transition safely between higher levels to ground: for use in homes, apartments, and in schools and with playground equipment.

Spectrum of Muscle Activity

Initially the child may turn sideways toward the lead limb so that the base of support is widened to the length of the foot as the lead limb steps down. As the child matures, the stance foot and the hip, knee, and trunk are maintained in an erect position.

Activity: *Ball Throwing: Overhead* (2–4 years)

Base of Support

Weight bearing on both feet.

Muscle Activity Pattern

Bilateral concentric shoulder flexion
Isometric shoulder horizontal adduction
Bilateral concentric elbow flexion
Isometric co-contraction of abdominals and back extensors
Bilateral concentric shoulder extension
Bilateral concentric elbow extension
Transfer of weight from heels to balls of the feet as ball passes over the head
Concentric abdominal contraction
Bilateral concentric contractions of wrist flexors that result in ulnar deviation

Functional Activity

Play skill.

Spectrum of Muscle Activity

Feet may be side by side, staggered, or increased weight bearing on the dominant foot (Fig. 6–29A). As the child becomes more proficient, movement can be more forceful and ballistic and you may begin to see ulnar deviation (Fig. 6–29B).

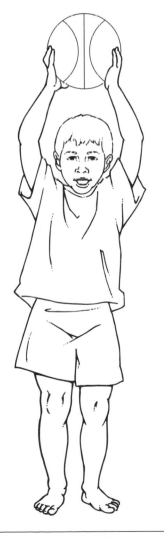

FIGURE 6–29A

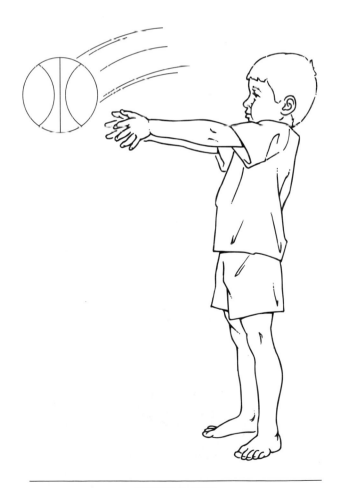

FIGURE 6–29B

Activity: *Ball Throwing: One-Handed* (43–53 months)

Base of Support

Plantar aspects of feet bilaterally. Foot on throwing side slightly posterior. Weight is transferred from posterior foot to anterior foot with follow-through (Fig. 6–30).

Muscle Activity Pattern

Preparation Phase
- Concentric contraction of hand intrinsics for gripping ball
- Isometric contraction of rotator cuff musculature for shoulder stabilization
- Concentric contraction of biceps
- Concentric contraction of shoulder flexors
- Posterior trunk rotation toward throwing arm
- Isometric contraction of throwing side abductors
- Isometric contraction of throwing side gluteals

Action Phase
- Concentric shoulder extension
- Concentric contraction of triceps
- Concentric contraction of wrist flexors
- Concentric contraction of obliques as trunk rotates forward
- Isometric contraction of contralateral abductors
- Isometric contraction of contralateral Quadriceps

Functional Activity

Upper-level ball skill.

Spectrum of Muscle Activity

Initially the child stands with feet side by side; the base of support is widened. There is little or no trunk rotation. At toddler age, the arm is drawn upward with little or no elbow flexion. During the action phase, the arm remains extended, with no wrist flexion. Trunk flexion may be seen as the ball is thrown. As the child's proficiency increases with age, weight is borne on the throwing side limb and then transferred to the contralateral limb as the ball is thrown forward.

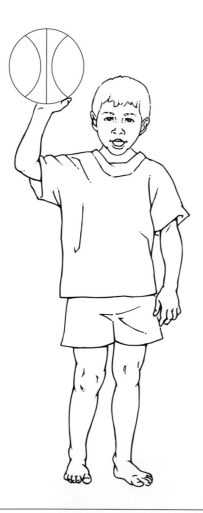

FIGURE 6–30

Activity: *Prehension: Palmar Supinate* (12-18 months)

Hand Position

Writing implement is held in a fisted hand; the wrist is slightly flexed and the forearm is supinated from midposition (Fig. 6-31).

Muscle Activity Pattern

Shoulder musculature active through flexion and extension with some horizontal adduction and abduction.

Activity: *Prehension: Digital Pronate* (2-3 years)

Hand Position

Writing implement is held with fingers. Wrist is ulnarly deviated and slightly extended; forearm is slightly pronated (Fig. 6-32).

Muscle Activity Pattern

Shoulder stabilization
Concentric contraction of biceps
Concentric contraction of triceps
Wrist stabilization via forearm musculature

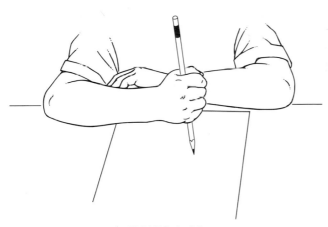

FIGURE 6-31

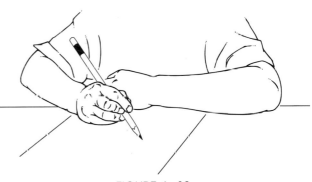

FIGURE 6-32

Activity: *Static Tripod* (3 1/2–4 years)

Hand Position

Writing implement is held with a crude approximation of thumb and index and middle fingers. Ring and little fingers are slightly flexed. There are no fine, localized movements of digits: the hand moves as a unit. The contralateral hand may be used to adjust the writing implement.

Muscle Activity Pattern

Concentric contraction of forearm finger flexors
Concentric contraction of intrinsic finger flexors
Concentric contraction of thumb adductor
Concentric contraction of wrist flexors and extensors

Activity: *Dynamic Tripod* (4 1/2–6 years)

Hand Position

The writing implement is held distally with precise opposition of distal phalanges of thumb and index and middle fingers. Ring and little fingers are flexed fully to form a stable support structure (Fig. 6–33). The wrist is slightly extended. The metacarpophalangeal (MCP) joints are stabilized during fine, localized movement of the proximal interphalangeal joints.

Muscle Activity Pattern

Concentric contraction of wrist extensors
Isometric contraction of intrinsics stabilizing MCP joints
Concentric contraction of flexor digitorum longus
Concentric contraction of extensor digitorum longus
Concentric contraction of thumb adductor
Concentric contraction of flexor hallucis longus

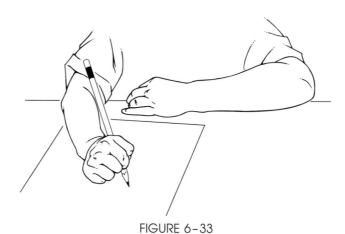

FIGURE 6–33

Case Study #3

Skylar is a 49-month-old girl with a medical diagnosis of Down syndrome and concordant hypotonia. She was seen at her special day preschool class for evaluation. Hearing was reported to be normal and vision has been corrected with glasses. Her mother is concerned that Skylar is not meeting motor milestones appropriate for her age.

Skylar's teacher reported that she is doing well in school, although she often refuses to perform tasks. She is able to physically access all areas of the classroom and campus that her curriculum demands. A psychological evaluation stated that she has scattered skills ranging from 29 to 38 months.

Observed Behaviors

Skylar was seated on the floor in the tailor's position when first seen during circle time. Her posture was slouched, consisting of capital extension, cervical flexion, increased thoracic kyphosis, decreased lumbar lordosis, and posterior pelvic tilt. Upon raising her hand, she reversed and maintained anterior pelvic tilt and lumbar lordosis for at least 15 seconds. She shifted her weight to the left, placed her left hand on the floor, and moved into a side-sitting position. When asked to place her name card in the appropriate position on the board, she transitioned to a quadruped position and moved through low kneel to high kneel (see Fig. 6–20A and B) to a half-kneel (see Fig. 6–20C) on the right leg. When moving to a stand from half-kneel, one hand was placed on the floor, the other on her knee. She shifted her center of mass between her hands and feet, lifted her bottom in the air, extended her spine, and moved to an upright position. She walked to the table for art time, grasped a crayon with her left hand, and transferred it to her right. She proceeded to scribble in a vertical manner using a digital pronate grasp (see Fig. 6–32).

During walking, she evidenced a lumbar lordosis, a slightly widened base of support, decreased hip and knee flexion, and low heel strike and toe-off, with a shortened step length. She bent to pick up a toy and side-stepped to the right (see Fig. 6–21) four steps, avoiding children playing on the floor, without loss of balance.

At recess, Skylar descended 6-inch steps, without a rail, in a pattern of two feet per stair. She hesitated at each step prior to lowering her foot to the next step. When asked to jump down from the last step she squatted slightly and made motions of jumping, but her feet did not leave the ground. When offered two-handed support, she jumped, but landed one foot at a time (see Fig. 6–24A and B). Once on the ground, she proceeded to jump from two feet repeatedly. She attained a height of approximately 2 inches (see Fig. 6–23A and B). She flexed her hips and knees minimally and her arms were maintained at medium guard.

When asked to climb up the steps, Skylar refused and ran across the playground to a group of her peers. She took a ball from another child and threw it against the fence from an overhead position (see Fig. 6–29A and B). Her feet were aligned in the frontal plane, the ball held directly over her head, and thrown with minimal elbow flexion and extension.

After 10 minutes, Skylar returned to the therapist and attempted to imitate standing on one foot (see Fig. 6–22A and B). She lifted her left leg briefly, but leaned her trunk to her right with her non–weight-bearing leg extended to the left. She immediately reached out for support.

After recess, the entire class returned to the room. Skylar ascended the steps (see Fig. 6–28) without a rail, in a reciprocal pattern (one foot per stair). Her base of support was slightly widened with oscillation of her center of mass in the frontal plane.

Analysis

Milestone	Figure	Grade
Low kneel to high kneel	6–20A and B	F
High kneel to half-kneel	6–20C	F
Side step	6–21	F
Stands on one foot	6–22B	NF
Jumps from two feet	6–23A and B	WF
Jumps off step	6–24A and B	WF
Ball throwing: overhead	6–29A and B	WF
Stair walking upstairs	6–28	F
Stair walking downstairs	6–28	WF
Digital pronate	6–32	F

Skylar has a physical developmental age of approximately 3 years old. She is independent and functional with all floor transitional skills (i.e., rolling, moving to sit, moving to quadruped, moving through high kneel to half-kneel). She performs these tasks functionally and with a Good to Fair approximation of appropriate muscle synergies.

When moving to stand, Skylar performed the task in an immature fashion. She transferred her weight posteriorly and positioned her center of mass over her base of support prior to elevating her bottom. This strategy decreases the demand on the Quadriceps, gluteals, and abductors. A typical presentation for this chronological age is to shift weight toward the right, moving the center of mass fluidly between the two limbs, accepting a greater portion of the body weight onto the right leg, and extending the left leg while elevating the center of mass with the right.

Skylar's gross motor skills associated with the lower extremities are immature and reveal signs of muscle weakness. During ambulation, Skylar presents with an immature, albeit functional, gait pattern. Her step length is shortened with decreased hip and knee flexion. These strategies decrease the eccentric demand on both the hamstrings and the Quadriceps. A widened base of support and shortened step length afford her increased stability, decreasing the demand placed on the abductors during single-limb stance. Decreased eccentric control of

Case Study #3 (Continued)

the Quadriceps is also evident as Skylar descends stairs. She hesitates prior to descending each step and is unable to maintain the demand required of the Quadriceps to utilize a reciprocal pattern. Skylar is not yet efficient at jumping from two feet. Her base of support continues to be widened to maintain her center of mass between her feet, with little compensation necessary through the trunk. Her preparation for flight is minimal, decreasing the eccentric demand on the Quadriceps. She is unable to jump off a step. While standing on one foot, Skylar was unable to maintain the position, other than momentarily. She was able to lift the non–weight-bearing leg, but adjusted her center of mass, as described above, to decrease the demand placed on the abductors of the weight-bearing limb. A compensation for decreased abductor

strength also is seen as Skylar ascends the stairs. Her base of support is widened and the center of mass oscillates between the weight-bearing limbs.

When throwing the ball from an overhead position, Skylar lacks a mature position of her base of support. Her feet were aligned in the frontal plane, shoulder-width apart, demonstrating a reluctance to narrow her base of support during a dynamic activity. When holding the ball overhead, she maintained her arms in an extended position, keeping the ball in line with her center of mass. A mature presentation of this skill is performed with one foot placed slightly in front of the other with a transfer of weight from the back to the front foot. The ball is held behind the head with flexion at the elbow, which is extended during the ballistic phase of the action.

References

1. Neisworth JT, Bagnato SJ. Assessment in early childhood special education. A typology of dependent measures. *In* Odom SL, Karnes MB (eds). *Early Intervention for Infants and Children with Handicaps: An Empirical Base.* Baltimore: Paul H Brookes, 1988.
2. Hanft BE, Pilkington KO. Therapy in natural environments: The means of end goal for early intervention. Infants Young Child 12: 1–13, 2000.
3. Piper MC, Darrah J. *Motor Assessment of the Developing Infant.* Philadelphia: WB Saunders, 1994.
4. Knobloch H, Pasamanick B. Revised Gesell and Amatruda Developmental Neurological Examination. 1974.
5. Bayley N. *Bayley Scales of Infant Development.* San Antonio: Harcourt Brace, 1993.
6. Folio M, Fewell R. *Peabody Developmental Scales.* Allen, TX: DLM Teaching Resources, 1983.
7. Evans HE, Glass L. *Perinatal Medicine* Hagerstown, MD: Harper & Row, 1976.

CHAPTER 7

Assessment of Muscles Innervated by Cranial Nerves

This chapter describes the muscles innervated by motor branches of the cranial nerves and describes test methods of assessing the muscles of the eyelid, face, jaw, tongue, soft palate, posterior pharyngeal wall, and larynx. It also covers the extraocular muscles. The tests are appropriate for patients whose neurologic deficits are either central or peripheral. The only requirement for the patient to participate in the test is the ability to follow simple directions.

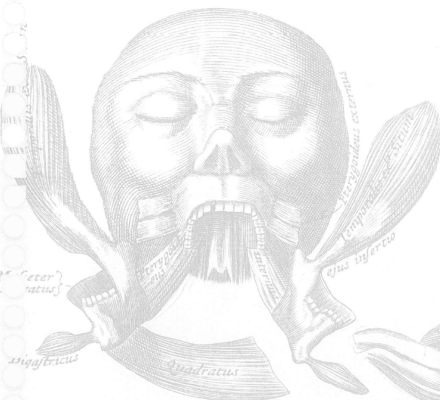

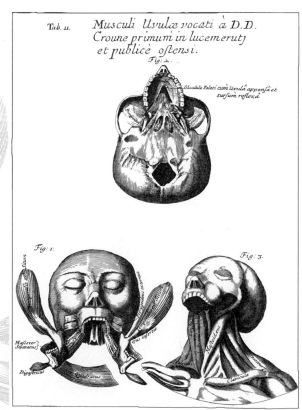

INTRODUCTION TO TESTING AND GRADING

Muscles innervated by the cranial nerves are not amenable to the classic methods of manual muscle testing and grading. In many, if not most, cases they do not move a bony lever, so manual resistance as a means of evaluation of their strength and function is not always the primary procedure.

The therapist needs to become familiar with the cranial nerve muscles in normal persons. Their appearance, strength, excursion, and rate of motion are all variables that are unlike the other skeletal muscles, which are more familiar. As for the infant and young child, the best way to assess the gross function of these muscles is to observe the child while crying, sucking, etc. In any event, experience with assessment requires considerable practice with both normal persons and a wide variety of patients with suspected and known cranial nerve motor deficits emanating from both upper and lower motor neuron lesions.

An anecdote from the personal experience of one of the authors (JM) involves a patient who was being evaluated for bulbar function because of a motor neuron disease. A "strange" structure appeared in the back of the throat when the patient opened wide to say "Ah-h-h." As it turned out, there was no tumor, no foreign object, and no structural deformity. The "strange" structure was the epiglottis, not commonly observed in many people.

The issue of symmetry is particularly important in testing the ocular, facial, tongue, jaw, pharyngeal, and palate muscles. The symmetry of these muscles, except for the laryngeal muscles, is visible to the examiner. Asymmetry is more readily detected just by observation in these than in the limb muscles and should always be documented.

In all tests in this chapter, the movements or instructions may not be entirely familiar to the patient, so each test should be demonstrated and the patient should be allowed to practice. In the presence of unusual or unexpected test results, the examiner should inquire about prior facial reconstructive (e.g., cosmetic) surgery.

General Grading Procedures

The distinction to be made in testing the muscles described in this chapter is to ascertain their relative functional level with respect to their intended activity. The scoring system, therefore, is a functional one, and motions or function are graded as follows:

F: Functional; appears normal or only slight impairment

WF: Weak functional; moderate impairment that affects the degree of active motion

NF: Nonfunctional; severe impairment

0: Absent

Universal Precautions in Bulbar Testing

In testing the muscles of the head, oral cavity, and throat the examiner frequently encounters body fluids such as saliva, tears, and bronchotracheopharyngeal secretions. The precaution of wearing gloves should always be followed. If the patient has any infectious disease or if there are copious secretions, the examiner should be masked and gowned as well as gloved.

The examiner should be cautious about standing directly in front of a patient who has been instructed to cough. This also is true in the case of the patient who has an open tracheostomy.

When a tongue blade is used, it should be sterile and care should be used about where it is placed between tests on a given patient.

Patient and Examiner Positions for All Tests

The short-sitting position is preferred. The head and trunk should be supported as necessary to maintain normal alignment or to accommodate deformities. If the patient cannot sit for any reason, use the supine position, which will not influence testing of the head and eye muscles. When the muscles of the oral cavity and throat are tested, however, the head should be elevated. The examiner stands or sits in front of the patient but slightly to one side. A stool on casters is preferred so the therapist can move about the patient quickly and efficiently.

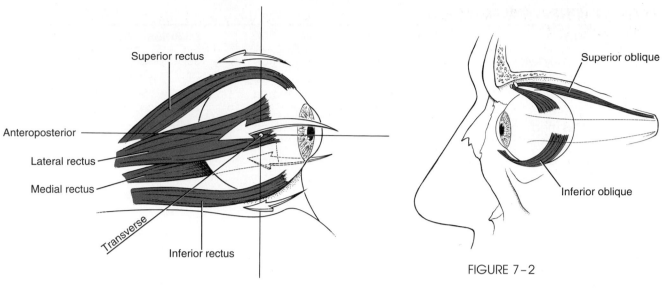

FIGURE 7-1

FIGURE 7-2

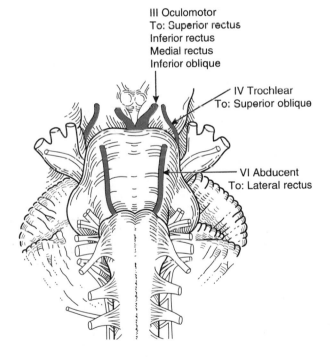

FIGURE 7-3

Table 7-1 EXTRAOCULAR MUSCLES

I.D.	Muscle	Origin	Insertion
6	Rectus superior	Sphenoid bone (via common annular tendon)	Superior anterior sclera (via tendinous expansion)
7	Rectus inferior	Sphenoid bone (via common annular tendon)	Inferior sclera (via tendinous expansion)
8	Rectus medialis	Sphenoid bone (via common annular tendon)	Medial sclera (via tendinous expansion)
9	Rectus lateralis	Sphenoid bone (via common annular tendon)	Lateral sclera (via tendinous expansion)
10	Obliquus superior oculi (Superior oblique)	Sphenoid bone (body) Tendon of Rectus superior	Frontal bone (via a frontal bone pulley) Trochlea to the superolateral sclera behind the equator on the supralateral surface
11	Obliquus inferior oculi (Inferior oblique)	Maxilla (orbital surface)	Lateral sclera behind the equator of the eyeball on lateral posterior quadrant

The six extraocular muscles of the eye (Figs. 7–1 and 7–2) move the eyeball in directions that depend on their attachments and on the influence of the movements themselves. It is probable that no muscle of the eye acts independently, and because these muscles cannot be observed, palpated, or tested individually, much of the knowledge of their function is derived from some variety of dysfunction. The extraocular muscles are innervated by cranial nerves III (oculomotor), IV (trochlear), and VI (abducent) (Fig 7–3).

The Axes of Eye Motion

The eyeball rotates in the orbital socket around one or more of three primary axes (Fig. 7–4), which intersect in the center of the eyeball.[1]

Vertical axis: Around this axis the lateral motions (abduction and adduction) take place in a horizontal plane.

Transverse axis: This is the axis of rotation for upward and downward motions.

Anteroposterior axis: Motions of rotation in the frontal plane occur around this axis.

The neutral position of the eyeball occurs when the gaze is straight-ahead and far away. In this neutral position the axes of the two eyes are parallel. Normally, the motions of the two eyes are conjugate, that is, coordinated, and the two eyes move together.

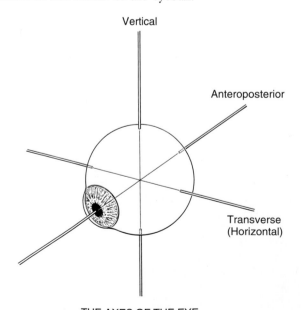

Vertical

Anteroposterior

Transverse (Horizontal)

THE AXES OF THE EYE

FIGURE 7-4.
The three primary axes of the eye.

Eye Motions

The extraocular muscles seem to work as a continuum; as the length of one changes, the length and tension of the others are altered, giving rise to a wide repertoire of movement.[2,3] Despite this continuous commonality of activity, the function of the individual muscles can be simplified and understood in a manner that does not detract from accuracy but simplifies the test procedure.

Conventional clinical testing assigns the following motions to the various extraocular muscles[1-3] (Fig. 7-5):

6. Rectus superior (III, Oculomotor)

Primary Movement: Elevation of the eyeball; movement is upward and inward.

Secondary Movements

1. Rotation of the adducted eyeball so the upper end of the vertical axis is inward (see Fig. 7–4)
2. Adduction of the eyeball to a limited extent

7. Rectus inferior (III, Oculomotor)

Primary Movement: Depression of the eyeball; movement is downward and inward.

Secondary Movements

1. Adduction of the eye
2. Rotation of the adducted eyeball so the upper end of the vertical axis is outward

8. Rectus medialis (III, Oculomotor)

Primary Movement: Adduction of the eyeball.

Secondary Movements: None.

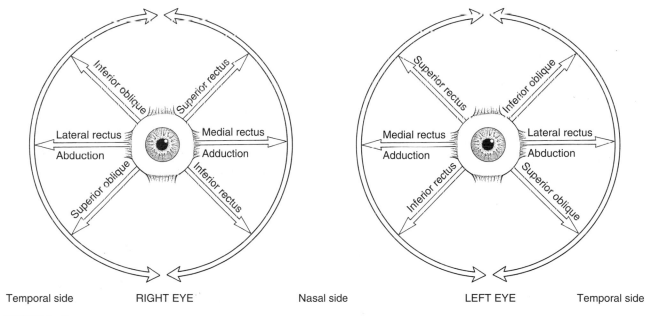

FIGURE 7–5.
Extraocular muscles and their actions. The six extraocular muscles enable each eye to move in a circular arc, usually accompanied by head movements, though head position is static during testing. The traditional pairing of extraocular muscles is an oversimplification of their movement patterns. In any ocular rotation all six muscles change length. The reference point for description of the motions of the extraocular muscles is the center of the cornea.

Eye Motions Continued

9. Rectus lateralis (VI, Abducent)

Primary Movement: Abduction of the eyeball.

Secondary Movements: None. VI nerve lesions limit lateral movement. In paralysis the eyeball is turned medially and cannot be abducted.

10. Obliquus superior (IV, Trochlear)

Primary Movement: Depression of the eye

Secondary Movements

1. Abduction of the eyeball.
2. IV nerve lesions limit depression, but abduction may be intact because abduction is the VI nerve.

11. Obliquus inferior (III, Oculomotor)

Primary Movement: Elevation of the eye, particularly from adduction; movement is upward and outward.

Secondary Movements

1. Abduction of the eyeball.
2. Rotation of the eyeball so the vertical axis is outward.
3. Note: In paralysis the eyeball is deviated downward and somewhat laterally; it cannot move upward when in abduction.
4. Note: In a III nerve lesion, the eye is outward and cannot be brought in. (This is often referred to irreverently as the "bum's eye," that is, down-and-out.) Such a lesion also results in ptosis, or drooping of the upper eyelid.[2,3]

Eye Tracking

Eye movements are tested by having the patient look in the cardinal directions (numbers in parentheses refer to tracks shown in Fig. 7–6).[2] All pairs in tracking are antagonists.

Laterally (1)	Upward and laterally (5)
Medially (2)	Upward and medially (7)
Upward (3)	Downward and medially (6)
Downward (4)	Downward and laterally (8)

Ask the patient to follow the examiner's slowly moving finger (or a pointer or flashlight) in each of the following tests. The object the patient is to follow should be at a comfortable reading distance. First, one eye is tested and then the other, covering the nontest eye. After single testing, both eyes are tested together for conjugate movements. Each test is started in the neutral position of the eye.

The range, speed, and smoothness of the motion should be observed as well as the ability to sustain lateral and vertical gaze.[2-4] The physical therapist will not be able to use these observational methods to distinguish movement deviations accurately because accuracy requires the sophisticated instrumentation used in ophthalmology. The tracking movements will appear normal or abnormal, but little else will be possible.

Position of Patient: Head and eyeball in neutral alignment, looking straight-ahead at examiner's finger to start. Head must remain static. If the patient turns the head while tracking the examiner's finger, the head will have to be held still with the examiner's other hand or by an assistant.

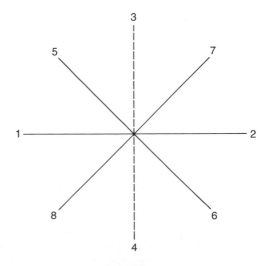

FIGURE 7–6

Eye Tracking Continued

Instructions to Patient: "Look at my finger. Follow it with your eyes" (Fig. 7–7).

Test: Test each eye separately by covering first one eye and then the other. Then test both eyes together.

Examples of two bilateral tests show conjugate motion in the two eyes when tracking upward and to the right (Fig. 7–8) and when tracking downward and to the left (Fig. 7–9).

Criteria for Grading

F: Immediate tracking in a smooth motion over the full range. Completes full excursion of the test movement.

WF and NF: Not possible to distinguish accurately from Grade F or Grade 0 without detailed diplopia testing (by ophthalmologist).

0: Tracking motion in a given test absent.

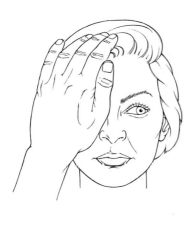
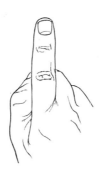

FIGURE 7–7

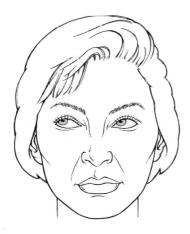

FIGURE 7–8.
Patient tracks upward and to the right. The patient's right eye shows motion principally with the Superior rectus; the left eye shows motion principally with the Inferior oblique.

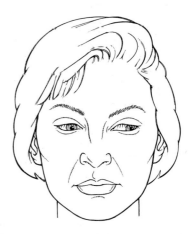

FIGURE 7–9.
Patient tracks downward and to the left. The right eye movement reflects principally the Superior oblique; the left eye shows motion principally with the Inferior rectus.

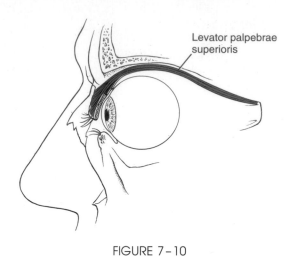

FIGURE 7-10

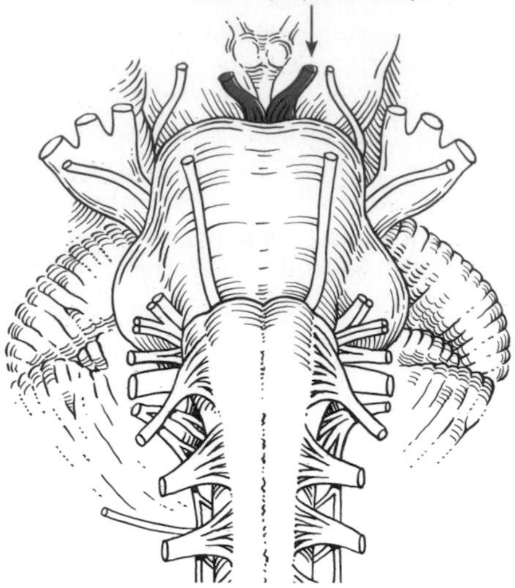

III Oculomotor
To: Levator palpebrae superioris

FIGURE 7-11

Table 7-2 MUSCLES OF THE EYELIDS AND EYEBROWS

I.D.	Muscle	Origin	Insertion
3	Levator palpebrae superioris	Sphenoid bone (lesser wing, inferior aspect) Roof of orbital cavity	Aponeurosis of orbital septum Superior tarsus of upper eyelid via aponeurosis Upper eyelid skin Sheath of Rectus superior
4	Orbicularis oculi (has three parts)	**Orbital Part** Frontal bone (nasal part) Maxilla (frontal process) Medial palpebral ligament	Blends with Occipitofrontalis and Corrugator supercilii Skin of the eyebrow
		Palpebral Part Medial palpebral ligament Frontal bone above and below ligament	Fibers form lateral palpebral raphe
		Lacrimal Part Lacrimal fascia Lacrimal bone (crest)	Tarsi (superior and inferior) of eyelids
5	Corrugator supercilii	Frontal bone (superciliary arch)	Deep skin of eyebrow (above supraorbital margin)

The face should be observed for mobility of expression, and any asymmetry or inadequacy of muscles should be documented. A one-sided appearance when talking or smiling, a lack of tone (with or without atrophy), the presence of fasciculations, asymmetrical or frequent blinking, smoothness of the face, or excessive wrinkling are all clues to VII nerve involvement.

The facial muscles (except for motions of the jaw) convey all emotions via voluntary and involuntary movements.

Eye Opening (3. Levator palpebrae superioris)

Opening the eye by raising the upper eyelid is a function of the Levator palpebrae superioris (see Fig. 7–10). The muscle should be evaluated by having the patient open and close the eye with and without resistance. The function of this muscle is assessed by its strength in maintaining a fully opened eye against resistance.

The patient with an oculomotor (III) nerve lesion will lose the function of the levator muscle, and the eyelid will droop in a partial or complete ptosis. (A patient with cervical sympathetic pathology may have a ptosis but will be able to raise the eyelid voluntarily.) Ptosis is evaluated by observing the amount of the iris that is covered by the eyelid.

In the presence of a facial (VII) nerve lesion the levator sign may be present.[2] In this case, the patient is asked to look downward and then slowly close the eyes. A positive levator sign is noted when the upper eyelid on the weak side moves upward because the action of the Levator palpebrae superioris is unopposed by the Orbicularis oculi.

Test: Patient attempts to keep the eyelids open against manual resistance (Fig. 7–12). Both eyes are tested at the same time. **NEVER PRESS ON THE EYEBALL FOR ANY REASON!**

Manual Resistance: The thumb or index finger is placed lightly over the opened eyelid above the lashes, and resistance is given in a downward direction (to close the eye). The examiner is cautioned to avoid depressing the eyeball into the orbit while giving resistance.

Instructions to Patient: "Open your eyes wide. Hold it. Don't let me close them."

Criteria for Grading

F: Completes normal range of movement and holds against examiner's light manual resistance. Iris will be fully visible.

WF: Can open eye but only partially uncovers the iris and takes no resistance. Patient may alternately open and close the lids, but excursion is small. The Frontalis muscle also may contract as the patient attempts to open the eye.

NF: Unable to open the eye, and the iris is almost completely covered.

0: No eyelid opening.

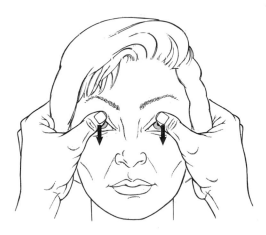

FIGURE 7–12

Peripheral vs. Central Lesions of the Facial (VII) Nerve

Involvement of the facial nerve may result from a lesion that affects the nerve or the nucleus, i.e., *a peripheral lesion*. Motor functions of the face also may be impaired after a central or supranuclear lesion. These two sites of interruption of the VII nerve lead to dissimilar clinical problems.[5]

The peripheral lesion results in a flaccid paralysis of all the muscles of the face *on the side of the lesion* (Occipitofrontalis, Corrugator, Orbicularis oculi, nose and mouth muscles). The affected side of the face becomes smooth, the eye remains open, the lower lid sags, and blinking does not completely close the eye; the nose is depressed and may deviate to the opposite side. The cheek muscles are flaccid, so the cheek appears hollow and the mouth is drawn to one side. Eating and drinking are difficult because chewing and retention of fluids and saliva are impaired. Speech sounds, especially vowels or sounds that require pursing of the lips, are slurred.

When the VII nerve is affected central to the nucleus, there is paresis of the muscles of the lower face but sparing of the muscles of the upper face. This occurs because the nuclear center that controls the upper face has both contralateral and ipsilateral supranuclear connections, whereas that which controls the lower face has only contralateral supranuclear innervation. For this reason, a lesion in one cerebral hemisphere causes paresis of the lower part of the face *on the contralateral side* and there is sparing of the upper facial muscles. This may be called a "central VII syndrome."

One notable difference between peripheral and central disorders is that peripheral lesions often (but certainly not always) result in paralysis of all facial muscles; central lesions leave some function even of the involved muscles and are, therefore, a paretic and not a paralytic problem.

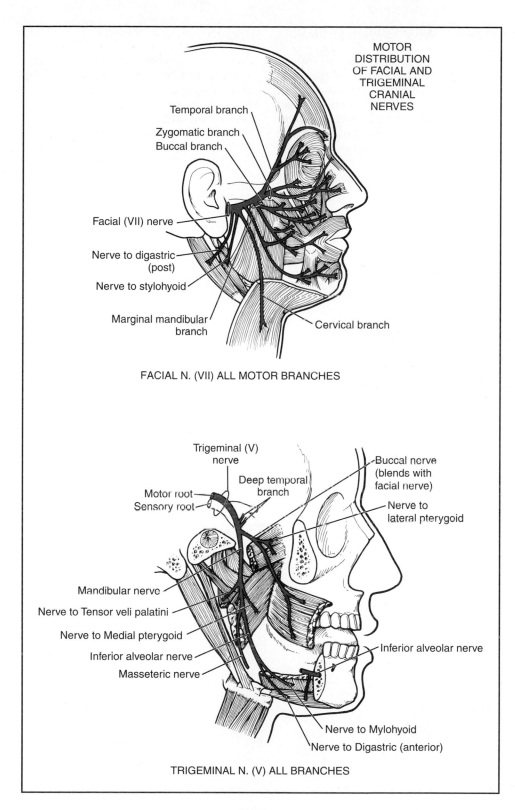

MOTOR DISTRIBUTION OF FACIAL AND TRIGEMINAL CRANIAL NERVES

Temporal branch
Zygomatic branch
Buccal branch
Facial (VII) nerve
Nerve to digastric (post)
Nerve to stylohyoid
Marginal mandibular branch
Cervical branch

FACIAL N. (VII) ALL MOTOR BRANCHES

Trigeminal (V) nerve
Deep temporal branch
Motor root
Sensory root
Buccal nerve (blends with facial nerve)
Nerve to lateral pterygoid
Mandibular nerve
Nerve to Tensor veli palatini
Nerve to Medial pterygoid
Inferior alveolar nerve
Masseteric nerve
Inferior alveolar nerve
Nerve to Mylohyoid
Nerve to Digastric (anterior)

TRIGEMINAL N. (V) ALL BRANCHES

PLATE 8

Closing the Eye (4. Orbicularis oculi)

The Orbicularis oculi muscle is the sphincter of the eye[1] (Fig. 7–13). Its lids are innervated by the facial (VII) nerve (temporal branch and zygomatic branch) (Figs. 7–14 and 7–15). Its palpebral portion closes the eyelids gently, as in blinking and sleep. The orbital portion of the muscle closes the eyes with greater force, as in winking. The lacrimal portion draws the eyelids laterally and compresses them against the sclera to receive tears. All portions act to close the eyes tightly (Fig. 7–16). Observation of the patient without specific testing will detect weakness of the Orbicularis because the blink will be delayed on the involved side.

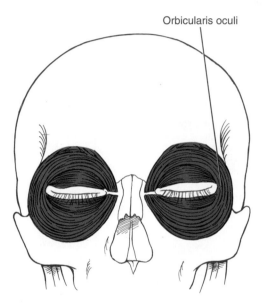

Orbicularis oculi

FIGURE 7–13

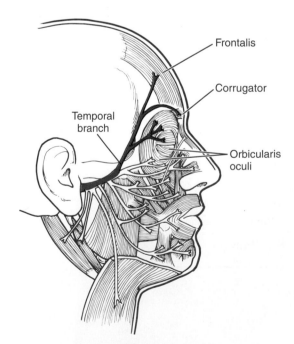

Frontalis

Corrugator

Temporal branch

Orbicularis oculi

FACIAL N. TEMPORAL BRANCH

FIGURE 7–14

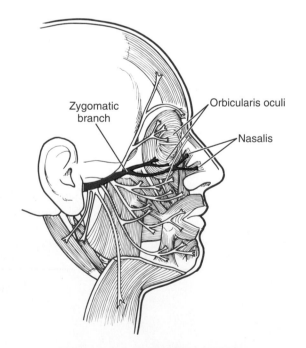

Zygomatic branch

Orbicularis oculi

Nasalis

FACIAL N. (VII) ZYGOMATIC BRANCH

FIGURE 7–15

Closing the Eye (4. Orbicularis oculi) Continued

Test: Observe the patient opening and closing the eyes voluntarily, first together and then singly (Fig. 7–16). (Single-eye closing is not a universal skill.) Patient closes eyes tightly, first together, then singly.

Rather than using resistance, the examiner may look at the depth to which the eyelashes are buried in the face when the eyes are closed tightly, noting whether the lashes are deeper on the uninvolved side.

Manual Resistance: Place the thumb and index finger below and above (respectively) each closed eye using a light touch (Fig. 7–17). The examiner attempts to open the eyelids by spreading the thumb and index finger apart. **REMINDER: NEVER PRESS ON THE EYEBALL FOR ANY REASON.**

Instructions to Patient: "Close your eyes as tightly as you can. Hold them closed. Don't let me open them" OR "Close your eye against my finger."

Criteria for Grading

F: Closes eyes tightly and holds against examiner's resistance. Iris may not be visible.

WF: Takes no resistance to eye closure; closure may be incomplete, but only a small amount of the sclera and no iris should be visible. There may be closure of the eye, but the eyelid on the weaker side may be delayed in contrast to the quick closure on the normal side.

NF: Unable to close eyes so that the iris is completely covered. (These patients may need artificial eyedrops to prevent drying of the eye.)

0: No evidence of Orbicularis oculi activity.

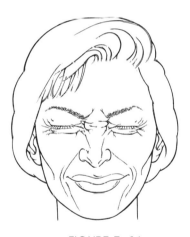

FIGURE 7–16

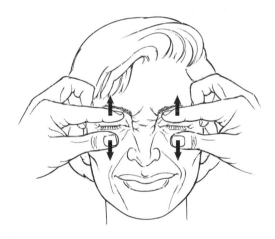

FIGURE 7–17

Helpful Hints

If in closing the eyes tightly, the eyeball rotates upward, the patient is exerting effort to perform the test correctly. This upward rotation of the eyeball is called Bell's phenomenon. If the patient is not exerting effort, all protestations to the contrary, the eyeball will remain in the neutral position. This observation may give the physical therapist a clue to other testing done with this kind of patient.

Frowning (5. Corrugator supercilii)

To observe the action of the Corrugator muscle (Fig. 7–18; see also Fig. 7–14), the patient is asked to frown. Frowning draws the eyebrows down and medially, producing vertical wrinkling of the forehead.

Test: Patient is asked to frown; the eyebrows are drawn down and together (Fig. 7–19).

Manual Resistance: The examiner uses the thumb (or index finger) of each hand placed gently at the nasal end of each eyebrow and attempts to move the eyebrows apart (smooths away the frown) (Fig. 7–20).

Instructions to Patient: "Frown. Don't let me erase it."

Criteria for Grading

F: Completes normal range (wrinkles are prominent) and holds against slight resistance.

WF: Frowns, but wrinkles are shallow and not too obvious; is unable to take resistance.

NF: Slight motion detected.

0: No frown.

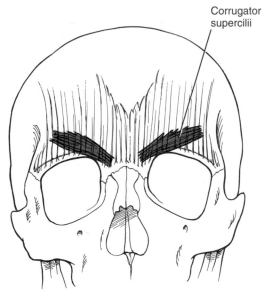

FIGURE 7–18

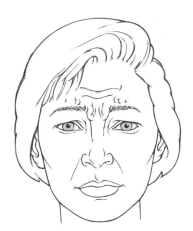

FIGURE 7–19

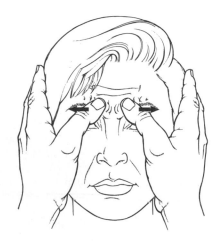

FIGURE 7–20

Raising the Eyebrows (1. Occipitofrontalis, frontalis part)

To examine the frontal belly of the Occipitofrontalis muscle (Fig. 7–21 and see Fig. 7–14) the patient is asked to create an expression of surprise where the forehead skin wrinkles horizontally. The occipital belly of the muscle is not tested usually, but it draws the scalp backward.

Test: Patient raises the eyebrows so that horizontal forehead lines appear (Fig. 7–22).

Manual Resistance: Examiner places the pad of a thumb above each eyebrow and applies resistance in a downward direction (smoothing the forehead) (Fig. 7–23).

Instructions to Patient: "Raise your eyebrows as high as you can. Don't let me pull them down."

Criteria for Grading

F: Completes movement; horizontal wrinkles are prominent. Tolerates considerable resistance.

WF: Wrinkles are shallow and easily erased by gentle resistance.

NF: Only slight motion detected.

0: No eyebrow raising.

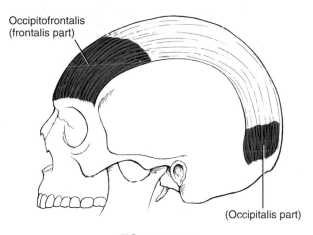

Occipitofrontalis
(frontalis part)

(Occipitalis part)

FIGURE 7–21

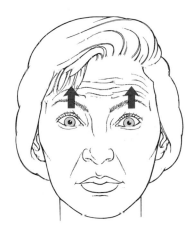

FIGURE 7–22

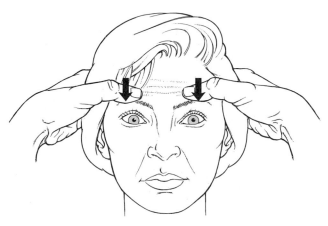

FIGURE 7–23

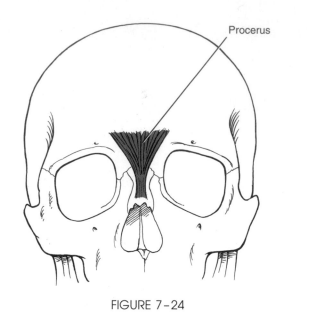

FIGURE 7-24

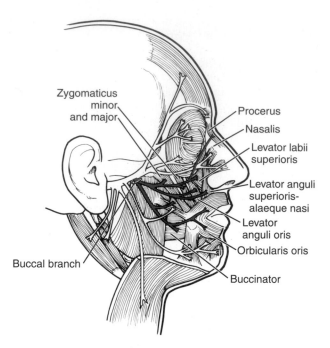

FACIAL N. (VII) BUCCAL BRANCH

FIGURE 7-25

Table 7-3 MUSCLES OF THE NOSE

I.D.	Muscle	Origin	Insertion
12	Procerus	Nasal bone apononeurosis Lateral nasal cartilage	Skin over lower forehead between eyebrows Joins Occipitofrontalis
13	Nasalis *Transverse part* (Compressor nares) *Alar part* (Dilator nares)	 Maxilla (above and lateral to incisive fossa) Maxilla (above lateral incisor) Alar cartilage	 Aponeurosis over bridge of nose Ala nasi cartilage at tip of nose Skin
14	Depressor septi*	Maxilla (above central incisor)	Nasal septum Alar cartilage

*The Depressor septi often is considered part of the Dilator nares.

The three muscles of the nose are all innervated by the facial (VII) nerve. The Procerus (Fig. 7–24) draws the medial angle of the eyebrows downward, causing transverse wrinkles across the bridge of the nose. The Nasalis (compressor nares) depresses the cartilaginous portion of the nose and draws the ala down toward the septum (see Fig. 7–15). The Nasalis (dilator nares) dilates the nostrils. The Depressor septi draws the alae downward, constricting the nostrils.

Of the three nose muscles only the Procerus is tested clinically. The others are observed with respect to nostril flaring and narrowing in patients who have such talent.

Wrinkling the Bridge of the Nose (12. Procerus)

Test: Patient wrinkles nose as if expressing distaste (Fig. 7–26).

Manual Resistance: The pads of the thumbs are placed beside the bridge of the nose, and resistance is given laterally (smoothing the creases) (Fig. 7–27).

Instructions to Patient: "Wrinkle your nose as if to say 'yuk.'"

Criteria for Grading

F: Prominent creases; patient tolerates some resistance.

WF: Shallow creases; patient yields to any resistance.

NF: Motion barely discernible.

0: No change of expression.

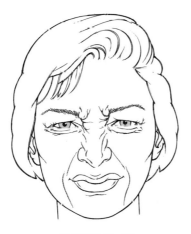

FIGURE 7–26

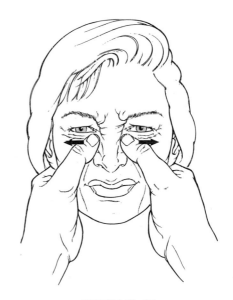

FIGURE 7–27

Helpful Hints

Isolated wrinkling of the nose is rare, and most patients bring in other facial muscles to perform this expressive movement.

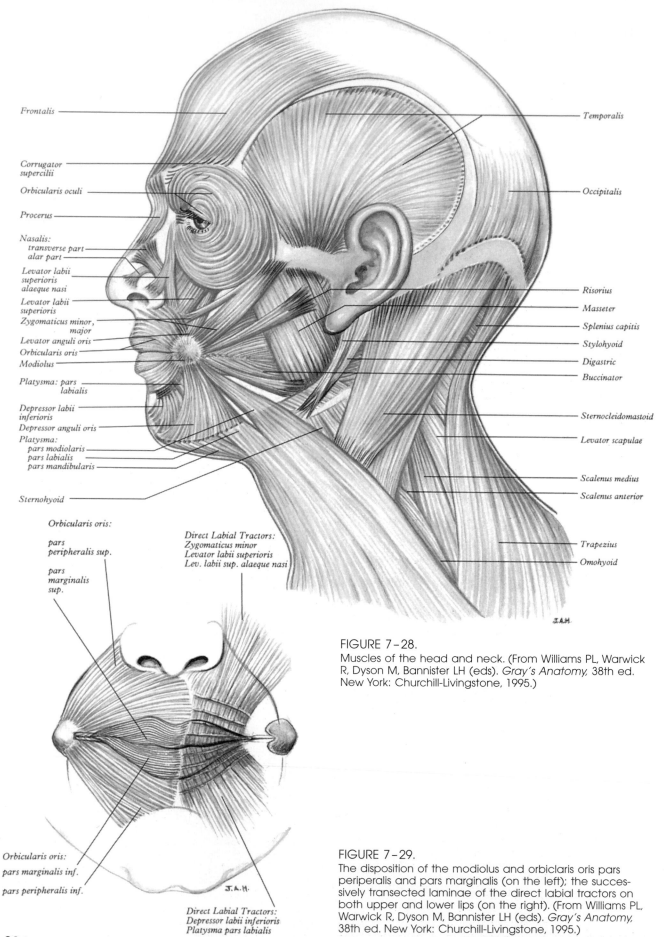

Frontalis

Corrugator
supercilii

Orbicularis oculi

Procerus

Nasalis:
  transverse part
  alar part

Levator labii
superioris
alaeque nasi

Levator labii
superioris

Zygomaticus minor,
  major

Levator anguli oris

Orbicularis oris

Modiolus

Platysma: pars
  labialis

Depressor labii
inferioris

Depressor anguli oris

Platysma:
  pars modiolaris
  pars labialis
  pars mandibularis

Sternohyoid

Temporalis

Occipitalis

Risorius

Masseter

Splenius capitis

Stylohyoid

Digastric

Buccinator

Sternocleidomastoid

Levator scapulae

Scalenus medius

Scalenus anterior

Trapezius

Omohyoid

FIGURE 7–28.
Muscles of the head and neck. (From Williams PL, Warwick R, Dyson M, Bannister LH (eds). *Gray's Anatomy*, 38th ed. New York: Churchill-Livingstone, 1995.)

Orbicularis oris:

pars
peripheralis sup.

pars
marginalis
sup.

Direct Labial Tractors:
Zygomaticus minor
Levator labii superioris
Lev. labii sup. alaeque nasi

Orbicularis oris:
pars marginalis inf.
pars peripheralis inf.

Direct Labial Tractors:
Depressor labii inferioris
Platysma pars labialis

FIGURE 7–29.
The disposition of the modiolus and orbiclaris oris pars periperalis and pars marginalis (on the left); the successively transected laminae of the direct labial tractors on both upper and lower lips (on the right). (From Williams PL, Warwick R, Dyson M, Bannister LH (eds). *Gray's Anatomy*, 38th ed. New York: Churchill-Livingstone, 1995.)

Table 7-4 MUSCLES OF THE MOUTH

I.D.	Muscle	Origin	Insertion
15	Levator labii superioris	Orbit of eye (inferior) Maxilla Zygomatic bone	Upper lip (no bony attachment)
17	Levator anguli oris	Maxilla (canine fossa)	Modiolus
18	Zygomaticus major	Zygomatic bone	Modiolus
24	Depressor labii inferioris	Mandible (between symphysis and mental foramen)	Skin and mucosa of lower lip Modiolus Blends with its paired muscle from opposite side and with Orbicularis oris
25	Orbicularis oris Accessory muscles: Incisivus labii superioris Incisivus labii inferioris	Modiolus No bony attachment	Modiolus Labial connective tissue Submucosa
26	Buccinator	Between maxilla and mandible (alveolar processes opposite molar teeth) Pterygomandibular raphe	Modiolus Submucosa of cheek and lips
21	Mentalis	Mandible (incisive fossa)	Skin over chin
23	Depressor anguli oris	Mandible (mental tubercle and oblique line)	Modiolus

Others

I.D.	Muscle
16	Levator labii superiorus alaeque nasi
19	Zygomaticus minor
20	Risorius
22	Transverse menti
88	Platysma

The Modiolus

The arrangement of the facial musculature often causes confusion and misunderstanding. This is not surprising since there are 14 small bundles of muscles running in various directions, with long names and unsupported functional claims. Of all the muscles of the face, those about the mouth may be the most important because they have responsibility for both ingestion of food and for speech.

One major source of confusion is the relationship between the muscles around the mouth. The common description until recently was of uninterrupted circumoral muscles. In fact, the Orbicularis oris muscle is not a complete ellipse but rather contains fibers from the major extrinsic muscles that converge on the buccal angle, as well as intrinsic fibers.[1,6,7] The authors and others do not describe complete ellipses, but most drawings illustrate such.[6]

The area on the face that has a large concentration of converging and diverging fibers from multiple directions lies immediately lateral and slightly above the corner of the mouth. Using the thumb and index finger on the outer skin and inside the mouth and compressing the tissue between them will quickly identify the knotlike structure known as the *modiolus*.[8–10]

The modiolus (from the Latin meaning nave of a wheel) is described as a muscular or tendinous node, a rather concentrated attachment of many muscles.[8–9] Its basic shape is conical (though this is oversimplified); it is about 1 cm thick and is found in most people about 1 cm lateral to the buccal angle. Its shape and size vary considerably with gender, race, and age. The muscular fibers enter and exit on different planes, superficial and deep, with some spiraling, but essentially they constitute a three-dimensional complexity.

Different classifications of modiolar muscles exist, but basically 9 or 10 facial muscles are associated with the structure:[9]

Radiating out from	Retractors of the upper lip
Levator anguli oris	Levator labii superioris
Orbicularis oris	Levator labii superioris alaeque nasi
Depressor anguli oris	Zyomaticus minor
Zygomaticus major	*Retractors and depressors of the lower lip*
Buccinator	Mentalis
	Depressor labii inferioris

Frequently associated are the special fibers of the Orbicularis oris (Incisive superior, Incisive inferior), Platysma, and Risorius (the latter is not a constant feature in the facial musculature).

The Orbicularis oris and the Buccinator form an almost continuous muscular sheet, which can be fixed in a number of positions by the Zygomaticus major, Levator anguli oris, and Depressor anguli oris (the latter three being the "stays" used to immobilize the modiolus in any position).

When the modiolus is firmly fixed, the Buccinator can contract to apply force to the cheek teeth; the Orbicularis oris can contract against the arch of the anterior teeth, thus sealing the lips together and closing the mouth tightly.[9] Similarly, control of the modiolar active and stay muscles enables accurate and fine control of lip movements and pressures in speech.

There are many muscles associated with the mouth, and all have some distinctive function, except perhaps the Risorius. Rather than detail a test for each, only definitive tests will be presented for the Buccinator and the Orbicularis oris (the sphincter of the mouth). The function of the remaining muscles is illustrated, and individual testing is left to the examiner. All muscles of the mouth are innervated by the facial (VII) nerve.

Lip Closing (25. Orbicularis oris)

This circumoral muscle (see Figs. 7–28 and 7–29) serves many functions for the mouth. It closes the lips, protrudes the lips, and holds the lips tight against the teeth. Furthermore, it shapes the lips for such functional uses as kissing, whistling, sucking, drinking, and the infinite shaping for articulation in speech. (For innervation see Fig. 7–25.)

Test: Patient compresses and protrudes the lips (Fig. 7–30).

Resistance: In deference to hygiene, a tongue blade rather than a finger is used to provide resistance. The flat side of the blade is placed diagonally across both the upper and lower lips, and resistance is applied inward toward the oral cavity (Fig. 7–31).

Instructions to Patient: "Purse your lips. Hold it. Push against the tongue blade."

Criteria for Grading

F: Completely seals lips and holds against relatively strong resistance.

WF: Closes lips but is unable to take resistance.

NF: Has some lip movement but is unable to bring lips together.

0: No closure of the lips.

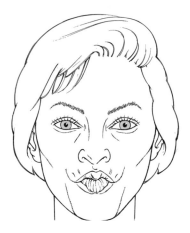

FIGURE 7–30

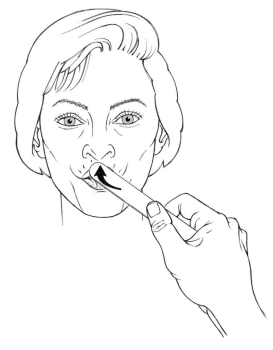

FIGURE 7–31

Cheek Compression (26. Buccinator)

The Buccinator (see Fig. 7–28) is a prime muscle used for positioning food for chewing and for controlling the passage of the bolus. It also compresses the cheek against the teeth and acts to expel air when the cheeks are distended (blowing). (For innervation see Fig. 7–25.)

Test: Patient compresses the cheeks (bilaterally) by drawing them into the mouth (Fig. 7–32).

Resistance: A tongue blade is used for resistance. The blade is placed inside the mouth, its flat side lying against the cheek (Fig. 7–33). Resistance is given by levering the blade inward against the cheek (at the angle of the mouth), which will cause the flat blade to push the test cheek outward.

Alternatively, the gloved index fingers of the examiner may be used to offer resistance. In this case, the index fingers are placed in the mouth (the left finger to the inside of the patient's left cheek and vice versa). The fingers are used simultaneously to try to push the cheeks outward. Use caution in this form of the test for patients with cognitive impairment (lest they bite!) or with those who have a bite reflex.

Instructions to Patient: "Suck in your cheeks. Hold. Don't let me push them out."

Criteria for Grading

F: Performs movement correctly and holds against strong resistance.

WF: Performs movement but is unable to hold against any resistance.

NF: Movement is detectable but not complete.

0: No motion of cheeks occurs.

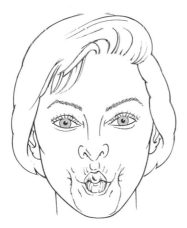

FIGURE 7–32

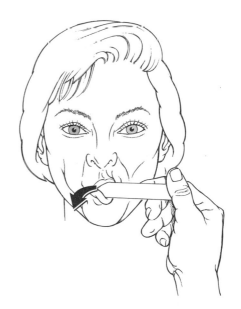

FIGURE 7–33

Other Oral Muscles

17. Levator anguli oris (for innervation see Fig. 7–25)

This muscle elevates the angles of the mouth and reveals the teeth in smiling. When used unilaterally, it conveys the expression of sneering (Fig. 7–34). The muscle creates the nasolabial furrow, which deepens in expressions of sadness and with aging.

15. Levator labii superioris (see Figs. 7–25, 7-28, and 7–29)

This muscle raises and pushes out the upper lip and modifies the nasolabial fold (or furrow), which runs from the end of the nose to flatten out over the cheek. It is a prominent feature of the subnasal area in many people and deepens in sadness and sometimes anger.

16. Levator labii superior alaeque nasi (see Fig. 7–25)

These two Levator labii muscles (15 and 16) elevate the upper lip (Fig. 7–35). The labii superioris also protracts the upper lip, and the alaeque nasi dilates the nostrils.

18. Zygomaticus major (see Fig. 7–28)

The major Zygomaticus muscles draw the angles of the mouth upward and laterally as in laughing (Fig. 7–36).

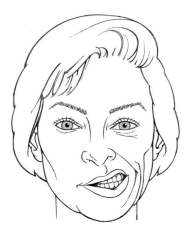

FIGURE 7–34

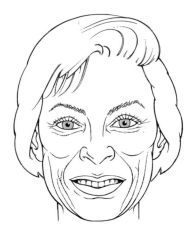

FIGURE 7–36

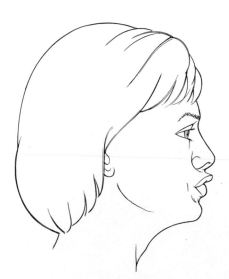

FIGURE 7–35

Other Oral Muscles Continued

21. Mentalis (see Fig. 7–37)

The Mentalis protrudes the lower lip as in pouting or sulking (Fig. 7–38).

23. Depressor anguli oris (see Fig. 7–37)

The anguli oris crosses the midline to meet with its fellow muscles of the opposite side, forming the "mental sling". It draws down the angle of the mouth, giving an appearance of deep sadness (see Fig. 7–38).

88. Platysma

These muscles depress the lower lip and the buccal angle of the mouth to give an expression of grief or sadness (Fig. 7–39). The Platysma draws the lower lip backward, producing an expression of horror, and it pulls up the skin of the neck from the clavicle (evoking the expression of "egad!"). This muscle may be tested by asking the patient to open the mouth against resistance or bite the teeth together tightly (see also Fig. 7–40).

24. Depressor labii inferioris

This muscle draws the lower lip down and laterally, producing an expression of melancholy or irony (Fig. 7–41).

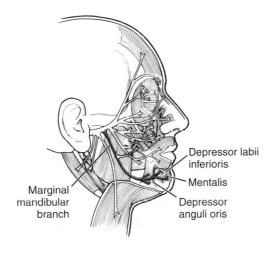

FACIAL N. (VII) MARGINAL MANDIBULAR BRANCH

FIGURE 7–37

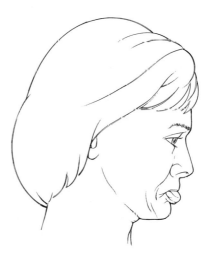

FIGURE 7–38

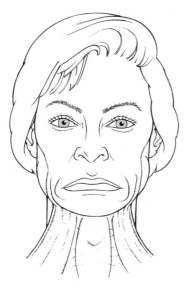

FIGURE 7–39

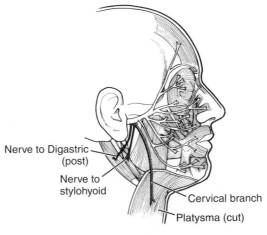

FACIAL N. (VII) CERVICAL BRANCH

FIGURE 7–40

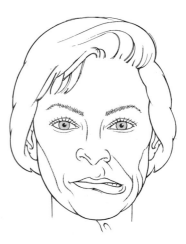

FIGURE 7–41

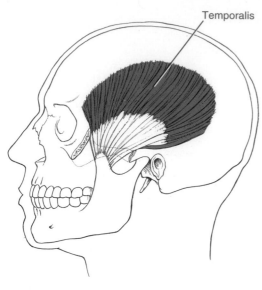

FIGURE 7-42

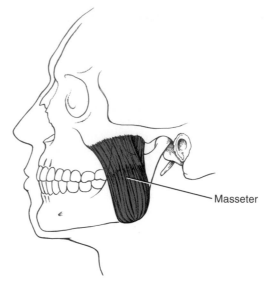

FIGURE 7-43

Table 7-5 MUSCLES OF MASTICATION

I.D.	Muscle	Origin	Insertion
28	Masseter (has three layers)		
	Superficial	Zygomatic bone (maxillary process)	
		Maxilla zygomatic arch (inferior border)	Mandible (posterior and lateral ramus)
	Intermediate	Zygomatic arch (medial part of anterior 2/3)	Mandible (ramus)
	Deep	Zygomatic arch (posterior 1/3)	Mandible (ramus)
29	Temporalis	Temporal bone (whole fossa) Temporal fascia (deep surface)	Mandible (tendon to coronoid process; ramus near last molar)
30	Lateral pterygoid (has two heads)		*Both heads*
	Superior	Sphenoid bone (greater wing and its crest)	Mandible (condylar neck)
	Inferior	Sphenoid bone (lateral pterygoid plate)	Temporomandibular joint (articular capsule and disc)
31	Medial pterygoid	Sphenoid bone (lateral pterygoid plate, medial surface) Palatine bone (pyramidal process) Maxilla (tuberosity)	Mandible (ramus and angle)
75	Mylohyoid	Mandible (length of mylohyoid line)	Hyoid bone (front of body)
76	Stylohyoid	Temporal bone (styloid process)	Hyoid bone (body at junction with greater cornu)
77	Geniohyoid	Mandible (symphysis menti)	Hyoid bone (anterior aspect)
78	Digastric (has two bellies joined by tendon)		
	Posterior belly	Temporal bone (mastoid notch)	Hyoid bone and greater cornu (two bellies meet in intermediate tendon which passes in a fibrous sling attached to hyoid bone)
	Anterior belly	Mandible (digastric fossa)	

Others

Infrahyoids (2)

| 84 | Sternothyroid |
| 86 | Sternohyoid |

Muscles of Mastication (28. Masseter, 29. Temporalis, 30. Lateral pterygoid, 31. Medial pterygoid)

The mandible is the only moving bone in the skull, and mandibular motion is largely related to chewing and speech. The muscles that control the jaw are all near the rear of the mandible (on the various surfaces and processes of the ramus), where they contribute considerable force for chewing and biting.[1] The muscles of mastication move the mandible forward (protraction) and backward (retraction), as well as shift it laterally. Excursion of the mandible is customarily limited somewhat, except in trained singers, who learn to open the mouth very wide to add to their vocal repertoire. The velocity of motions used for chewing is relatively slow, but for speech motions it is very rapid.

The muscles of mastication are all innervated by the motor division of the V (trigeminal) nerve (see Plate 8, page 299). The Masseter elevates and protrudes the mandible. The Temporalis elevates and retracts the mandible. The Lateral pterygoids, (Fig. 7–44) acting in concert, protrude and depress the mandible; when one acts alone, it causes lateral movement to the opposite side. The Medial pterygoids (see Fig. 7–44) acting together elevate and protrude the mandible along with the Lateral pterygoids, but acting alone they draw the mandible forward with deviation to the opposite side (as in chewing). The suprahyoid muscles (see Figs. 7–45 and 7–46), acting via the hyoid bone, aid in jaw depression when the hyoid is fixed. The infrahyoids are weak accessories to jaw depression.

Lesions of the motor division result in weakness or paralysis of the motions of elevating, depressing, protruding, and rotating the mandible. In a unilateral lesion the jaw deviates to the weak side; in a bilateral lesion the jaw sags and is "paralyzed." The jaw should be examined for muscle tone, atrophy (jaw contour), and fasciculations.

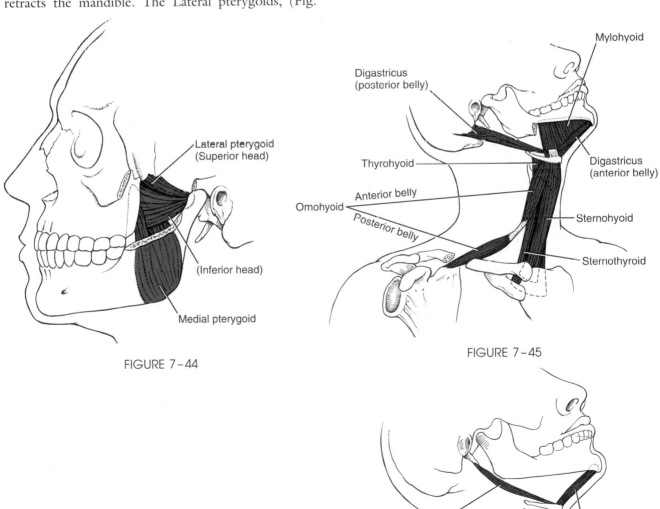

FIGURE 7–44

FIGURE 7–45

FIGURE 7–46

Jaw Opening (Mandibular Depression)
(30. Lateral pterygoid, 75–78. Suprahyoid Muscles)

Note: Prior to testing the jaw muscles, the temporo-mandibular joint should be checked for tenderness and crepitus. If either is present, manual testing is avoided, and jaw opening and closing are simply observed.

Test: Patient opens the mouth as far as possible and holds against manual resistance.

Manual Resistance: One hand of the examiner is cupped under the chin; the other hand is placed on the crown of the head for stabilization (Fig. 7–47). Resistance is given in a vertical upward direction in an attempt to close the jaw.

Instructions to Patient: "Open your mouth as wide as you can. Hold it. Don't let me close it."

Criteria for Grading

F: Completes available range and holds against strong resistance. Indeed, this muscle is so powerful that in the normal person it can rarely be overcome with manual resistance. The mouth opening should accommodate three (sometimes four) stacked fingers (in an average-sized person), or 35 to 40 mm. There should be no deviation except downward.

WF: Can open mouth to accommodate two or fewer stacked fingers and can take some resistance.

NF: Minimal motion occurs. The Lateral pterygoid can be palpated with a gloved finger inside the mouth, with the tip directed posteriorly past the last upper molar to the condyloid process of the ramus of the mandible. No resistance is tolerated.

0: No voluntary mandibular depression occurs.

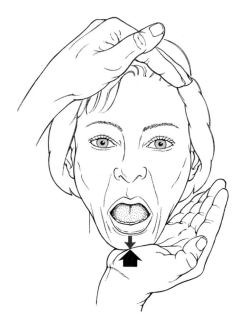

FIGURE 7–47

Jaw Closure (Mandibular Elevation) (28. Masseter, 29. Temporalis, 31. Medial pterygoid)

Test: Patient clenches jaws tightly (for innervation see Plate 8, page 299).

Manual Resistance: The chin of the patient is grasped between the thumb and index finger of the examiner and held firmly in the thumb web. The other hand is placed on top of the head for stability. Resistance is given vertically downward in an attempt to open the closed jaw (Fig. 7–48).

Instructions to Patient: "Clench (or hold) your teeth together as tightly as you can, keeping your lips relaxed. Hold it. Don't let me open your mouth."

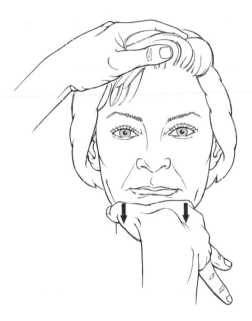

FIGURE 7–48

Criteria for Grading

F: Patient closes mouth (jaw) tightly. Examiner should not be able to open the mouth. This is a very strong muscle group. Consider circus performers who hang by their teeth!

WF: Patient closes jaw, but examiner can open the mouth with less than maximal resistance.

NF: Patient closes mouth but tolerates no resistance. The Masseter and Temporalis muscles are palpated on both sides. The Masseter is palpated under the zygomatic process on the lateral cheek above the angle of the jaw. The Temporalis muscle is palpated over the temple at the hairline, anterior to the ear and superior to the zygomatic bone.

0: Patient cannot completely close the mouth. This is more of a cosmetic problem (drooling, for example) than a significant clinical one.

In unilateral involvement, the jaw deviates to the strong side during attempts to close the mouth.

Alternate Test Procedure
The patient is asked to bite hard on a tongue blade with the molar teeth. Comparison of the depth of the bite marks from each side of the jaw is an indication of strength. If the examiner can pull out the tongue blade while the patient is biting, there is weakness of the Masseter, Temporalis, and Lateral pterygoid muscles. (Note: This method of testing should never be used with a patient who has a bite reflex or the patient may break the blade and be injured by the splinters.)

Lateral Jaw Deviation (30. Lateral pterygoid, 31. Medial pterygoid)

When the patient deviates the jaw to the right, the acting muscles are the right Lateral pterygoid and the left Medial pterygoid. Deviation to the left is supported by the left Lateral pterygoid and the right Medial pterygoid.

With weakness of the pterygoids, when the patient opens the mouth there will be deviation to the side of the weakness.

The patient moves the jaw side to side against resistance. In V nerve involvement the patient can move the jaw to the paralyzed side but not to the unaffected side.

Test: Patient deviates jaw to the right and then to the left (for innervation see Plate 8, page 299).

Manual Resistance: One hand of the examiner is used for resistance and is placed with the palmar side of the fingers against the jaw (Fig. 7–49). The other hand is placed with the fingers and palm against the opposite temple to stabilize the head. Resistance is given in a lateral direction to move the jaw toward the midline.

Criteria for Grading

F: The range of motion for jaw lateral deviation is variable. Deviation is assessed by comparing the relationship between the upper and lower incisor teeth when the jaw is moved laterally from the midline. Do not assess deviation by the position of the lips. A pencil or ruler lined up vertically with the center of the nose may indicate mandibular deviation.

Most people can move the center point of the lower incisors laterally over three upper teeth (approximately 10 mm).[5] The patient tolerates strong resistance.

WF: Motion is decreased to lateral movement across one upper tooth, and resistance is minimal.

N: Minimal deviation occurs, and no resistance is taken.

0: No motion occurs.

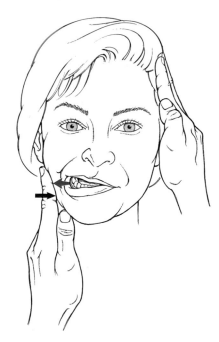

FIGURE 7–49

Jaw Protrusion (30. Lateral pterygoids, 31. Medial pterygoids)

The Medial and Lateral pterygoids act to protrude the jaw, which gives the face a pugnacious expression. The protrusion causes a malocclusion of the teeth, the lower teeth projecting beyond the upper teeth. With a unilateral lesion, the protruding jaw deviates to the weak side.

Test: Patient protrudes jaw so the lower teeth project beyond the upper teeth (for innervation see Plate 8, page 299).

Manual Resistance: This is a powerful motion. The examiner stabilizes the head with one hand placed behind the head (Fig. 7–50). The hand for resistance cups the chin in the thumb web with the thumb and index finger grasping the mandible. Resistance is given horizontally backward.

Instructions to Patient: "Push your jaw forward. Hold it. Don't let me push it back."

Criteria for Grading

F: Completes a range that moves the lower teeth in front of the upper teeth and can hold against strong resistance. There is sufficient space between the teeth in most people to see a gap between the upper and lower teeth.

WF: Moves jaw slightly forward but there is no discernible gap between the upper and lower teeth, and the patient tolerates only slight resistance.

NF: Minimal motion is detected, and the patient takes no resistance.

0: No motion and no resistance occur.

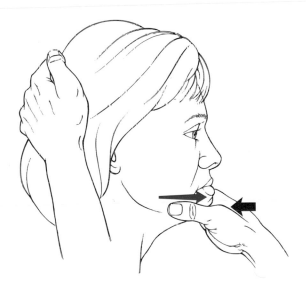

FIGURE 7–50

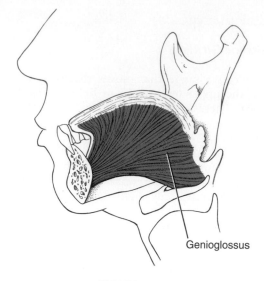

FIGURE 7-51

Genioglossus

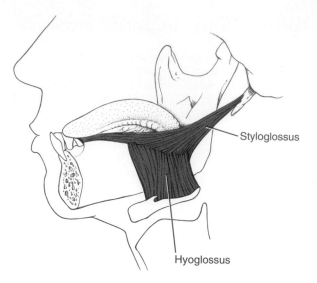

Styloglossus

Hyoglossus

FIGURE 7-52

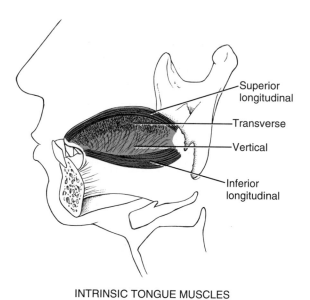

Superior
longitudinal

Transverse

Vertical

Inferior
longitudinal

INTRINSIC TONGUE MUSCLES

FIGURE 7-53

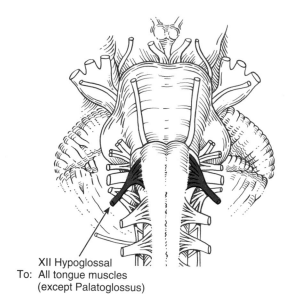

XII Hypoglossal
To: All tongue muscles
(except Palatoglossus)

FIGURE 7-54

Table 7-6 MUSCLES OF THE TONGUE

I.D.	Muscle	Origin	Insertion
Extrinsic Muscles			
32	Genioglossus	Mandible (symphysis menti on inner surface of superior mental spine)	Hyoid bone (upper anterior side) Tongue (posterior, and ventral surfaces) Blends with middle pharyngeal constrictor
33	Hyoglossus	Hyoid bone (greater cornu and side of body)	Tongue (merges on side with intrinsics)
34	Chondroglossus	Hyoid bone (lesser cornu and medial body)	Tongue (blends with intrinsic muscles on side)
35	Styloglossus	Temporal bone (styloid process, near apex) Stylomandibular ligament	Tongue (side then blends with intrinsics)
36	Palatoglossus	Soft palate (anterior)	Tongue (side to blend with Transverse lingual)
Others			
75–78	Suprahyoid muscles		
Intrinsic Muscles			
37	Superior longitudinal	Tongue (oblique and longitudinal fibers on root and superior surface)	Tongue (to lingual margins)
38	Inferior longitudinal	Root of tongue (inferior surface)	Tongue (at tip) Hyoid bone (body) Blends with Styloglossus
39	Transverse lingual	Median lingual septum	Tongue (dorsum and lateral margins) (Blends with Palatopharyngeus)
40	Vertical	Tongue (dorsum, anterolateral)	Tongue (ventral surface)

The extrinsic and intrinsic muscles of the tongue except the Palatoglossus are innervated by the hypoglossal (XII) cranial nerve, a pure motor nerve. One XII nerve innervates half of the tongue (unilaterally). The hypoglossal nucleus, however, receives both crossed (mostly) and uncrossed (to a lesser extent) upper motor neuron fibers from the lowest part of the precentral gyrus via the internal capsule. Lesions of the XII nerve or its central connections may cause tongue paresis or paralysis.

Description of Tongue Muscles

The paired extrinsic muscles pass from the skull or the hyoid bone to the tongue. The intrinsic muscles rise and end within the tongue. The bulk of the tongue structure is muscle.

The principal muscle of the tongue is the Genioglossus. It is a triangular muscle whose apex arises from the apex of the mandible, which is hard and immobile; its base inserts into the base of the tongue, which is soft and mobile. The Genioglossus (Fig. 7–51) is the principal tongue protractor, and it has crossed supranuclear innervation. The posterior fibers of the paired Genioglossi draw the root of the tongue forward; a single Genioglossus pushes the tongue toward the opposite side. The anterior fibers of the paired muscles draw the tongue back into the mouth after protrusion and depress it. The Genioglossi acting together also depress the central part of the tongue, making it a tube.

The Hyoglossi (paired) (Fig. 7–52) and the Chondroglossi retract and depress the sides of the tongue, making the superior surface convex. The two Styloglossi (see Fig. 7–52) draw the tongue upward and backward and elevate the sides, causing a dorsal transverse concavity.

The Suprahyoid muscles influence the movements of the tongue via their action on the hyoid bone.

The intrinsic tongue muscles (Fig. 7–53) are similarly innervated by the XII nerve (Fig. 7–54). The Superior longitudinal muscle shortens the tongue and curls its tip upward; the Inferior longitudinal shortens the tongue and curls its tip downward. Their combined function is to alter the shape of the tongue in almost infinite variations to provide the tongue with the versatility required for speech and swallowing.

One test of a tongue motion used by therapists is called "channeling" in which the tongue is curled longitudinally; this motion may be considered to assist in sucking and directing the bolus of food into the pharynx. The difficulty presented with this motion, however, is that it is not a constant motion but rather a dominantly inherited trait that only 50 percent of the population can perform. Testing it is all right as long as the inability to perform the motion is not considered a neurologic deficiency.

Examination of the Tongue

The tongue is a restless muscle, and when testing it, minor deviations are best ignored.[4] The test should start with observation of the tongue at rest on the floor of the mouth and then with the tongue protruded. The tongue is observed as it is curled up and down over the lip and then when the margins are elevated; both motions should be performed both slowly and rapidly. In all tests the ability to change the shape of the tongue is observed, but especially in tipping and channeling. One listens for difficulty in enunciation, especially of consonants.

The examiner must become familiar with the contour and mass of the normal tongue. The tongue should be examined for atrophy, which is evidenced by decreased mass, corrugations on the sides, and longitudinal furrowing. Unilateral atrophy is easy to detect and is usually accompanied by deviation to that side. When there is bilateral atrophy, the tongue will protrude weakly if at all, and deviation also will be weak.

Fasciculations are easily visible in the tongue at rest (the surface of the tongue appears to be in constant motion) and can be separated from the normal tremulous motions that occur in the protruded tongue. The "tremors" that are a part of supranuclear lesions disappear when the tongue is at rest in the mouth, whereas the fasciculations of motor neuron disease such as amyotrophic lateral sclerosis continue. The hyperkinesias of parkinsonism are exaggerated when the tongue is protruded or during talking.

The therapist proceeds to examine protrusion and deviation of the tongue at slow and fast speeds. The normal tongue can move in and out (in the midline) with vigor and usually protrudes quite far beyond the lips.[11] The tongue deviates to the side of a weakness whether the cause of that weakness is a disturbance of the upper motor neuron (supranuclear disturbance) or the lower motor neuron (infranuclear disturbance).

Unilateral Weakness of the Tongue: At rest in the mouth, the tongue with a unilateral weakness may deviate slightly to the uninvolved side because of the unopposed action of the Styloglossus.[11] The protruded tongue will deviate to the weak side and show weakness or inability to deviate to the normal side. Tipping may be normal because the intrinsic

muscles are preserved. These functions may be impossible to evaluate if the clinical picture includes facial and jaw muscle weakness.

Early in the course of the disorder, before the onset of atrophy, the weak side of the tongue may appear enlarged and may ride higher in the mouth. After the onset of atrophy the weak side becomes smaller, furrowed, and corrugated on the lateral edge. A unilateral weakness of the tongue may result in few functional problems, and speech and swallowing may be minimally disturbed if at all.

Bilateral Paresis: In persons with bilateral lesions, the tongue cannot be protruded or moved laterally. There will be indistinct speech, and swallowing may be difficult. Some patients experience interference with breathing when swallowing is impaired because the tongue may fall back into the throat. Total paralysis of the tongue muscles is rare (except in brain stem lesions or advanced motor neuron disease).

Supranuclear versus Infranuclear Lesions: In the presence of a supranuclear XII nerve lesion (central), the protruded tongue will deviate to the side of the weakness, which is the side opposite to the cerebral lesion. There is no atrophy of the tongue muscles. The tongue muscles also may evidence spasticity.[11]

In dyskinetic states (athetosis, chorea, seizures, and so on) the tongue may protrude involuntarily as well as deviate to the opposite side. This is accompanied by other generally slow involuntary tongue movements that make speech thick and slow and difficult to understand.

Patients with hemiparesis following a vascular lesion (a unilateral corticobulbar lesion) may have a variety of bulbar symptoms, including tongue muscle dysfunction. In common with other bulbar manifestations, these symptoms generally are moderate and subside with time or are well compensated, so that little functional disability persists.[5] Only in patients with a second stroke or a bilateral stroke (because these muscles have bilateral cortical innervation) will the bulbar signs persist.

Inability to flick the tongue in and out of the mouth quickly (after some practice) may indicate a bilateral supranuclear lesion. In an infranuclear (peripheral) nerve lesion, the tongue will deviate to the side of the weakness, which also is the side of the lesion. There will be atrophy of the tongue muscles. Bilateral atrophy most commonly is caused by motor neuron disease. The tongue also may be weak in myasthenia gravis (fatiguing after a series of protrusions), but there will be no atrophy.

The distinction between a lower motor neuron lesion and an upper motor neuron lesion of the XII nerve depends on the presence of supporting evidence of other upper motor neuron signs and on the presence of classic lower motor neuron signs such as hemiatrophy, unilateral fasciculations, and obvious deviation to the side of the paralysis when the tongue is protruded.[4]

Tongue Protrusion, Deviation, Retraction, Posterior Elevation, Channeling, and Curling

Test for Protrusion (32. Genioglossus, Posterior Fibers)

Patient protrudes tongue so that the tip extends out beyond the lips.

Manual Resistance: Examiner uses a tongue blade against the tip of the tongue and provides resistance in a backward direction to the forward motion of the tongue (Fig. 7–55).

Instructions to Patient: "Stick out your tongue. Hold it. Don't let me push it in."

Test for Tongue Deviation (32. Genioglossus and Other Muscles)

Patient protrudes tongue and moves it to one side and then to the other.

Manual Resistance: Using a tongue blade, resist the lateral tongue motion along the side of the tongue near the tip (Fig. 7–56). Resistance is given in the direction opposite to the attempted deviation.

Instructions to Patient: "Stick out your tongue and move it to the right." (Repeat for left side.)

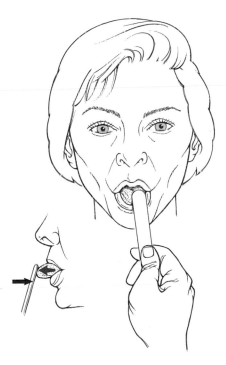

FIGURE 7–55

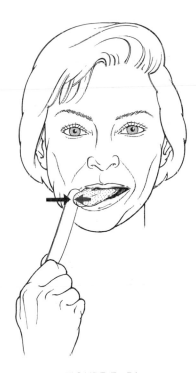

FIGURE 7–56

Tongue Protrusion, Deviation, Retraction, Posterior Elevation, Channeling, and Curling Continued

Test for Tongue Retraction (32. Genioglossus (anterior fibers), 35. Styloglossus)

Patient retracts tongue from a protruded position.

Manual Resistance: Holding a 3 × 4 gauze pad, securely grasp the anterior tongue by its upper and under sides (Fig. 7–57). Resist retraction by holding the tongue firmly and gently pulling it forward. (The tongue is very slippery, but be careful not to pinch.)

Instructions to Patient: (Tell patient you are going to grasp the tongue.) "Stick out your tongue. Now pull your tongue back. Don't let me keep it out."

Test for Posterior Elevation of the Tongue (36. Palatoglossus, 35. Styloglossus)

Patient elevates (i.e., "humps") the dorsum of the posterior tongue.

Manual Resistance: Examiner places tongue blade on the superior surface of the tongue over the anterior one-third. Placing the blade too far back will initiate an unwanted gag reflex (Fig. 7–58). Resistance is applied in a down and backward direction, as in levering the tongue blade down, using the bottom teeth as a fulcrum (Fig. 7–59).

Instructions to Patient: This is a difficult motion for the patient to understand. After directions are given, time is allowed for practice.

Begin the test by rocking the tongue blade back and forth so the patient experiences pressure on the middle to the back of the tongue.

"Push against this stick."

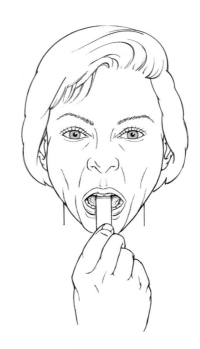

FIGURE 7–58

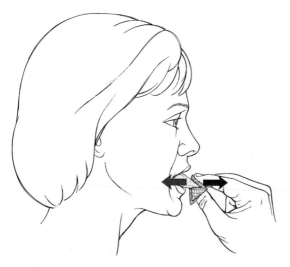

FIGURE 7–57

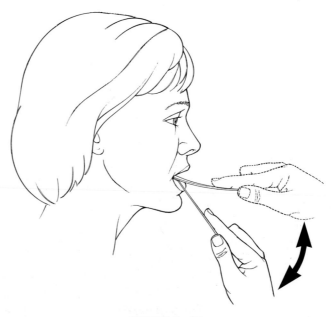

FIGURE 7–59

Tongue Protrusion, Deviation, Retraction, Posterior Elevation, Channeling, and Curling Continued

Test for Channeling the Tongue (32. Genioglossus, 37–40. Intrinsic tongue muscles)

Patient draws tongue downward and rolls sides up to make a longitudinal channel or tube, which is part of sucking and directing a bolus of food into the pharynx (Fig. 7–60). Inability to perform this motion should not be recorded as a deficit because the motion is a dominantly inherited trait, and its presence or absence should be treated as such.

Manual Resistance: None

Instructions to Patient: Demonstrate tongue motion to the patient. "Make a tube with your tongue."

Test for "Tipping" or Curling the Tongue (37, 38. Superior and Inferior longitudinals)

Patient protrudes tongue and curls it upward to touch the philtrum and then downward to the chin (Fig. 7–61).

Manual Resistance: None

Instructions to Patient: "Touch above your upper lip with your tongue."
"Touch your tongue to your chin."

Criteria for Grading Tongue Motions

F: Patient completes available range and holds against resistance.

Protrusion: Tongue extends considerably beyond lips.

Deviation: Tongue reaches some part of the cheek or the lateral sulcus (pocket between teeth and cheek).
Retraction: Tongue returns to rest position in mouth against resistance.
Elevation: Tongue rises so that superior surface reaches the hard palate against considerable resistance; it blocks the oral cavity from the oropharynx.
Tipping: Tongue protrudes and touches area between upper lip and nasal septum (philtrum).

WF
Protrusion: Tongue reaches margin of lips.
Deviation: Tongue reaches corner(s) of mouth.
Retraction: Tongue returns to rest posture but with slight resistance.
Elevation: Tongue reaches hard palate with slight resistance, and oral cavity is blocked from oropharynx.
Tipping: Tongue protrudes and curls but does not reach philtrum.

NF
Protrusion: Minimal protrusion and tongue does not clear mouth.
Deviation: Tongue protrudes and deviates slightly to side.
Retraction: Tongue tolerates no resistance and retracts haltingly.
Elevation: Tongue moves toward hard palate but does not occlude oropharynx from oral cavity.

0

All motions: None

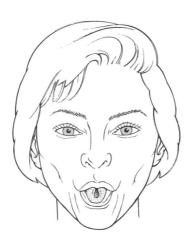

FIGURE 7–60

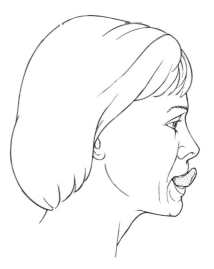

FIGURE 7–61

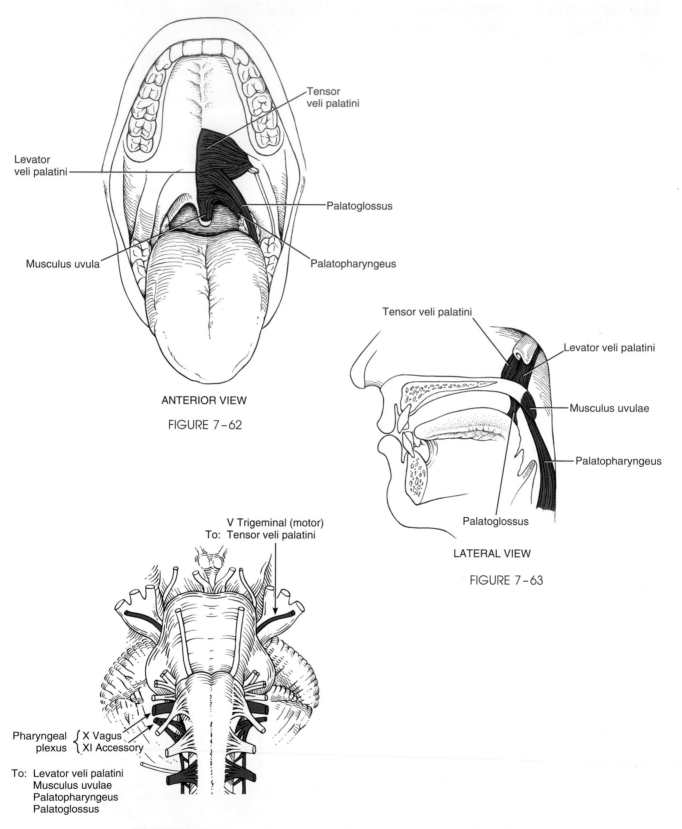

Tensor
veli palatini

Levator
veli palatini

Palatoglossus

Musculus uvula

Palatopharyngeus

ANTERIOR VIEW

FIGURE 7–62

Tensor veli palatini

Levator veli palatini

Musculus uvulae

Palatopharyngeus

Palatoglossus

LATERAL VIEW

FIGURE 7–63

V Trigeminal (motor)
To: Tensor veli palatini

Pharyngeal {X Vagus
plexus {XI Accessory

To: Levator veli palatini
Musculus uvulae
Palatopharyngeus
Palatoglossus

FIGURE 7–64

Table 7-7 MUSCLES OF THE PALATE

I.D.	Muscle	Origin	Insertion
46	Levator veli palatini	Temporal bone Tympanic fascia Auditory (pharyngotympanic) tube (cartilage)	Palatine aponeurosis (Interlaces with its contralateral muscle to form a sling)
47	Tensor veli palatini	Auditory (pharyngotympanic) tube (cartilage, anterior) Sphenoid bone (spine and Pterygoid process (scaphoid fossa))	Palatine aponeurosis Palatine bone (crest)
48	Musculus uvulae	Palatine bone (posterior nasal spine) Palatine aponeurosis (dorsal)	Uvula mucosa and connective tissue
49	Palatopharyngeus	Soft palate (pharyngeal aspect) Palatine aponeuroris Hard palate (posterior border)	Thyroid cartilage (posterior border) Pharynx (wall; crosses midline to join its contralateral muscle)

The muscles of the palate are innervated by the pharyngeal plexus (derived from the X [vagus] and XI [accessory] cranial nerves) (Fig. 7–64), with the single exception of the Tensor veli palatini, which derives its motor supply from the trigeminal (V) nerve (see Plate 8, page 299).

The Tensor veli palatini elevates the soft palate, and paralysis of this muscle results in slight deviation of the uvula toward the unaffected side with its tip pointing toward the involved side. Weakness of the Tensor as an elevator of the palate may be masked if the pharyngeal muscles innervated by the pharyngeal plexus are intact.[1,11–13] In any event, the Levator veli palatini is a more important elevator of the palate than the Tensor.[12,13]

The Levator veli palatini also pulls the palate upward and backward to block off the nasal passages in swallowing. The Musculus uvulae shortens and bends the uvula to aid in blocking the nasal passages for swallowing. The Palatopharyngeus draws the pharynx upward and depresses the soft palate.

In the presence of a unilateral vagus (X) nerve lesion, the Levator veli palatini (Fig. 7–64) and the Musculus uvulae on the involved side are weak. There is a resultant lowering or flattening of the palatal arch, and the median raphe deviates toward the uninvolved side. With phonation, the uvula deviates to the uninvolved side.

With a bilateral vagus lesion, the palate cannot be elevated for phonation, but it does not sag because of the action of the Tensor veli palatini (V nerve).[12] The nasal cavity is not blocked off from the oral cavity with the bilateral lesion, which may lead to nasal regurgitation of liquids. Also, during speaking, air escapes into the nasal cavity, and the change in resonance gives a peculiar nasal quality to the voice. Dysphagia may be severe.

Description of the Palate

The palate, or roof of the oral cavity, is viewed with the mouth fully open and the tongue protruding (Fig. 7–65). The palate has two parts: the hard palate is the vault over the front of the mouth, and the soft palate is the roof over the rear of the oral cavity.[1]

The hard palate is formed from the maxilla (palatine processes) and the horizontal plates of the palatine bones. Its boundaries are: anterolaterally, the alveolar arch and

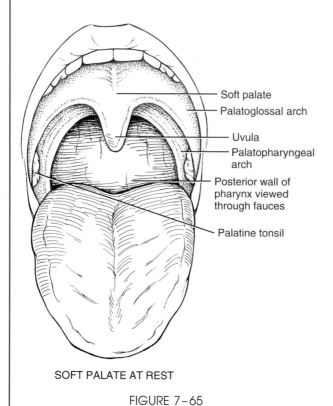

Soft palate

Palatoglossal arch

Uvula

Palatopharyngeal arch

Posterior wall of pharynx viewed through fauces

Palatine tonsil

SOFT PALATE AT REST

FIGURE 7–65

gums of the teeth, and posteriorly, the soft palate. The frontal mucosa is thick, pale, and corrugated; the posterior mucosa is darker, thinner, and not corrugated. The superior surface of the palate forms the nasal floor.

The soft palate is really a rather mobile soft tissue flap suspended from the hard palate, which slopes down and backward.[1] Its superior border is attached to (or continuous with) the posterior margin of the hard palate, and its sides blend with the pharyngeal wall. The inferior wall of the soft palate hangs free as a border between the mouth and the pharynx. The conical uvula drops from its posterior border.

The palatal arches are two curved folds of tissue containing muscles that descend laterally from the base of the uvula on either side. The anterior of these, the *palatoglossal arch*, holds the Palatoglossus and descends to end in the lateral sides of the tongue. The posterior fold, the *palatopharyngeal arch*, contains the Palatopharyngeus muscle and descends on the lateral wall of the oropharynx.[1,6] The palatine tonsils lie in a triangular notch between the diverging palatoglossal and palatopharyngeal arches.

The pharyngeal isthmus (or margin of the fauces) lies between the border of the soft palate and the posterior pharyngeal wall. The fauces forms the passageway between the mouth and the pharynx that includes the lumen as well as its boundary structures. The fauces closes during swallowing as a result of the elevation of the palate and contraction of the palatopharyngeal muscles (acting like a sphincter) and by elevation of the dorsum of the posterior tongue (Palatoglossus).

In examining the soft palate, observe the position of the palate and uvula at rest and during quiet breathing and then during phonation. If the palatine arches elevate symmetrically, minor deviations of the uvula are insignificant (for one thing, uvular changes often follow tonsillectomy).[11] Check for the presence of dysarthria and dysphagia (both liquids and solids).

Normally the uvula hangs in the midline and elevates in the midline during phonation.

Elevation and Adduction of the Soft Palate (46. Levator veli palatini, 47. Tensor veli palatini, 36. Palatoglossus, 48. Musculus uvulae)

Test: Patient produces a high-pitched "Ah-h-h" to cause the soft palate to elevate and adduct (the arches come closer together, narrowing the fauces) (Fig. 7–66).

To see the palate and fauces adequately, the examiner may need to place a tongue blade lightly on the tongue and use a flashlight to illuminate the interior of the mouth. Placing the tongue blade too far back or too heavily on the tongue may initiate a disagreeable gag reflex.

When this test does not give the desired information, the examiner may have to stimulate a gag reflex. Light touch stimulation, done slowly and gradually with an applicator (preferably) or tongue blade placed on the posterior tongue or soft palate, will evoke a reflex and produce the desired motion when phonation fails to do so.

Remember that the gag reflex is not a constant finding. Some normal people do not have one, and many people have an exaggerated reflex.

Resistance: None.

Instructions to Patient: "Use a high-pitched (soprano) tone to say 'Ah-a-a-a'."

Criteria for Grading (Derived from Observation of Uvular and Arch Motion)

F: Uvula moves briskly and elevates while remaining in the midline. The palatoglossal and palatopharyngeal arches elevate and adduct to narrow the fauces.

WF: Uvula moves sluggishly and may deviate to one or the other side. Uvula deviation is toward the uninvolved side (Fig. 7–67). The arches may elevate slightly and asymmetrically.

NF: Almost imperceptible motion of both the uvula and the arches occurs.

0: No motion occurs, and the uvula is flaccid and pendulous.

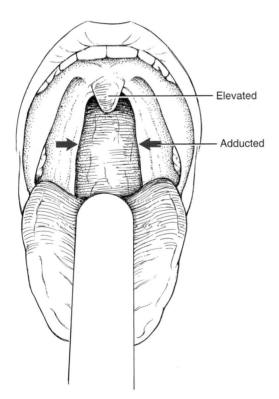

SOFT PALATE DURING TEST

FIGURE 7–66

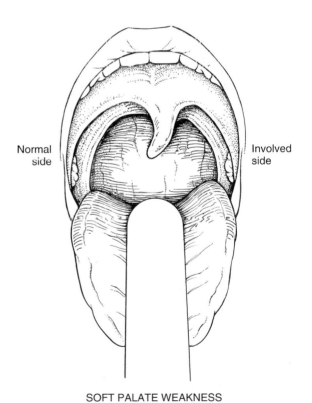

SOFT PALATE WEAKNESS

FIGURE 7–67

Occlusion of the Nasopharynx (49. Palatopharyngeus)

Test: Aiming at the examiner's finger, the patient blows through the mouth with pursed lips to occlude the nasopharynx via the Palatopharyngeus. Place a slim mirror above the upper lip (horizontally blocking off the mouth) to check for air escape from the nostrils (the mirror clouds). Alternatively, place a small feather fixed to a small plastic platform right under the nose; the motion of the feather is used to detect air leakage.

Nasal speech is a sign of inability to close off the nasopharynx.

Resistance: None

Instructions to Patient: "Blow on my finger."

Criteria for Grading

F: No leakage of air through the nose.

WF: Minimal leakage of air. Slight mirror clouding or feather ruffling.

NF-0: Heavy mirror clouding or brisk feather ruffles.

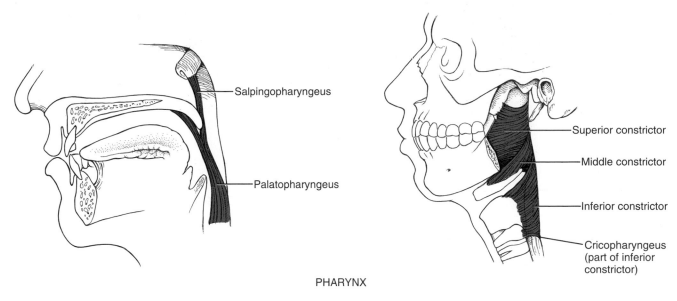

Salpingopharyngeus

Palatopharyngeus

PHARYNX

FIGURE 7–68

Superior constrictor

Middle constrictor

Inferior constrictor

Cricopharyngeus (part of inferior constrictor)

FIGURE 7–69

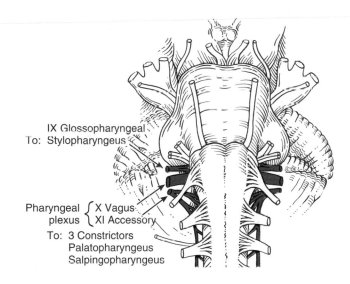

IX Glossopharyngeal
To: Stylopharyngeus

Pharyngeal { X Vagus
plexus { XI Accessory
To: 3 Constrictors
Palatopharyngeus
Salpingopharyngeus

FIGURE 7–70

Table 7-8 MUSCLES OF THE PHARYNX

I.D.	Muscle	Origin	Insertion
41	Inferior constrictor	Cricoid cartilage Thyroid cartilage (oblique line) Hyoid bone, inferior cornu	Pharynx (posterior median fibrous raphe)
42	Middle constrictor	Hyoid bone (lesser horn anterior); (greater horn entire upper border) Stylohyoid ligament	Pharynx (posterior median fibrous raphe)
43	Superior constrictor	Sphenoid (Medial pterygoid plate) Pterygoid hamulus Mandible (mylohyoid line) Tongue (side)	Pharynx (median fibrous raphe) Occipital bone (basilar part of pharyngeal tubercle)
44	Stylopharyngeus	Temporal bone (styloid process medial base)	Thyroid cartilage (some fibers merge with constrictor muscles and Palatopharyngeus)
45	Salpingopharyngeus	Auditory tube (inferior cartilage)	Blends with Palatopharyngeus

The function of the pharyngeal muscles is tested by observing their contraction during phonation and their elevation of the larynx during swallowing. The pharyngeal reflex also should be invoked and the nature of the muscle contraction noted. The manner in which the patient handles solid and liquid foods, as well as the quality and character of speech, should be described.

The motor parts of the glossopharyngeal (IX) cranial nerve (Fig. 7–70) go to the pharynx but probably innervate only the Stylopharyngeus muscle. The Stylopharyngeus elevates the upper lateral and posterior walls of the pharynx in swallowing.[18]

The remaining pharyngeal muscles (Inferior, Middle, and Superior constrictors, Palatopharyngeus, and Salpingopharyngeus) are innervated by the pharyngeal plexus composed of elements from the vagus (X) and accessory (XI) cranial nerves. The three constrictor muscles flatten and contract the pharynx in swallowing and are important participants in forcing the bolus of food into the esophagus, thereby initiating peristaltic activity in the gut. The Salpingopharyngeus blends with the Palatopharyngeus and elevates the upper portion of the pharynx.[1] Because the pharynx acts as a resonator box for sound, impairment of the pharyngeal muscles will alter the voice.

The Inferior constrictor has two parts, which often are referred to as if they were separate muscles.[1] One, the Cricopharyngeus, blends with the circular esophageal fibers to act as a distal pharyngeal sphincter in swallowing. These fibers prevent air from entering the esophagus during respiration and reflux of food from the esophagus back into the pharynx. It has been reported that when the system is at rest, the Cricopharyngeus is actively contracted to prevent air from entering the esophagus.[15] When a swallow is initiated, some form of neural inhibition causes the Cricopharyngeus to relax.[15,16] At the same time, the hyoid bone and the larynx elevate and move anteriorly, and the constrictor muscles act in a peristaltic manner, the sum of which permits passage of the bolus.[15]

The upper part of the Inferior constrictor is the Thyropharyngeus, which acts to propel the bolus of food downward.[1]

In unilateral lesions of the vagus (X) nerve, laryngeal elevation is decreased on one side, and in bilateral lesions it is decreased on both sides.

Constriction of the Posterior Pharyngeal Wall

Test: Patient opens mouth wide and says "Ah-h-h" with a high-pitched tone.

This sound causes the posterior pharyngeal wall to contract (the soft palate adducts and elevates as well).

Because it is difficult to observe the posterior wall of the pharynx, use a flashlight to illuminate the interior of the mouth. A tongue blade will probably be needed to keep the tongue from obstructing the view, but care must be taken not to initiate a gag reflex.

Patients with weakness may have an accumulation of saliva in the mouth. Ask the patient to swallow, or, if this does not work, use mouth suctioning. If the patient has a nasogastric tube it will descend in front of the posterior wall and may partially obstruct a clear view.

If there is little or no motion of the pharyngeal wall, the examiner will have to stimulate the pharyngeal reflex to ascertain contractile integrity of the Superior constrictor and other muscles of the pharyngeal wall. Patients do not like this reflex test.

The Pharyngeal Reflex Test: The pharyngeal reflex is tested by applying a stimulus with an applicator to the posterior pharyngeal wall or adjacent structures (Fig. 7–71). The stimulus should be applied bilaterally. If positive, elevation and constriction of the pharyngeal muscles will occur along with retraction of the tongue.

Criteria for Grading

F: Brisk contraction of the posterior pharyngeal wall.

WF: Decreased movement or sluggish motion of the pharyngeal wall.

NF: Trace of motion (easily missed).

0: No contractility of the pharyngeal wall.

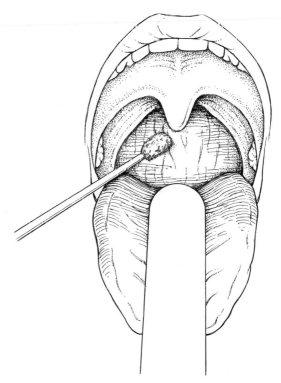

SOFT PALATE JUST PRIOR TO TOUCH

FIGURE 7–71

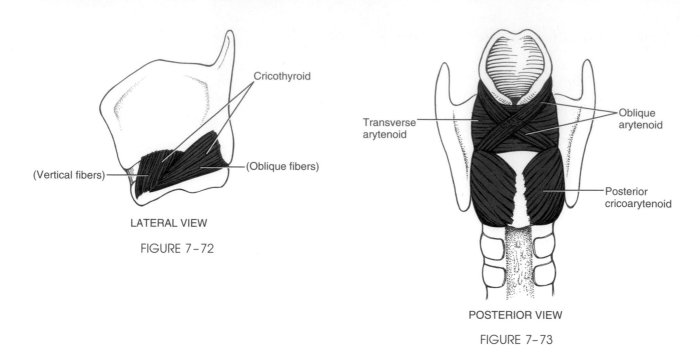

Cricothyroid

(Vertical fibers)

(Oblique fibers)

LATERAL VIEW

FIGURE 7–72

Transverse arytenoid

Oblique arytenoid

Posterior cricoarytenoid

POSTERIOR VIEW

FIGURE 7–73

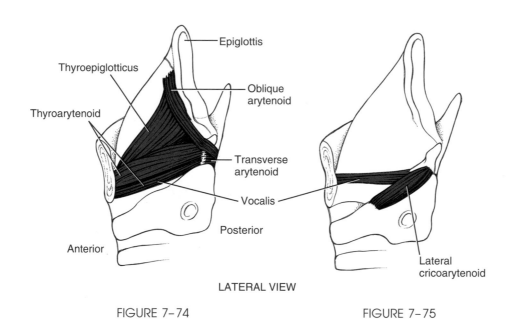

Epiglottis

Thyroepiglotticus

Oblique arytenoid

Thyroarytenoid

Transverse arytenoid

Vocalis

Posterior

Anterior

LATERAL VIEW

FIGURE 7–74

Lateral cricoarytenoid

FIGURE 7–75

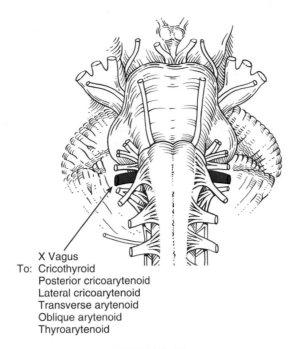

X Vagus
To: Cricothyroid
Posterior cricoarytenoid
Lateral cricoarytenoid
Transverse arytenoid
Oblique arytenoid
Thyroarytenoid

FIGURE 7-76

Table 7-9 MUSCLES OF THE LARYNX

I.D.	Muscle	Origin	Insertion
50	Cricothyroid	Cricoid cartilage (external aspect of arch)	Thyroid lamina Thyroid cartilage
51	Posterior cricoarytenoid	Cricoid cartilage (posterior surface)	Arytenoid cartilage (posterior on same side)
52	Lateral cricoarytenoid	Cricoid cartilage (arch)	Arytenoid cartilage (anterior on same side)
53	Transverse arytenoid (unpaired muscle)	Crosses transversely between the two arytenoid cartilages	Lateral border of both arytenoids Fills posterior concave surface between two arytenoids
54	Oblique arytenoids	Arytenoid cartilage (posterior) Cross back of larynx obliquely	Arytenoid cartilage (apex) on opposite side
55	Thyroarytenoid (Vocalis muscle formed by band of fibers off lateral vocal process)	Thyroid cartilage (angle and lower half) Cricothyroid ligament	Arytenoid cartilage (anterior base) Vocal process (lateral)
Others			
84-87	Infrahyoid muscles		
84	Sternothyroid		
85	Thyrohyoid		
86	Sternohyoid		
87	Omohyoid		

Examination of the muscles of the larynx includes assessing the quality and nature of the voice, noting any abnormalities of phonation or articulation; impairment of coughing (see accompanying sidebar); and any problems with respiration. Also important is the rate of opening and closing of the glottis.

Some general definitions are in order. *Phonation* is the production of vocal sounds without the formation of words; phonation is a function of the larynx[5] *Articulation,* or the formation of words, is a joint function of the larynx along with the pharynx, palate, tongue, teeth, and lips.

The laryngeal muscles all are innervated by the recurrent branches of the X (vagus) cranial nerve with the exception of the Cricothyroid, which receives its motor innervation from the superior laryngeal nerve. The laryngeal muscles regulate the tension of the vocal cords and open and close the glottis by abducting and adducting the vocal cords. The vocal cords normally are open (abducted) during inspiration and adducted while speaking or during coughing.

The Cricothyroids (paired) are the principal tensors owing to their action in lengthening the vocal cords.[1,5,11] The Posterior cricoarytenoids (paired) are the main abductors and glottis openers; the Lateral cricoarytenoids (paired) are the main adductors and glottis closers. The Thyroarytenoids (paired) shorten and relax the vocal cords by drawing the arytenoid cartilages forward. The unpaired Arytenoid (transverse and oblique heads) draws the arytenoid cartilages together; the oblique head acts as the sphincter of the upper larynx (called the aryepiglottic folds), and the transverse head acts as the sphincter of the lower larynx.

Paralysis of the laryngeal muscles on one side does not cause an appreciable change in the voice in contrast to the difficulty resulting from bilateral weakness. Loss of the Cricothyroids leads to loss of the high tones and the voice sounds deep and hoarse and fatigues readily, but respiration is normal. Loss of the Thyroarytenoids bilaterally changes the shape of the glottis and results in a hoarse voice, but again, respiration is normal.

With bilateral paralysis of the Posterior cricoarytenoids, both vocal cords will lie close to the midline and cannot be abducted, leading to severe dyspnea and difficult inspiratory effort (inspiratory stridor).[5] Expiration is normal.

In bilateral adductor paralysis (lateral Cricoarytenoids), inspiration is normal because abduction is unimpaired. The voice, however, is lost or has a whisper quality.

With unilateral loss of both abduction and adduction the involved vocal cords are motionless, and the voice is low and hoarse. In bilateral loss all vocal cords are quiescent, and speech and coughing are lost. Marked inspiratory stress occurs, and the patient is dyspneic.

The Functional Anatomy of Coughing

Cough is an essential procedure to maintain airway patency and to clear the pharynx and bronchial tree when secretions accumulate. A cough may be a reflex or voluntary response to irritation anywhere along the airway downstream from the nose.

The cough reflex occurs as a result of stimulation of the mucous membranes of the pharynx, larynx, trachea, or bronchial tree. These tissues are so sensitive to light touch that any foreign matter or other irritation initiates the cough reflex. The sensory (afferent) limb of the reflex carries the impulses set up by the irritation via the glossopharyngeal and vagus cranial nerves to the fasciculus solitarius in the medulla, from which the motor impulses (efferent) then move out to the muscles of the pharynx, palate, tongue, and larynx as well as to those of the abdominal wall, chest, and Diaphragm. The reflex response is a deep inspiration (about 2.5 liters of air) followed quickly by a forced expiration during which the glottis closes momentarily, trapping air in the lungs.[14] The Diaphragm contracts spasmodically, as do the abdominal muscles and intercostal muscles. This raises intrathoracic pressure (to above 200 mmHg) until the vocal cords are forced open, and the explosive outrush of air expels mucus and foreign matter. The expiratory airflow at this time may reach a velocity of 70 mph.[17] Important to the reflex action is the fact that the bronchial tree and laryngeal walls collapse because strong compression of the lungs causes an invagination such that the high linear velocity of airflow moving past and through these tissues dislodges mucus or foreign particles, thus producing an effective cough.

The three phases of cough—inspiration, compression, and forced expiration—are mediated by the muscles of the thorax and abdomen, as well as of the pharynx, larynx, and tongue. The deep inspiratory effort is supported by the Diaphragm, Intercostals, and the Arytenoid abductor muscles (the Posterior cricoarytenoids), permitting inhalation of upward of 1.5 liters of air.[16] The Palatoglossus and Styloglossus elevate the tongue and close off the oropharynx from the nasopharynx.

The compression phase requires the Lateral cricoarytenoid muscles to adduct and close the glottis.

The strong expiratory movement is augmented by strong contractions of the thorax muscles, particularly the Latissimus dorsi and the oblique and transverse abdominal muscles. The abdominal muscles raise intra-abdominal pressure, forcing the relaxing Diaphragm up and drawing the lower ribs down and medially. Elevation of the Diaphragm raises intrathoracic pressure to about 200 mmHg, and the explosive expulsion phase begins with forced abduction of the glottis.

Elevation of the Larynx in Swallowing

Test: The larynx elevates during swallowing. The examiner lightly grasps the larynx with the thumb and index finger on the anterior throat to determine the fact of elevation and its extent (Fig. 7–77). **DO NOT PRESS DIRECTLY ON THE FRONT OF THE LARYNX AND NEVER USE MUCH PRESSURE ON THE NECK.**

Resistance: None

Instructions to Patient: "Swallow."

Criteria for Grading

F: Larynx elevates at least 20 mm in most people.[18] The motion is quick and controlled.

WF: Laryngeal excursion may be normal or slightly limited. The motion is sluggish and may be irregular.

NF: Excursion is perceptible but less than normal. Aspiration may occur.

0: No laryngeal elevation occurs. (Aspiration will result in this event.)

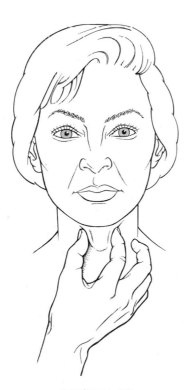

FIGURE 7–77

Vocal Cord Abduction and Adduction (51. Posterior cricoarytenoids, 52. Lateral cricoarytenoids)

In this test the examiner is looking for hoarseness, pitch and tone range, breathlessness, breathiness, nasal-quality speech, dysarthria, and articulation or phonation disturbances.

Test and Instructions to Patient: The patient is asked to respond to four different commands to determine the nature of airflow control during respiration, vocalization, and coughing.

1. "State your name." Patient should be able to say his or her name completely without running out of breath.
2. "Sing several notes in the musical scale" (do, re, mi, etc.) first at a low pitch and then at a higher pitch. Patient should be able to sustain a tone (even when "can't carry a tune") and vary the pitch.
3. "Repeat five times a hard staccato, interrupted sound: 'Akh, Akh, Akh.'" Examiner must demonstrate this sound to the patient. Patient should make and break sounds crisply with a definite halt between each sound in the series.
4. "Cough."

Evaluation of Cough in the Context of Laryngeal Function: Refer to the accompanying sidebar on cough. Examiner determines whether the patient has a voluntary and effective cough. A voluntary cough is initiated on command. A reflex cough, because it cannot be initiated on command, must be evaluated when it occurs, which may be outside of the test session. The reflex cough occurs in response to irritation of the membranes of the postnasal air passages.

An effective or functional cough, voluntary or reflex, clears secretions from the lungs or airways. A functional cough is dependent on the coordination of the respiratory and laryngeal muscles.

Control of inspiration must be sufficient to fill the lungs with the necessary volume of air to produce a cough. Effective expiration of air during a cough is dependent on forceful contraction of the abdominal muscles. The vocal cords must adduct tightly to prevent air loss. Adduction of the vocal cords must be maintained prior to the expulsion of air.

A nonfunctional cough resulting from laryngeal deficiency sounds like clearing the throat or a low guttural sound, or there may be no cough sound at all.

The kinesiology of swallowing is the subject of continued controversy. Many of the rapid actions described as sequential are close to simultaneous events. The means of studying swallowing are limited to a great extent by the limitations inherent in palpation, following ingested food. Videofluoroscopy, manometry, and acoustic measures improve assessment accuracy.

MUSCLE ACTIONS IN SWALLOWING

Ingestion of Food and Formation of Bolus (Oral Preparatory Phase)

- The food or liquid is placed in the oral cavity, and the Orbicularis oris contracts to maintain a labial seal and to prevent drooling. The Palatoglossus maintains a posterior seal by maintaining the tongue against the soft palate, which prevents leakage too early into the pharynx.[19]
- Foods are broken down mechanically by integrated action of the muscles of the tongue, jaw, and cheeks.
- Liquids: Intrinsic tongue muscles squirt fluids into the back of the mouth. The Mylohyoid raises and bulges the back of the tongue into the oropharynx. Lips must be closed to retain fluids.
- Solids: Muscles of the tongue and cheek (Buccinator) place the food between the teeth, which bite, crush, and grind it via action of the muscles of mastication (see Table 7–5). The food, when mixed with saliva (by the tongue intrinsics), forms a bolus behind the tip of the tongue.
- The tongue muscles (see Table 7–6) raise the anterior tongue and press it against the hard palate, which pushes the bolus back into the fauces.

The Oral Phase

- In this phase of swallowing the bolus is squeezed against the hard palate by the tongue, the lip seal is maintained, and the Buccinator continues to prevent pocketing or lodging of food in the lateral sulci.
- The tongue is drawn up and back by the Styloglossus.
- The palate muscles (see Table 7–7) depress the soft palate down onto the tongue to "grip" the bolus.
- The hyoid bone and the larynx are elevated and moved forward by the Suprahyoid muscles.
- The palatal arches are adducted by the paired Palatoglossi.
- The bolus is driven back into the oropharynx.
- As a prelude to the act of swallowing, the hyoid bone is raised slightly, and this action is accompanied by a quiescence of all muscle action: chewing, talking, food movement in the mouth, capital and cervical motion, facial movements. Even respiration is momentarily arrested.[16,19]
- The soft palate is raised (Levator veli palatini) and tightened (Tensor veli palatini) to be firmly fixed against the posterior pharyngeal wall. This leads to a tight closure of the pharyngeal isthmus (Palatopharyngeus and Superior constrictor), which prevents the bolus from rising into the nasopharynx.

The Engulfing Actions Through the Pharynx (Pharyngeal Phase)

- The epiglottis moves upward and forward, coming to a halt at the root of the tongue, and literally bends backward (possibly because of the weight of the bolus) to cover the laryngeal inlet. The bolus of food slides over its anterior surface. (The epiglottis in the human is not essential to swallowing, which is normal even in the absence of an epiglottis.[1])
- The fauces narrow (Palatoglossi).
  Note: The pharyngeal isthmus is at the border of the soft palate and the posterior pharyngeal wall and is the communication between the nasal and oral parts of the pharynx. Its closure is effected by the approximation of the two Palatopharyngeus muscles and the Superior constrictor, which form a palatopharyngeal sphincter.
- The larynx and pharynx are raised up behind the hyoid (Salpingopharyngeus, Stylopharyngeus, Thyrohyoid, and Palatopharyngeus).
- The arytenoid cartilages are drawn upward and forward (Oblique arytenoids and Thyroarytenoids), and the aryepiglottic folds approximate, which prevents movement of the bolus into the larynx.
- During swallowing the thyroid cartilage and hyoid bone are approximated, and there is a general elevation of the pharynx, larynx, and trachea. This causes the many laryngeal folds to bulge posteriorly into the laryngeal inlet, thus narrowing it during swallowing.[19,20]
- The bolus then slips further over the epiglottis, and partly by gravity and partly by the action of the constrictor muscles it passes into the lowest part of the pharynx. Passage is aided by contraction of the Palatopharyngei, which elevate and shorten the pharynx, thus angling the posterior pharyngeal wall to allow the bolus to slide easily downward.[21]
- The laryngeal passage is narrowed by the aryepiglottic folds (Posterior cricoarytenoids, Oblique arytenoids, and Transverse arytenoids), which close the laryngeal vestibule (glottis) and also form lateral channels to direct the bolus toward the esophagus.
- When the Posterior cricoarytenoids are weak or paralyzed, the laryngeal inlet is not closed off in

swallowing, the aryepiglottic folds move medially, and fluid or food enters the larynx (aspiration).

The Esophageal Phase

- At the beginning of this phase the compressed bolus is in the distal pharynx. The Inferior constrictor pushes the bolus inferiorly (peristaltic action) to enter the esophagus. The distal fibers of the Inferior constrictor, called the Cricopharyngeus, are a distal sphincter and therefore must relax to allow the bolus to pass, but the mechanism of this action is in dispute.[21,22]
- After the passage of the bolus the intrinsic tongue muscles move saliva around the mouth to cleanse away debris.

TESTING SWALLOWING

Swallowing is tested only when there is good cause to suspect that the swallowing mechanisms are faulty. Do not make an a priori assumption that the presence of a nasogastric tube, a gastrostomy, or a liquid diet precludes swallowing. The examiner also should review information from the patient's history and current chart to identify the site of the lesion, the presence of upper respiratory tract infections, and similar facts, which will assist the direction of the evaluation.

When a patient has a tracheostomy, a suctioning machine is essential, and expertise with its use is required.

The examiner will have some prior information about patients from direct observation, such as how they handle saliva (swallowing it or drooling), whether and how they manage liquids and solids at mealtime, reports from nursing staff and family, and the nature of reported problems about swallowing. These all will suggest a starting point for testing.

In most swallowing tests use a bib around the patient's neck to prevent soiling. Remember to protect yourself from sudden aspirates! Damp washcloths or tissues should be available for clean-up.

Position of Patient: Sitting preferred, supine if necessary, but head and trunk should be elevated to at least 30°. Maintain head and neck in neutral position.

Position of Therapist: Sitting in front of and slightly to one side of the patient.

Table 7-10 COMMON SWALLOWING PROBLEMS AND MUSCLE INVOLVEMENT

Problem	Possible Anatomical Cause
Drooling	Weakness of Orbicularis oris
Pocketing in the lateral sulci	Weakness of the Buccinator and intrinsic and extrinsic tongue muscles
Decreased ability to break down food mechanically during the oral preparatory phase	Weakness of the muscles of mastication
Decreased ability to form bolus	Weakness of the intrinsic and extrinsic tongue muscles Weakness of the Buccinator
Decreased ability to maintain bolus in the oral cavity during the oral preparatory phase	Weakness of the Palatoglossus or Styloglossus or both
Nasal regurgitation	Weakness of the Palatopharyngeus, Levator veli palatini, or Tensor veli palatini, individually or severally
Posterior pharyngeal wall residual after the swallow	Weakness of the pharyngeal constrictor(s) muscles
Coughing or choking prior to the swallow	Food may spill into an unprotected airway secondary to: 1. Weakness of the intrinsic or extrinsic tongue muscles resulting in decreased ability to form a bolus (lack of bolus formation may result in spillage of the oral contents without initiation of a swallow) 2. Weakness of the Palatoglossus and Styloglossus resulting in decreased ability to maintain the bolus in the oral cavity prior to initiation of a swallow
Coughing or choking during the swallow	Weakness of the muscles responsible for closing the true vocal folds, false vocal folds, and aryepiglottic folds
Coughing or choking after the swallow	Decreased strength of the Genioglossus resulting in decreased tongue retraction with vallecular residual, which spills after the swallow into an unprotected airway Pharyngeal constrictor weakness with residual spillage from the pharyngeal walls after the swallow into an unprotected airway Decreased cricopharyngeal opening with overflow from the piriform sinus after the swallow into an unprotected airway

PRELIMINARY PROCEDURES TO DETERMINE CLINICALLY THE SAFETY OF INGESTION OF FOOD OR LIQUIDS

Test Sequence 1

Laryngeal Elevation: Examiner lightly grasps the larynx between the thumb and index finger on the anterior surface of the throat. Ask the patient to swallow. Ascertain if there is laryngeal elevation and its extent (see Fig. 7–77).

Criteria for Grading

F: Larynx elevates at least 20 mm. Motion is quick and controlled.

WF: Laryngeal excursion may be normal or slightly limited. The motion may be sluggish or appear irregular.

NF: Elevation is perceptible but significantly less than normal.

0: No laryngeal elevation occurs.

Implications of Grade: If the patient is graded F (Functional) or WF (Weak functional), proceed with the swallowing assessment. If the patient is graded NF (Nonfunctional) or 0 and does not have a tracheostomy, discontinue the swallowing assessment. For patients with a tracheostomy, add a blue vegetable dye to the bolus to facilitate identification of any aspirated bolus during suctioning.

Test Sequence 2

Initial Ingestion of Water

Prerequisites: The patient has a grade of F or WF on Test Sequence 1.

There also must be at least a grade of WF or higher on the tests for posterior elevation of the tongue (see pages 322 and 323) and constriction of the posterior pharyngeal wall (see page 331).

Procedure: There are several ways to get water into the mouth to test swallowing. It does not matter which is used.

The first trial of swallowing begins with a small amount (1 to 3 mL) of water. The rationale is that should the patient not be able to swallow the water correctly and it is aspirated, the lungs can absorb this small quantity without penalty. There also is evidence accumulating that differences in the pH of water can cause damage to the lungs, so the small amount of water is very important. Each procedure should be repeated at least three or four times.

1. If the patient is cognitively clear, offer a glass or cup containing a tiny amount of water and allow the patient to sip. The test is successful if the water can be swallowed with one attempt, the swallow is inaudible, and the water is swallowed without any choking or coughing. If successful, proceed to Test Sequence 3.
2. If the patient cannot sip from a cup, offer a straw and ask the patient to suck a small amount. The shorter and wider the straw, the easier the task. If the swallowing attempt is successful as described in (1) above, proceed to Test Sequence 3.
3. If the patient cannot sip or suck, trap water in a straw and place the straw in the side of the patient's mouth between the cheek and lower teeth. Tell the patient you are going to release the water and request a swallow. If successful, proceed to Test Sequence 3.
4. If the patient is not cognitively clear, control the amount of water available. This is most readily done by trapping water in a straw to give to the patient.
5. For the patient who cannot handle fluid, try thickening the water with gelatin to a consistency of thin gruel or thick pea soup.

Outcomes: If any of these trials are successful, proceed cautiously to a trial of pureed food. If none of these tests are successful and the patient does not have a tracheostomy, DO NOT give the patient food by mouth until further testing (e.g., fluoroscopy) can be conducted.

If the procedures with water are not successful and the patient has a tracheostomy (through which aspirated food can be suctioned), proceed cautiously to the use of pureed food, which usually is easier to swallow than water.

Test Sequence 3

Pureed Food

The most palatable commercial pureed foods are the pureed baby food fruits. The pureed meats and vegetables are totally unseasoned, which is unfamiliar and usually unpalatable to adults. Avoid milk products initially because they thicken the saliva. Ask about patient food preferences and try to use something enjoyable.

A suctioning machine is essential if the patient has a tracheostomy. It is recommended that the food be colored with vegetable dye (blue is readily seen and is not confused with body secretions or fluids) so that any aspiration can be readily detected as the color appears in tracheostomy secretions.

Criteria for Initiating Trials with Pureed Foods

1. Laryngeal elevation is Functional (F) or Weak functional (WF).

PRELIMINARY PROCEDURES TO DETERMINE CLINICALLY THE SAFETY OF INGESTION OF FOOD OR LIQUIDS

2. Posterior pharyngeal wall constriction is at least WF.
3. Patient has been successful in handling water in Test Sequence 2 or by observation.
4. Patient *must* have a functional cough (voluntary or reflex) or a tracheostomy. Some patients have a depressed gag reflex, but cough is the essential component in swallowing. The examiner cannot assume that a hyperactive gag reflex is synonymous with a functional cough.
5. The patient must have adequate cognition to attend to feeding.
6. There cannot be any respiratory problem present, such as aspiration pneumonia, that might be compromised by additional aspiration.

Procedures

1. Place a small amount (1/2 teaspoon) of food on the front of the tongue. Ask the patient to swallow, and observe ability to manipulate food in the mouth to position it for swallowing. Allow the patient to place the food in the mouth if possible because this will better coordinate feeding with the respiratory cycle.
2. If the patient cannot move the food in the mouth, push it back slightly with a tongue blade, being careful not to initiate a gag reflex. Ask the patient to swallow, while lightly palpating the larynx to check laryngeal elevation.
3. Ask the patient to open the mouth, and check to see that food has indeed been swallowed and that none of it has pooled in the pharyngeal isthmus or oral cavity.
4. To check for a clear airway, ask the patient to repeat three sequential crisp sounds: "Agh, Agh, Agh." Any gurgling indicates that food is in the airway and ask the patient to swallow again.

Repeat this procedure a number of times and check each response.

After four or five trials with pureed food, pause for about 10 minutes to ascertain that the patient does not have delayed coughing because of food collecting in the pharynx, larynx, or trachea. A blue aspirate from the tracheostomy tube may occur sometime after the actual ingestion of food.

Outcomes: If the patient has no immediate or delayed coughing, choking, or positive aspirate after swallowing and the airway is clear, the test is successful.

If the patient repeatedly coughs, chokes, or has a positive aspirate, this is solid evidence that there is inadequacy of swallowing, and the test should be terminated and no other food administered.

For patients who have been on a nasogastric tube and have demonstrated the ability to swallow water and pureed food without aspiration, proceed with feeding the pureed food until at least three-fourths of the jar has been consumed. For the next meal, order a tray of pureed food. Observe the patient during eating; look for any problems and assess fatigue.

Use of a Mechanical Soft Diet: A mechanical soft diet (ground meat, ground vegetables if fibrous or hard) should be substituted for regular-consistency food for patients with any of the following: lack of teeth or dentures, poor intraoral control for chewing, fatigue during mastication (e.g., postpolio or Landry-Guillain-Barré syndrome), limited jaw range of motion, limited attention span to complete the oral preparatory phase.

References

Cited References

1. Williams PL, Warwick R, Dyson M, et al. *Gray's Anatomy,* 38th ed. New York: Churchill-Livingstone, 1995.
2. Walsh FB. *Walsh & Hoyt's Clinical NeuroOphthalmology,* 5th ed. Baltimore: Williams & Wilkins, 1998.
3. Bender MB, Rudolph SH, Stacy CB. The neurology of the visual and oculomotor systems. In Joynt RJ (ed). *Clinical Neurology.* Philadelphia: JB Lippincott, 1993.
4. Van Allen MW. *Pictorial Manual of Neurologic Tests.* Chicago: Year Book, 1969.
5. Haerer AF. *DeJong's The Neurologic Examination,* 5th ed. Philadelphia: JB Lippincott, 1992.
6. Clemente CD. *Gray's Anatomy,* 30th ed. Philadelphia: Lea & Febiger, 1991.
7. Jenkins DB. *Hollingshead's Functional Anatomy of the Limbs and Back,* 7th ed. Philadelphia: WB Saunders, 1998.
8. DuBrul EL. *Sicher and DuBrul's Oral Anatomy,* 8th ed. St. Louis: Ishiyaku EuroAmerica, 1988.
9. Nairn RI. The circumoral musculature: Structure and function. Br Dent J 138:49–56, 1975.
10. Lightoller GH. Facial muscles: The modiolus and muscles surrounding the rima oris with remarks about the panniculus adiposus. J Anat 60:1–85, 1925.
11. Brodal A. *Neurological Anatomy in Relation to Clinical Medicine.* London: Oxford University Press, 1981.
12. Misuria VK. Functional anatomy of the tensor palatini and levator palatini muscles. Ann Otolaryngol 102:265, 1975.
13. Keller JT, Saunders MC, Van Loveren H, Shipley MT. Neuroanatomical considerations of palatal muscles: Tensor and levator palatini. J Cleft Palate. 21:70–75, 1984.
14. Guyton AC. *Textbook of Medical Physiology,* 10th ed. Philadelphia: WB Saunders, 2000.
15. Miller AJ. Neurophysiological basis of swallowing. Dysphagia 1:91–100, 1986.
16. Doty R. Neural organization of deglutition. In *Handbook of Physiology,* Section 6, Alimentary Canal. Washington, DC: American Physiologic Society, 1968.
17. Starr JA. Manual techniques of chest physical therapy and airway clearance techniques. In Zadai CC. Pulmonary Management in Physical Therapy. *Clinics in Physical Therapy.* New York: Churchill-Livingstone, 1992.
18. Jacob P, Kahrilas PJ, Logemann JA, et al. Upper esophageal sphincter opening and modulation during swallowing. Gastroenterology 97:1469–1478, 1989.
19. Logemann JA. *Evaluation and Treatment of Swallowing Disorders.* San Diego: College-Hill Press, 1997.
20. Bosma J. Deglutition: Pharyngeal stage. Physiol Rev 37:275–300, 1957.
21. Buthpitiya AG, Stroud D, Russell COH. Pharyngeal pump and esophageal transit. Dig Dis Sci 32:1244–1248, 1987.
22. Kilman WJ, Goyal RK. Disorders of pharyngeal and upper esophageal sphincter motor function. Arch Intern Med 136:592–601, 1976.

Other Readings

Cunningham DP, Basmajian JV. Electromyography of genioglossus and geniohyoid muscles during deglutition. Anat Rec 165: 401–409, 1969.
Hrycyshyn AW, Basmajian JV. Electromyography of the oral stage of swallowing in man. Am J Anat 133:333–340, 1972.
Isley CL, Basmajian JV. Electromyography of the human cheeks and lips. Anat Rec 176:143–147, 1973.
Miller AJ. The Neuroscientific Principles of Swallowing and Dysphagia. (Dysphagia Series.) San Diego: Singular Publishing Group, 1998.
Palmer JB, Tanaka E, Ensrud E. Motion of the posterior pharyngeal wall in human swallowing: A quantitative videofluorographic study. Arch Phys Med Rehabil 11:1520–1526, 2000.
Vitti M, Basmajian JV. Electromyographic investigation of procerus and frontalis muscles. Electromyogr Clin Neurophysiol 16:227–236, 1976.
Vitti M, Basmajian JV, Ouelette PL, et al. Electromyographic investigation of the tongue and circumoral muscular sling with fine-wire electrodes. J Dent Res 54:844–849, 1975.
Zablotny CM, Evaluation and management of swallowing dysfunction. In Montgomery J. *Physical Therapy for Traumatic Brain Injury.* New York: Churchill-Livingstone, 1995.
Zafar H. Integrated jaw and neck function in man. Studies of mandibular and head-neck movements during jaw opening-closing tasks. Swed Dent J Suppl 143.1–41, 2000.

CHAPTER

8

Upright
Motor Control

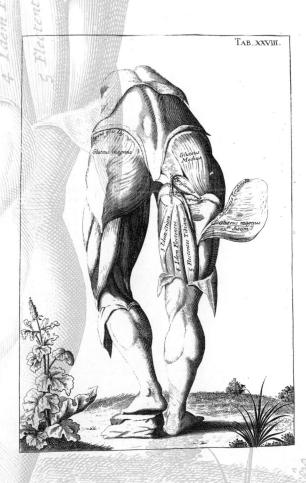

TAB. XXVIII.

The manual muscle tests described in Chapters 2 through 5 of this book are not germane to the evaluation of muscle activity when there is dysfunction of the central nervous system (CNS). In patients with CNS disorders, the muscles have normal innervation, but their control is disturbed because of damage to the CNS, either in the brain or in the spinal cord. These persons have upper motor neuron disorders that are characterized by one or any combination of the following:

Abnormal limb movement patterns
Disturbed muscle tone (spasticity, rigidity)
Aberrations in the selection, amplitude, or timing of synergistic muscle activity, duration, and rate (velocity) of activity in individual muscles
Impaired tactile sensation: paresthesias, anesthesias, or hypesthesias
Disturbed proprioception and kinesthesia
Impaired spatial discrimination
Impaired body image
Disturbed central balance mechanisms and abnormal postural reactions
Abnormal reflex activity

Analysis of a patient with some combination of these problems is a complex task. Manual muscle testing was not designed for such patients and should not be used to evaluate them.[1] *Manual muscle testing was (and is) designed to evaluate patients with a lower motor neuron disorder manifested by flaccid weakness or paralysis.* Its use in persons with CNS dysfunction yields spurious clinical results that have little or no relevance to function. Indeed, muscle testing scores in patients with lower motor neuron disorders do not necessarily relate to, or predict, function.

An obvious exclusion from this blanket assertion is patients with both CNS and lower motor neuron disorders. Two good examples are the patient with a spinal cord injury and the patient with amyotrophic lateral sclerosis.

Evaluation of muscle performance, however, is an important tool of the physical therapist in treating the patient with CNS derangement. One such tool was developed to test lower extremity control during standing.[2] It can be used in patients who have selective control, patterned motion, or a combination of the two.

Selective control is the ability to move a single joint without activating movement in an adjacent or neighboring joint of the same extremity. For example, the patient should be able to flex the elbow without incurring simultaneous motion at the shoulder or wrist.

Patterned motion is the inability to perform a fractionated motion (i.e., wrist extension without movement at the elbow or fingers). For example, following a stroke or brain injury a flexor pattern of movement is common in the upper extremity, as follows (the pattern is named after the prevailing motion at the elbow):

Shoulder abduction or extension
Elbow flexion
Forearm supination
Wrist and finger flexion

It is also common to see an extensor pattern of motion in the lower extremity:

Hip extension
Knee extension
Plantar flexion and inversion

These patterns are fairly stereotyped, but studies reveal multiple variations in the participating muscles and their amplitude in a "typical" flexion or extensor pattern.[3–5]

The upright motor control test was designed to incorporate the effects of upright posture and weight bearing.[2] It simulates the activity required for walking (i.e., flexion, which includes the factor of speed, and extension, which assesses joint stability.) Intertester reliability has been established at 96 percent agreement for the flexion portion of the test and 90 percent agreement for the extension portion of the test.[2] Validity with respect to prediction of gait performance from test data has not been published.

THE TEST FOR UPRIGHT CONTROL

One examiner and an assistant are required to conduct this evaluation properly. The assistant should be a physical therapist or a person who has received extensive instruction in methods of positioning himself or herself and the patient to provide appropriate (neither too little nor too much) stabilization and support. The patient must be able to understand all test instructions, as verified by appropriate responses to verbal commands or demonstration. The patient also must require no more than the assistance of one person for either single- or double-limb stance.

The test itself has two major sections: the flexion control test and the extension control test. Each of these sections has three parts, one each for the hip, the knee, and the ankle.

FLEXION CONTROL TEST (IN PARTS 1, 2, 3)

The purpose of this portion of the upright motor control test is to ascertain flexion control of the non–weight-bearing extremity (i.e., for limb advancement in the swing phase of gait).

The test is conducted bilaterally unless there is unequivocal evidence that one side is without neurologic deficit. The assistant provides manual balance support by holding the patient's hand, positioning his or her arm so that the hand is at about the level of the greater trochanter. The support is given on the side contralateral to that being tested and should be sufficient for the patient to maintain standing balance during this segment of the test.

For the patient who has bilateral lower extremity involvement, external stabilization for contralateral hip and knee extension may be required during the single-limb flexion test. This can be done manually by preventing knee flexion and holding the patient in hip extension; an external support such as a "knee immobilizer" may be used.

The examiner may stand in front of and facing the patient, or, if the patient has side confusion, he or she may stand slightly in front but facing in the same direction. The examiner demonstrates each test part as many times as necessary to ensure patient understanding. The patient then is allowed no more than two practice trials to avoid fatigue.

The actual data collection (graded trial) is limited to one trial per limb segment. Just prior to grading, the patient's test limb should be positioned in neutral at both hip and knee (0° at the hip and 0° at the knee). If the patient cannot reach neutral, a position of maximal extension range should be used.

Part 1: Hip Flexion

Instructions to Patient: "Stand as straight as you can. Bring your knee up toward your chest, as high and as fast as you can."

Grading: The hip flexion motion must occur at the hip joint. Do not allow substitution or other contamination of the motion such as backward lean or pelvic tilt (see Table 8–1).

Table 8–1 HIP FLEXION

Score	Criteria
Weak (W)	No motion, or patient actively flexes less than 30°. Three repetitions through any range that requires, as a group, more than 10 sec to complete.
Moderate (M)	Actively completes an arc of hip flexion from 0° (or maximal extension angle) to between 30° and 60° three times within 10 sec.
Strong (S)	Actively completes an arc of hip flexion from 0° (or maximal extension angle) to more than 60° three times within 10 sec.

Part 2: Knee Flexion

Instructions to Patient: "Stand as straight as you can. Bring your knee up toward your chest three times, as high and as fast as you can."

Grading: See Table 8–2.

Table 8–2 KNEE FLEXION

Score	Criteria
Weak (W)	No motion, or knee flexes less than 30°. Completes three repetitions through any range but requires, as a group, more than 10 sec.
Moderate (M)	Actively completes an arc of knee flexion from 0° to between 30° and 60° three times within 10 sec.
Strong (S)	Knee flexes more than 60° three times within 10 sec.

Part 3: Ankle Flexion (Dorsiflexion)

Instructions to Patient: "Stand as straight as you can. Bring your knee and foot up toward your chest as high and as fast as you can."

Grading: See Table 8–3.

Table 8–3 DORSIFLEXION

Score	Criteria
Weak (W)	No motion, or actively dorsiflexes to less than a right angle. (Examiner is cautioned not to confuse forefoot or toe extension with true ankle motion.) Completes three repetitions through any range but requires, as a group, more than 10 sec.
Moderate (M)	This grade is not used because range of dorsiflexion is so limited and very little dorsiflexion is used in the swing phase of gait.
Strong (S)	Actively dorsiflexes to a right angle or greater three times in 10 sec.

EXTENSION CONTROL TEST (IN PARTS 4, 5, AND 6)

The purpose of this portion of the upright motor control test is to ascertain extension control of a single weight-bearing extremity (i.e., for single-limb stance in gait).

Instructions and procedures for the test are similar to those used in the flexion control test. The examiner demonstrates each segment sufficiently to ensure patient understanding but allows only two practice trials per segment to avoid fatigue. Only one graded trial per segment is permitted.

The starting position for this test is double-limb stance with both limbs in neutral alignment or the patient's maximal available extension range. The patient is required to bring the nontest limb off the floor; if this is not possible, help in flexing the nontest limb should be provided by the assistant.

The assistant helps to stabilize or provide hand support as described under each test part.

If the patient has a fixed equinus contracture that is greater than the neutral ankle position, the contracture must be accommodated by placing a hard wedge under the heel. The purpose of the wedge is to align the tibia into a vertical position.

If a stable plantigrade platform cannot be maintained (with manual support or with an ankle-foot orthosis), the examiner should give a score of UT (Unable to Test) at the hip and knee. The ankle score should be noted as E (Excessive). That is to say, if excessive tone precludes the foot from assuming a position flat on the floor, the extension control test cannot be conducted.

Part 4: Hip Extension

Positioning and Stabilization: The examiner is positioned beside the patient to offer hand support and to ensure that the patient begins from a position of neutral alignment or from the patient's maximal hip extension range (Fig. 8–1).

The assistant provides manual stabilization to maintain neutral knee extension and a stable ankle. Remember that plantigrade positioning of the foot is required.

Instructions to Patient: "Stand on both legs as straight as you can."

"Now stand as straight as you can on just your right/left leg." (Note: This is the weaker limb if the test is to be unilateral.)

"Lift this leg up [point to or touch desired leg] . . . keep standing as straight as you can."

Grading: When the patient is balanced on the test limb, the examiner gradually decreases the amount of hand support to determine the degree of hip control (Table 8–4).

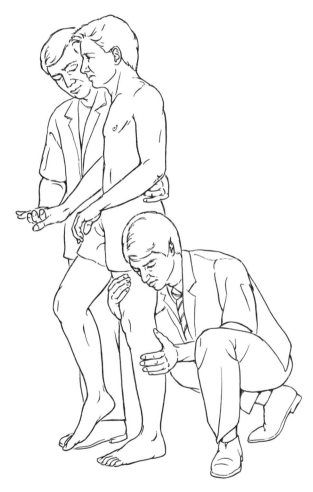

FIGURE 8–1
Hip extension test. The patient, aligned in neutral, raises the nontest limb. The examiner (on patient's right) maintains trunk and limb alignment in neutral, and if the knee or ankle or both are unstable, manual support is provided by the assistant, as illustrated.

Table 8-4 HIP EXTENSION

Score	Criteria
Weak (W)	Uncontrolled trunk flexion on hip occurs. (Examiner must prevent continued forward motion of the trunk by providing additional hand support.)
Moderate (M)	Patient is unable to maintain trunk completely erect or at the end of the available hip extension range. The patient is, however, able to stop the forward trunk momentum. Alternatively, the trunk wobbles back and forth or the patient hyperextends the trunk on the hip.
Strong (S)	Patient maintains trunk erect or at the end of the available hip extension range.

Part 5: Knee Extension

Positioning and Stabilization: The assistant is positioned behind the patient to provide hand support for balance and to maintain the trunk erect on the hip (Fig. 8–2).

The examiner positions the patient's knees in 30° of flexion bilaterally. If the patient is unable to maintain both feet flat on the floor with approximately 30° of knee flexion, a hard wedge should be placed under the heel to compensate for the limited dorsiflexion range of motion.

Instructions to Patient: "Stand on both feet with your knees bent. Keep your knees bent and lift your right/left leg." (Note: the raised leg should be the stronger limb.)

If the patient can support body weight on a flexed knee during single-limb support without further collapse into flexion, proceed to the test for Strong (S) (Table 8–5).

Grading: See Table 8–5. When a knee flexion contracture is present, the grade awarded can never exceed Moderate (M).

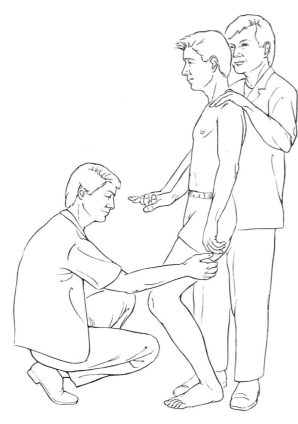

FIGURE 8–2
Knee extension test. The patient stands with both feet in plantigrade position. The examiner, kneeling in front, gives manual cues to the patient to flex both knees to 30°. The assistant stands behind the patient to offer balance support to one of the patient's hands and uses the other hand to cue the patient to maintain erect posture.

Table 8–5 KNEE EXTENSION

Score	Criteria
Weak (W)	Patient is unable to maintain body weight on a flexed knee; therefore, the knee continues to collapse into flexion or the heel rises.
Moderate (M)	Patient supports body weight on a flexed knee without either further collapse into flexion or heel rise.
Strong (S)	Patient supports body weight on a flexed knee and on request straightens that knee to the end of available knee extension range. Hyperextension is allowed.
Excessive (E)	It is not possible to position the knee in flexion because of severe extensor thrust or extensor tone.
Unable to Test (UT)	Absence of plantigrade foot or other condition renders test invalid.

Part 6: Ankle Extension (Plantar Flexion)

The purpose of this part of the extension test is to identify ankle control relative to maintaining a vertical tibial position.

If the patient has a knee flexion contracture in the test limb, the test cannot be conducted in a correct manner. With the knee flexed, the quadriceps muscle group can maintain single-limb stance despite the presence or absence of activity at the ankle.

Positioning and Stabilization: The assistant is positioned behind the patient to maintain the trunk in an erect posture over the hip (Fig. 8–3). The examiner is positioned to prevent knee hyperextension (i.e., ankle plantar flexion).

The passive range of ankle motion must be measured with the knee extended. If necessary, accommodate lack of dorsiflexion range (as occurs with a plantar flexion contracture) by placing a hard wedge under the heel. This will place the ankle in more plantar flexion, thus providing some relative dorsiflexion range for the purpose of this test.

Instructions to Patient: "Stand on both legs as straight as you can. Lift and hold up your right/left leg." (Note: The raised leg should be the stronger limb.)

If the patient can control the tibia with the knee in neutral, proceed to ask for a heel rise while the knee is kept at 0°:

"Keep your knee straight and go up on your toes as high as you can."

Grading: See Table 8–6.

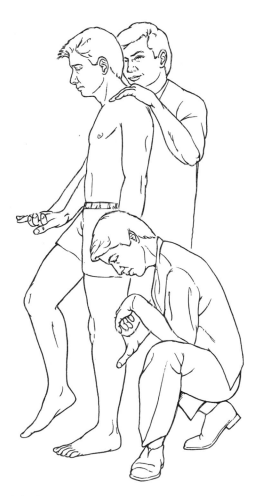

FIGURE 8–3
Ankle extension test. The patient stands erect in plantigrade position, then raises the nontest limb. The examiner kneels alongside or slightly behind to keep the knee from hyperextending. The assistant stands behind the patient to offer balance support and to cue the patient to maintain erect posture.

Table 8-6 PLANTAR FLEXION

Score	Criteria
Weak (W)	Patient is unable to maintain knee in neutral position; knee collapses into flexion and the ankle into dorsiflexion so that the tibia is displaced forward. Alternatively, the knee or ankle segment wobbles back and forth between flexion and extension or hyperextension. The presence of an extensor thrust that cannot be controlled by examiner also may indicate lack of adequate ankle control.
Moderate (M)	Patient can control the knee in a neutral (0°) position and the ankle in a neutral (90°) position so that the tibia is vertical.
Strong (S)	Patient maintains knee at neutral and lifts heel off floor on command. (Any degree of heel rise while maintaining the knee at neutral is acceptable.)
Excessive (E)	Severity of equinus or varus is so great that patient cannot maintain a stable plantigrade ankle.
Unable to Test (UT)	Patient has a knee flexion contracture.

References

1. Lovett RW, Martin EG. Certain aspects of infantile paralysis and a description of a method of muscle testing. JAMA 66:729–733, 1916.
2. Montgomery J. Assessment and treatment of locomotor deficits in stroke. *In* Duncan P, Radke M (eds): *Stroke Rehabilitation*. St Louis: Mosby–Year Book, 1987.
3. Perry J, Giovan P, Harris LJ, et al. The determinants of muscle action in the hemiparetic lower extremity. Clin Orthop 131:71–89, 1978.
4. Sawner K, LaVigne JM. *Brunnstrom's Movement Therapy in Hemiplegia*. Philadelphia: JB Lippincott, 1992.
5. Knutsson E, Richards C. Different types of disturbed motor control in gait of hemiparetic patients. Brain 102:405–430, 1979.

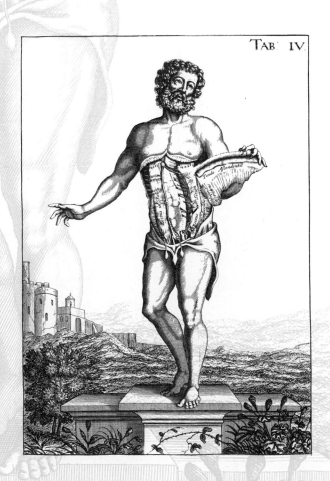

CHAPTER 9

*Ready
Reference
Anatomy*

USING THIS READY REFERENCE

This chapter of the book is intended as a quick source of information about muscles, their anatomical description, participation in motions, and innervation. This information is not intended to be comprehensive, and for depth of subject matter the reader is referred to any of the major texts of human anatomy. We relied on the American[1] and British[2] versions of *Gray's Anatomy* as principal references but also used *Sobotta's Atlas*[3] Clemente,[4] Netter,[5] Hollingshead,[6] Jenkins,[6] Grant,[7] and Moore,[8] among others. The final arbiter in all cases was the 38th edition of *Gray's Anatomy* (British) by Williams et al.[2]

The variations in text descriptions of individual muscles remain exceedingly diverse so at times we have consolidated information to provide abstracted descriptions.

Origins, insertions, descriptions, and functions of individual muscles often are abbreviated but should allow the reader to place the muscle correctly and visualize its most common actions; this in turn may help the reader to recall more detailed anatomy.

Nomina Anatomica nomenclature for the muscles appears in brackets when a more common usage is listed.

Muscle Reference (ID) Numbers

Each skeletal muscle in the body has been given a number that is used with that muscle throughout the book. The order of numbering is derived from the regional sequence of muscles used in Part 2 of this reference. The numbering should, however, permit the reader to refer quickly to any one of the summaries or to cross-check information between summaries. In the first part of the ready reference section (and also inside the front cover) the muscles are listed in alphabetical order, and this is followed by a list of muscles by region (also inside the back cover). In each muscle test the participating muscles also are preceded by their assigned identification (reference) number.

PART 1. ALPHABETICAL LIST OF MUSCLES

A

159 Abductor digiti minimi (hand)
215 Abductor digiti minimi (foot)
224 Abductor hallucis
171 Abductor pollicis brevis
166 Abductor pollicis longus
180 Adductor brevis
225 Adductor hallucis
179 Adductor longus
181 Adductor magnus
173 Adductor pollicis
144 Anconeus
27 Auriculares
201 Articularis genus

B

140 Biceps brachii
192 Biceps femoris
141 Brachialis
143 Brachioradialis
26 Buccinator
120 Bulbospongiosus

C

34 Chondroglossus
116 Coccygeus
139 Coracobrachialis
5 Corrugator supercilii
50 Cricothyroid [Cricothyroideus]
117 Cremaster

D

133 Deltoid [Deltoideus]
23 Depressor anguli oris
24 Depressor labii inferioris
14 Depressor septi
101 Diaphragm
78 Digastric [Digastricus]

E

2 Epicranius
149 Extensor carpi radialis brevis
148 Extensor carpi radialis longus
150 Extensor carpi ulnaris
158 Extensor digiti minimi

154 Extensor digitorum

212 Extensor digitorum brevis

211 Extensor digitorum longus

221 Extensor hallucis longus

155 Extensor indicis

168 Extensor pollicis brevis

167 Extensor pollicis longus

F

151 Flexor carpi radialis

153 Flexor carpi ulnaris

160 Flexor digiti minimi brevis (hand)

216 Flexor digiti minimi brevis (foot)

214 Flexor digitorum brevis

213 Flexor digitorum longus

157 Flexor digitorum profundus

156 Flexor digitorum superficialis

223 Flexor hallucis brevis

222 Flexor hallucis longus

170 Flexor pollicis brevis

169 Flexor pollicis longus

G

205 Gastrocnemius

190 Gemellus inferior

189 Gemellus superior

32 Genioglossus

77 Geniohyoid [Geniohyoideus]

182 Gluteus maximus

183 Gluteus medius

184 Gluteus minimus

178 Gracilis

H

33 Hyoglossus

I

176 Iliacus

66 Iliocostalis cervicis

89 Iliocostalis thoracis

90 Iliocostalis lumborum

41 Inferior pharyngeal constrictor [Constrictor pharyngis inferior]

38 Inferior longitudinal (tongue) [Longitudinalis inferior]

84–87 Infrahyoids (see Sternothyroid, Thyrohyoid, Sternohyoid, Omohyoid)

136 Infraspinatus

102 Intercostales externi

103 Intercostales interni

104 Intercostales intimi

164 Interossei, dorsal (hand) [Interossei dorsales]

219 Interossei, dorsal (foot) [Interossei dorsales]

165 Interossei, palmar or volar [Interossei palmarcs]

220 Interossei, plantar [Interossei plantares]

69 Interspinales cervicis

97 Interspinales thoracis

98 Interspinales lumborum

70 Intertransversarii cervicis

99 Intertransversarii thoracis

99 Intertransversarii lumborum

121 Ischiocavernosus

L

52 Lateral cricoarytenoid [Cricoarytenoideus lateralis]

30 Lateral pterygoid [Pterygoideus lateralis]

130 Latissimus dorsi

115 Levator ani

17 Levator anguli oris

15 Levator labii superioris

16 Levator labii superioris alaeque nasi

3 Levator palpebrae superioris

127 Levator scapulae

46 Levator veli palatini

107 Levatores costarum

60 Longissimus capitis

64 Longissimus cervicis

91 Longissimus thoracis

74 Longus capitis

79 Longus colli

163 Lumbricales (hand) [Lumbricals]

218 Lumbricales (foot) [Lumbricals]

M

28 Masseter

31 Medial pterygoid [Pterygoideus medialis]

21 Mentalis

42 Middle pharyngeal constrictor [Constrictor pharyngis medius]

94 Multifidi

48 Musculus uvulae

75 Mylohyoid [Mylohyoideus]

N

13 Nasalis

O

54 Oblique arytenoid [Arytenoideus obliquus]

59 Obliquus capitis inferior

58 Obliquus capitis superior

110 Obliquus externus abdominis

11 Obliquus inferior oculi

111 Obliquus internus abdominis

10 Obliquus superior oculi

188 Obturator externus [Obturatorius externus]

187 Obturator internus [Obturatorius internus]

1 Occipitofrontalis

87 Omohyoid [Omohyoideus]

161 Opponens digiti minimi

172 Opponens pollicis

4 Orbicularis oculi

25 Orbicularis oris

P

36 Palatoglossus

49 Palatopharyngeus

162 Palmaris brevis

152 Palmaris longus

177 Pectineus

131 Pectoralis major

129 Pectoralis minor

209 Peroneus brevis

208 Peroneus longus

210 Peroneus tertius

186 Piriformis

207 Plantaris

88 Platysma

202 Popliteus

51 Posterior cricoarytenoid [Cricoarytenoideus posterior]

12 Procerus

147 Pronator quadratus

146 Pronator teres

174 Psoas major

175 Psoas minor

114 Pyramidalis

Q

191 Quadratus femoris

100 Quadratus lumborum

217 Quadratus plantae

196–200 Quadriceps femoris (see Rectus femoris, Vastus intermedius, Vastus medialis longus, Vastus medialis oblique, Vastus lateralis)

R

113 Rectus abdominis

72 Rectus capitis anterior

73 Rectus capitis lateralis

56 Rectus capitis posterior major

57 Rectus capitis posterior minor

196 Rectus femoris

7 Rectus inferior

9 Rectus lateralis

8 Rectus medialis

6 Rectus superior

125 Rhomboid major [Rhomboideus major]

126 Rhomboid minor [Rhomboideus minor]

20 Risorius

71 Rotatores cervicis

96 Rotatores lumborum

95 Rotatores thoracis

S

45 Salpingopharyngeus

195 Sartorius

80 Scalenus anterior

81 Scalenus medius

82 Scalenus posterior

194 Semimembranosus

62 Semispinalis capitis

65 Semispinalis cervicis

93 Semispinalis thoracis

193 Semitendinosus

128 Serratus anterior

109 Serratus posterior inferior

108 Serratus posterior superior

206 Soleus

123 Sphincter ani externus

122 Sphincter urethrae

63 Spinalis capitis

68 Spinalis cervicis

92 Spinalis thoracis

61 Splenius capitis

67 Splenius cervicis

83 Sternocleidomastoid [Sternocleidomastoideus]

86 Sternohyoid [Sternohyoideus]

84 Sternothyroid [Sternothyroideus]

35 Styloglossus

76 Stylohyoid [Stylohyoideus]

44 Stylopharyngeus

132 Subclavius

105 Subcostales

134 Subscapularis

43 Superior pharyngeal constrictor [Constrictor pharyngis superior]

37 Superior longitudinal (tongue) [Longitudinalis superior]

145 Supinator

75-78 Suprahyoids (see Mylohyoid, Stylohyoid, Geniohyoid, Digastric)

135 Supraspinatus

T

29 Temporalis

2 Temporoparietalis

185 Tensor fasciae latae

47 Tensor veli palatini

138 Teres major

137 Teres minor

85 Thyrohyoid [Thyrohyoideus]

55 Thyroarytenoid [Thyroarytenoideus]

203 Tibialis anterior

204 Tibialis posterior

39 Transverse lingual [Transversus linguae]

112 Transversus abdominis

53 Transverse arytenoid [Arytenoideus transversus]

22 Transversus menti

119 Transversus perinei profundus

118 Transversus perinei superficialis

106 Transversus thoracis

124 Trapezius

142 Triceps brachii

U

48 Uvula (see Musculus uvulae)

V

198 Vastus intermedius

199 Vastus medialis longus

200 Vastus medialis oblique

197 Vastus lateralis

40 Vertical lingual [Verticalis linguae]

Z

18 Zygomaticus major

19 Zygomaticus minor

PART 2. LIST OF MUSCLES BY REGION

HEAD AND FOREHEAD

1 Occipitofrontalis
2 Temporoparietalis

EYELIDS

3 Levator palpebrae superioris
4 Orbicularis oculi
5 Corrugator supercilii

OCULAR MUSCLES

6 Rectus superior
7 Rectus inferior
8 Rectus medialis
9 Rectus lateralis
10 Obliquus superior
11 Obliquus inferior

NOSE

12 Procerus
13 Nasalis
14 Depressor septi

MOUTH

15 Levator labii superioris
16 Levator labii superioris alaeque nasi
17 Levator anguli oris
18 Zygomaticus major
19 Zygomaticus minor
20 Risorius
21 Mentalis
22 Transversus menti
23 Depressor anguli oris
24 Depressor labii inferioris
25 Orbicularis oris
26 Buccinator

EAR

27 Auriculares

JAW (MASTICATION)

28 Masseter
29 Temporalis
30 Lateral pterygoid
31 Medial pterygoid

TONGUE

32 Genioglossus
33 Hyoglossus
34 Chondroglossus
35 Styloglossus
36 Palatoglossus
37 Superior longitudinal
38 Inferior longitudinal
39 Transverse lingual
40 Vertical lingual

PHARYNX

41 Inferior pharyngeal constrictor
42 Middle pharyngeal constrictor
43 Superior pharyngeal constrictor
44 Stylopharyngeus
45 Salpingopharyngeus
49 Palatopharyngeus (see under *Palate*)

PALATE

46 Levator veli palatini
47 Tensor veli palatini
48 Musculus uvulae
36 Palatoglossus (see under *Tongue*)
49 Palatopharyngeus

LARYNX

50 Cricothyroid

51 Posterior cricoarytenoid

52 Lateral cricoarytenoid

53 Transverse arytenoid

54 Oblique arytenoid

55 Thyroarytenoid

55a Vocalis

55b Thyroepiglotticus

NECK

56 Rectus capitis posterior major

57 Rectus capitis posterior minor

58 Obliquus capitis superior

59 Obliquus capitis inferior

60 Longissimus capitis

61 Splenius capitis

62 Semispinalis capitis

63 Spinalis capitis

64 Longissimus cervicis

65 Semispinalis cervicis

66 Iliocostalis cervicis

67 Splenius cervicis

68 Spinalis cervicis

69 Interspinales cervicis

70 Intertransversarii cervicis

71 Rotatores cervicis

72 Rectus capitis anterior

73 Rectus capitis lateralis

74 Longus capitis

75 Mylohyoid

76 Stylohyoid

77 Geniohyoid

78 Digastricus

79 Longus colli

80 Scalenus anterior

81 Scalenus medius

82 Scalenus posterior

83 Sternocleidomastoid

84 Sternothyroid

85 Thyrohyoid

86 Sternohyoid

87 Omohyoid

88 Platysma

BACK

61 Splenius capitis (see under *Neck*)

67 Splenius cervicis (see under *Neck*)

66 Iliocostalis cervicis (see under *Neck*)

89 Iliocostalis thoracis

90 Iliocostalis lumborum

60 Longissimus capitis (see under *Neck*)

64 Longissimus cervicis (see under *Neck*)

91 Longissimus thoracis

63 Spinalis capitis

68 Spinalis cervicis

92 Spinalis thoracis

62 Semispinalis capitis (see under *Neck*)

65 Semispinalis cervicis (see under *Neck*)

93 Semispinalis thoracis

94 Multifidi

71 Rotatores cervicis

95 Rotatores thoracis

96 Rotatores lumborum

69 Interspinalis cervicis

97 Interspinalis thoracis

98 Interspinalis lumborum

70 Intertransversarii cervicis

99 Intertransversarii thoracis

99 Intertransversarii lumborum

100 Quadratus lumborum

THORAX (RESPIRATION)

101 Diaphragm

102 Intercostales externi

103 Intercostales interni

104 Intercostales intimi

105 Subcostales

106 Transversus thoracis

107 Levatores costarum

108 Serratus posterior superior

109 Serratus posterior inferior

ABDOMEN

110 Obliquus externus abdominis

111 Obliquus internus abdominis

112 Transversus abdominis

113 Rectus abdominis

114 Pyramidalis

PERINEUM

115 Levator ani

116 Coccygeus

117 Cremaster

118 Transversus perinei superficialis

119 Transversus perinei profundus

120 Bulbospongiosus

121 Ischiocavernosus

122 Sphincter urethrae

123 Sphincter ani externus

UPPER EXTREMITY

Shoulder Girdle

124 Trapezius

125 Rhomboid major

126 Rhomboid minor

127 Levator scapulae

128 Serratus anterior

129 Pectoralis minor

Vertebrohumeral

130 Latissimus dorsi

131 Pectoralis major

Shoulder

132 Subclavius

133 Deltoid

134 Subscapularis

135 Supraspinatus

136 Infraspinatus

137 Teres minor

138 Teres major

139 Coracobrachialis

Elbow

140 Biceps brachii

141 Brachialis

142 Triceps brachii

143 Brachioradialis

144 Anconeus

Forearm

145 Supinator

146 Pronator teres

147 Pronator quadratus

140 Biceps brachii (see under *Elbow*)

Wrist

148 Extensor carpi radialis longus

149 Extensor carpi radialis brevis

150 Extensor carpi ulnaris

151 Flexor carpi radialis

152 Palmaris longus

153 Flexor carpi ulnaris

Fingers

154 Extensor digitorum

155 Extensor indicis

156 Flexor digitorum superficialis

157 Flexor digitorum profundus

163 Lumbricales

164 Interossei, dorsal

165 Interossei, palmar

Little Finger and Hypothenar Muscles

158 Extensor digiti minimi

159 Abductor digiti minimi

160 Flexor digiti minimi brevis

161 Opponens digiti minimi

162 Palmaris brevis

Thumb and Thenar Muscles

166 Abductor pollicis longus

167 Extensor pollicis longus

168 Extensor pollicis brevis

169 Flexor pollicis longus

170 Flexor pollicis brevis

171 Abductor pollicis brevis

172 Opponens pollicis

173 Adductor pollicis

LOWER EXTREMITY

Hip and Thigh

174 Psoas major

175 Psoas minor

176 Iliacus

177 Pectineus

178 Gracilis

179 Adductor longus

180 Adductor brevis

181 Adductor magnus

182 Gluteus maximus

183 Gluteus medius

184 Gluteus minimus

185 Tensor fasciae latae

186 Piriformis

187 Obturator internus

188 Obturator externus

189 Gemellus superior

190 Gemellus inferior

191 Quadratus femoris

192 Biceps femoris

193 Semitendinosus

194 Semimembranosus

195 Sartorius

Knee

196-200 Quadriceps femoris

196 Rectus femoris

197 Vastus lateralis

198 Vastus intermedius

199 Vastus medialis longus

200 Vastus medialis oblique

201 Articularis genus

192 Biceps femoris

193 Semitendinosus

194 Semimembranosus

202 Popliteus

Ankle

203 Tibialis anterior

204 Tibialis posterior

205 Gastrocnemius

206 Soleus

207 Plantaris

208 Peroneus longus

209 Peroneus brevis

210 Peroneus tertius

Lesser Toes

211 Extensor digitorum longus

212 Extensor digitorum brevis

213 Flexor digitorum longus

214 Flexor digitorum brevis

215 Abductor digiti minimi

216 Flexor digiti minimi brevis

217 Quadratus plantae

218 Lumbricales

219 Interossei, dorsal

220 Interossei, plantar

Great Toe (Hallux)

221 Extensor hallucis longus

222 Flexor hallucis longus

223 Flexor hallucis brevis

224 Abductor hallucis

225 Adductor hallucis

PART 3. SKELETAL MUSCLES OF THE HUMAN BODY

MUSCLES OF THE FOREHEAD

The Epicranius (Two Muscles)

1 Occipitofrontalis

2 Temporoparietalis

1 OCCIPITOFRONTALIS

Muscle has two parts

Occipital part (Occipitalis)

Origin:
   Occiput (superior nuchal line, lateral 2/3)
   Temporal bone (mastoid process)

Insertion:
   Galea aponeurotica

Frontal part (Frontalis)

Origin:
   Superficial fascia over scalp
   No bony attachments
   Median fibers continuous with Procerus
   Intermediate fibers join Corrugator supercilii and Orbicularis oculi
   Lateral fibers also join Orbicularis oculi

Insertion:
   Galea aponeurotica
   Skin of eyebrows and root of nose

Description:
   Overlies the cranium from the eyebrows to the superior nuchal line on the occiput. The Epicranius consists of the Occipitofrontalis with its four thin branches on either side of the head; the broad aponeurosis called the galea aponeurotica; and the Temporoparietalis with its two slim branches. The medial margins of the two bellies join above the nose and run together upward and over the forehead.

   The Galea aponeurotica covers the cranium between the frontal belly and the occipital belly of the Epicranius and between the two occipital bellies over the occiput. It is adhered closely to the dermal layers (scalp), which allows the scalp to be moved freely over the cranium.

Function:
   Contracting together, both bellies draw the scalp up and back, thus raising the eyebrows (surprise!) and assisting with wrinkling the forehead
   Working alone, the frontal belly raises the eyebrow on the same side

Innervation:
   Facial (VII) nerve
      Temporal branches: to Frontalis
      Posterior auricular branch: to Occipitalis

2 TEMPOROPARIETALIS

Origin:
   Temporal fascia (superior and anterior to external ear, then fanning out and up over temporal fascia)

Insertion:
   Galea aponeurotica (lateral border)
   Into skin and temporal fascia somewhere high on lateral side of head

Description:
   A thin broad sheet of muscle in two bellies which lie on either side of head. Highly variable. See also description of Occipitofrontalis.

Function:
Tightens scalp
Draws back skin over temples
Raises auricula of the ear
In concert with Occipitofrontalis, raises the eyebrows, widens the eyes, and wrinkles the skin of the forehead (in expressions of surprise and fright)

Innervation:
Facial (VII) nerve (temporal branches)

MUSCLES OF THE EYELIDS AND EYEBROWS

3 Levator palpebrae superioris

4 Orbicularis oculi

5 Corrugator supercilii

3 LEVATOR PALPEBRAE SUPERIORIS

Origin:
Sphenoid bone (inferior surface of lesser wing)
Roof of orbital cavity

Insertion:
Into several lamellae:
Aponeurosis of the orbital septum
Superior tarsus (a small thin smooth fiber muscle on the inferior surface of the Levator palpebrae and skin of eyelids)
Upper eyelid skin
Sheath of the Rectus superior (and with it, blends with the superior fornix of the conjunctiva)

Description:
Thin and flat muscle lying posterior and superior to the orbit. At its origin it is tendinous, broadening out to end in a wide aponeurosis that splits into three lamellae. Connective tissue of the Levator fuses with adjoining connective tissue of the Rectus superior and this aponeurosis can be traced laterally to a tubercle of the zygomatic bone and medially to the medial palpebral ligament.

Function:
Raises upper eyelid

Innervation:
Oculomotor (III) nerve (superior division)

4 ORBICULARIS OCULI

Muscle has three parts

Origin:
Orbital part:
Frontal bone (nasal part)
Maxilla (frontal process in front of lacrimal groove)
Medial palpebral ligament
Palpebral part:
Medial palpebral ligament
Frontal bone just in front of and below the palpebral ligament
Lacrimal part:
Lacrimal fascia
Lacrimal bone (crest and lateral surface)

Insertion:
Orbital part: The fibers blend with nearby muscles. (Occipitofrontalis and Corrugator supercilii). Some fibers also insert into skin of eyebrow.
Palpebral part: Lateral palpebral raphe
Lacrimal part: Superior and inferior tarsi of the eyelids. Fibers form lateral palpebral raphe.

Description:
Forms a broad thin layer that fills the eyelids (see Fig. 7–13) and surrounds the circumference of the orbit but also spreads over the temple and cheek. Orbital fibers form complete ellipses. On the lateral side there are no bony attachments. The upper orbital fiber ellipses blend with the Occipitofrontalis and Corrugator supercilii muscles. Fibers also insert into the skin of the eyebrow forming a Depressor supercilii. Medially some ellipses reach the Procerus.
The inferior orbital ellipses blend with the Levator labii superioris alaeque nasi, Levator labii superioris, and the Zygomaticus minor.
The fibers of the palpebral part sweep across the upper and lower eyelids anterior to the orbital septum to form the lateral palpebral raphe. The ciliary bundle is composed of a small group of fibers behind the eyelashes.
The lacrimal part fibers lying behind the lacrimal sac (in the medial corner of the eye) divide into upper and lower slips which insert into the superior and inferior tarsi of the eyelids and the lateral palpebral raphe.

Function:
The Orbicularis oculi is the sphincter of the eye.
Orbital part: While closing the eye is mostly lowering of the upper lid, the lower lid also rises and both are under voluntary control and can work with greater force, as in winking.
Palpebral part: Closes lids in blinking (protective reflex) and for sleep (voluntary).
Lacrimal part: Draws the eyelids and lacrimal canals medially, compressing them against the globe of the eye to receive tears. Also compresses lacrimal sac during blinking.

Entire muscle contraction draws skin of forehead, temple, and cheek toward the medial angle of the eye, tightly closing the eye and displacing the lids medially. The folds formed by this action in later life form "crow's feet." The muscles around the eye are important because they cause blinking, which keeps the eye lubricated and prevents dehydration of the conjunctiva. The muscle also bunches up to protect the eye from excessive light.

Innervation:
Facial (VII) nerve (temporal and zygomatic branches)

5 CORRUGATOR SUPERCILII

Origin:
Frontal bone (superciliary arch, medial end)

Insertion:
Skin (deep surface) of eyebrow over middle of orbital arch

Description:
Fibers of this small muscle lie at the medial end of each eyebrow, deep to the Occipitofrontalis and Orbicularis oculi muscles with which it often blends.

Function:
Draws eyebrows down and medially, producing vertical wrinkles of the forehead between the eyes (frowning). This action also shields the eyes from bright sun.

Innervation:
Facial (VII) nerve (temporal branch)

OCULAR MUSCLES

6 Rectus superior

7 Rectus inferior

8 Rectus medialis

9 Rectus lateralis

10 Obliquus superior

11 Obliquus inferior

The Extraocular Muscles

There are seven extraocular muscles of the eye: the four Recti, the two Obliquii, and the Levator palpebrae. The Recti with the Obliquii can move the eyeball in infinite directions, while the Levator can raise the upper eyelid. In addition, there are Superior and Inferior tarsal muscles in the upper and lower eyelids; the superior is related to the Levator palpebrae superior, while the Inferior works with the Rectus inferior and Inferior oblique. The Orbicularis oculi also is an extraocular muscle but it is described with the facial muscles.

6–9 THE FOUR RECTI (Fig. 9-1)

Rectus superior, inferior, medialis, and lateralis

Origin:
At the back of the eye, the tendons of the four recti are attached to a common annular tendon. This tendon rings the superior, medial, and inferior margins of the optic foramen and attaches to the sphenoid bone (greater wing). It also adheres to the sheath of the optic nerve. The attachments of the four Recti circle the tendon on its medial, superior, and inferior margins. The ring around the optic nerve is completed by a lower fibrous extension (tendon of Zinn), which gives origin to the Rectus inferior, part of the Rectus medialis, and the lower head of origin of the Rectus lateralis. An upper fibrous expansion gives rise to the Rectus superior, part of the Rectus medialis, and the upper head of the Rectus lateralis.

Insertion:
Each of the Recti passes anteriorly in the position indicated by its name and inserts via a tendinous expansion into the sclera a short distance behind the cornea.

Description:
From their common origin around the margins of the optic canal these straplike muscles become wider as they pass anteriorly to insert on different points on the sclera (see Fig. 9–1) The Rectus superior is the smallest and thinnest and inserts on the superoanterior sclera under the orbital roof. The inferior muscle inserts on the inferoanterior sclera just above the orbital floor. The Rectus medialis is the broadest of the recti and inserts on the medial scleral wall well in front of the equator. The Rectus lateralis, the longest of the Recti, courses around the lateral side of the eyeball to insert well forward of the equator.

Function:
The ocular muscles rotate the eyeball in directions that depend on the geometry of their relationships and that can be altered by the eye movements themselves. Eye movements also are accompanied by head motions, which assist with the incredibly complex varieties of stereoscopic vision.

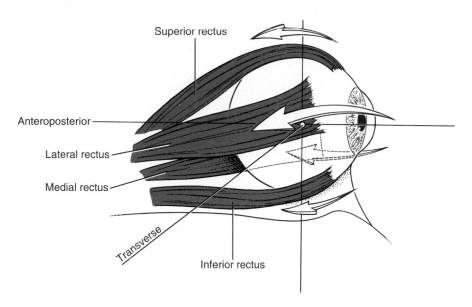

FIGURE 9-1
The four Recti, lateral view

The ocular muscles are not subject to direct study or routine assessment. It is essential to know that a change in the tension of one of the muscles alters the length-tension relationships of all six ocular muscles. It is likely that all six muscles are continuously involved, and consideration of each in isolation is not a functional exercise. The functional relationship between the four Recti and the two Obliquui may be considered as two differing synergies.

The Rectus superior, inferior, and medialis act together as adductors or convergence muscles.

The lateral Rectus, together with the two Obliquui, act as muscles of abduction or divergence.

Convergence generally is associated with elevation of the visual axis, and divergence with lowering of the visual axis.

Neurologists regularly test the ocular muscles when there is an isolated paralysis which gives greater insight into their functions.[9]

Superior rectus paralysis: Eye turns down and slightly outward. Upward motion is limited.

Medial rectus paralysis: Eyeball turns laterally and cannot deviate medially.

Inferior rectus paralysis: Eyeball deviates upward and somewhat laterally. It cannot be moved downward and the eye is abducted.

Lateral rectus paralysis: The eyeball is turned medially and cannot be abducted.

Inferior oblique paralysis: Eyeball is deviated downward and slightly medially, it cannot be moved upward when in abduction.

Superior oblique paralysis: Here there may be little deviation of the eyeball but downward motion is limited when the eye is adducted. There is no movement toward the midline of the face when looking downward in abduction (intorsion).[9]

Innervation:

Oculomotor (III) nerve: Rectus superior (superior division of III), inferior, and medialis, and Obliquus inferior (inferior division of III)

Abducent (VI) nerve: Rectus lateralis

Trochlear (IV) nerve: Obliquus superior

10 OBLIQUUS SUPERIOR OCULI

Origin:

Sphenoid bone (superior and medial to optic canal)

Rectus superior (tendon)

Insertion:

Frontal bone (via a round tendon that inserts through a pulley [a cartilaginous ring called the trochlea] that inserts in the trochlear fovea)

Sclera (behind the equator on the superolateral surface)

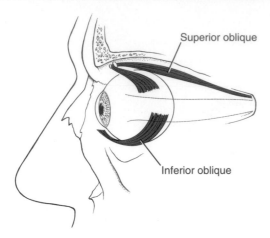

FIGURE 9–2
The oblique extraocular muscles

eyeball, passing under the Rectus lateralis to insert on the sclera beneath that muscle (see Figs. 9–1 and 9–2).

Function:
See under Obliquus superior (#10).

Innervation:
Oculomotor (III) nerve (inferior division)

MUSCLES OF THE NOSE

12 Procerus

13 Nasalis

14 Depressor septi

12 PROCERUS

Origin:
Nasal bone (dorsum of nose, lower part)
Nasal cartilage (lateral, upper part)

Insertion:
Skin over lower part of forehead between eyebrows
Joins Occipitofrontalis

Description:
From its origin over bridge of nose it courses straight upward to blend with Frontalis.

Function:
Produces transverse wrinkles over bridge of nose
Draws eyebrows downward

Innervation:
Facial (VII) nerve (buccal branch)

13 NASALIS

Transverse Part (Compressor nares)

Origin:
Maxilla (above and lateral to incisive fossa)

Insertion:
Aponeurosis over bridge of nose joining with muscle on opposite side

Alar Part (Dilator nares)

Origin:
Maxilla (above lateral incisor tooth)
Alar cartilage

Insertion:
Ala nasi
Skin at tip of nose

Description:
The superior oblique lies superomedially in the orbit (Fig. 9–2). It passes forward, ending in the round tendon that loops through the trochlear pulley, which is attached to the trochlear fovea. It then turns abruptly posterolaterally and passes thence to the sclera to end between the Rectus superior and the Rectus lateralis.

Function:
The superior oblique acts on the eye from above, whereas the inferior oblique acts on the eye directly below; the superior oblique elevates the posterior aspect of the eyeball, and the inferior oblique depresses it. The superior oblique, therefore, rotates the visual axis downward, whereas the inferior oblique rotates it upward, both motions occurring around the transverse axis.

Innervation:
Trochlear (IV) nerve

11 OBLIQUUS INFERIOR OCULI

Origin:
Maxilla (orbital surface, lateral to the lacrimal groove)

Insertion:
Sclera (lateral part) behind the equator of the eyeball between the insertions of the Rectus inferior and lateralis and near, but behind, the insertion of the Superior oblique

Description:
Located near the anterior margin of the floor of the orbit, it passes laterally under the eyeball between the Rectus inferior and the bony orbit. It then bends upward on the lateral side of the

Description:
> Muscle has two parts that cover the distal and medial surfaces of the nose. Fibers from each side rise upward and medially, meeting in a narrow aponeurosis near the bridge of the nose.

Function:
> *Transverse part:* Depresses cartilaginous portion of nose and draws alae toward septum
> *Alar part:* Dilates nostrils (during breathing it resists tendency of nares to close from atmospheric pressure).
> Noticeable in anger or labored breathing

Innervation:
> Facial (VII) nerve (buccal and zygomatic branches)

14 DEPRESSOR SEPTI

Origin:
> Maxilla (above and lateral to incisive fossa, i.e., central incisor)

Insertion:
> Nasal septum (mobile part) and alar cartilage

Description:
> Fibers ascend vertically from central maxillary origin. Muscle lies deep to the superior labial mucous membrane. It often is considered part of the dilator nares (of the Nasalis).

Function:
> Draws alae of nose downward (constricting nares)

Innervation:
> Facial (VII) nerve (buccal and zygomatic branches)

MUSCLES OF THE MOUTH

There are four independent quadrants, each of which has a pars peripheralis which lies along the junction of the red margin of the lip and skin and a pars marginalis which is found in the red margin of the lip (see Fig. 7–29). These two parts are supported by fibers from the Buccinator and Depressor anguli oris (upper lip) and from the Buccinator and Levator anguli oris (lower lip). These muscles are uniquely developed for speech.

> **15** Levator labii superioris
>
> **16** Levator labii superioris alaeque nasi
>
> **17** Levator anguli oris
>
> **18** Zygomaticus major

> **19** Zygomaticus minor
>
> **20** Risorius
>
> **21** Mentalis
>
> **22** Transversus menti
>
> **23** Depressor anguli oris
>
> **24** Depressor labii inferioris
>
> **25** Orbicularis oris
>
> **26** Buccinator

15 LEVATOR LABII SUPERIORIS

(Also called Quadratus labii superioris)

Origin:
> Orbit of eye (inferior margin)
> Maxilla
> Zygomatic bone

Insertion:
> Upper lip

Description:
> Converging from a rather broad place of origin on the inferior orbit, the fibers converge and descend into the upper lip between the other levator muscles and the Zygomaticus minor.

Function:
> Elevates and protracts upper lip.

Innervation:
> Facial (VII) nerve (buccal branch)

16 LEVATOR LABII SUPERIORIS ALAEQUE NASI

Origin:
> Maxilla (frontal process)

Insertion:
> Ala of nose
> Upper lip

Description:
> Muscle fibers descend obliquely lateral and divide into two slips: one to the greater alar cartilage of the nose and one to blend with the Levator labii superioris and Orbicularis oris (thence to the modiolus)

Function:
> Dilates nostrils
> Elevates upper lip

Innervation:
> Facial (VII) nerve (buccal branch)

Commentary on Facial Muscles

The muscles of the face are different from most skeletal muscles in the body because they are cutaneous muscles located in the deep layers of the skin and frequently have no bony attachments. All of them (scalp, eyelids, nose, lips, cheeks, mouth, and auricle) give rise to "expressions" and convey "thought," the most visible of the body language systems (Fig. 9–3).

The orbital muscles of the mouth are important for speech, drinking, and ingestion of solid foods.[10–12] Although the Buccinator is described in this section, it is not a muscle of expression but does serve an important role in regulating the position of, and action on, food in the mouth.

These muscles are continuously tonic to provide the facial skin with tension; the skin becomes baggy or flabby (resulting in, e.g., "crow's feet" or "wattles") when it is denervated or in the presence of the atrophic processes associated with aging. There are wide differences in these muscles among individuals and among racial groups, and to deal with such variations craniofacial and plastic surgeons often classify the facial muscles differently (e.g., in single vs. multiple heads) from the system presented here.

Continuous skin tension also gives rise to the gaping wounds that occur with facial lacerations, and surgeons take great care to understand the planes of the muscles to minimize scarring in the repair of such wounds.

The facial muscles all arise from the mesoderm of the second branchial (hyoid) arch. The muscles lie in all parts of the face and head but retain their innervation by the facial (VII) nerve.

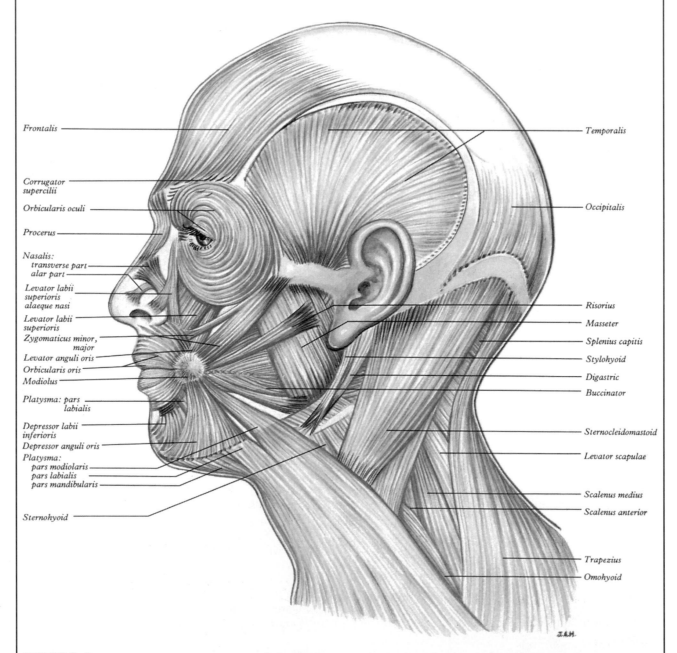

FIGURE 9–3
Muscles of the head and neck (superficial lateral view), including cicumorbital, buccolabial, nasal, epicranial, masticatory, and cervical groups. The articular muscles are omitted. Risorius, a variable muscle, here has two fasciculi, of which the lower one is unlabeled. The nature of the modiolus, the modiolar muscles, and their cooperation in facial movement is described in the text. The laminae of the direct labial tractors to both upper and lower lips have been transected to reveal the Orbicularis oris underneath. (From Williams PL (ed). *Gray's Anatomy,* 38th ed. London: Churchill Livingstone, 1999.)

17 LEVATOR ANGULI ORIS

Origin:
Maxilla (canine fossa)

Insertion:
Modiolus
Dermal attachment at angle of mouth

Description:
Muscle descends from maxilla, inferolateral to orbit, down to modiolus. It lies partially under
the Zygomaticus minor.

Function:
Raises angle of mouth and by so doing displays
teeth in smiling
Contributes to nasolabial furrow (from side of
nose to corner of upper lip). Deepens in sadness and aging.

Innervation:
Facial (VII) nerve (buccal branch)

18 ZYGOMATICUS MAJOR

Origin:
Zygomatic bone (lateral)

Insertion:
Modiolus[10-12]

Description:
Descends obliquely lateral to blend with other
modiolar muscles. A small and variable group
of superficial fascicles called the Malaris are
considered part of this muscle.

Function:
Draws angle of mouth lateral and upward (as in
laughing)

Innervation:
Facial (VII) nerve (buccal branch)

19 ZYGOMATICUS MINOR

Origin:
Zygomatic bone (malar surface) medial to origin
of Zygomaticus major

Insertion:
Upper lip; blends with Levator labii superioris
Modiolus[10-12]

Description:
Descends initially with Zygomaticus major, then
moves medially on top of Levator labii superioris, with which it blends.

Function:
Muscle of facial expression (as in sneering, expres-
sions of contempt, and smiling)
Elevates and curls upper lip, exposing the maxil-
lary teeth
Deepens nasolabial furrow

Innervation:
Facial (VII) nerve (buccal branch)

20 RISORIUS

Origin:
Masseteric fascia

Insertion:
Modiolus[10-12]

Description:
This muscle is so highly variable, even when present, it is possibly wrong to classify it as a separate muscle. When present, it passes forward almost horizontally. It may vary from a few fibers
to a wide, thin, superficial, fan-shaped sheet. It
is often considered the muscle of laughing, but
this is equally true of other modiolar muscles.

Function:
When present, retracts angle of mouth

Innervation:
Facial (VII) nerve (buccal branch)

21 MENTALIS

Origin:
Mandible (incisive fossa)

Insertion:
Skin over chin

Description:
Descends medially from its origin just lateral to
labial frenulum to center of skin of chin

Function:
Wrinkles skin over chin
Protrudes and raises lower lip (as in sulking or
drinking)

Innervation:
Facial (VII) nerve (marginal mandibular branch)

22 TRANSVERSUS MENTI

Origin:
Skin of the chin (laterally)

Insertion:
Skin of the chin
Blends with its contralateral muscle

Description:

As frequently absent as it is present. Very small muscle traverses chin inferiorly and therefore is called the mental sling. Often continuous with Depressor anguli oris.

Function:

Depresses angle of mouth; supports skin of chin

Innervation:

Facial (VII) nerve (marginal mandibular branch)

23 DEPRESSOR ANGULI ORIS

Origin:

Mandible (mental tubercle and oblique line)

Insertion:

Modiolus

Description:

Ascends in a curve from its broad origin below tubercle of mandible to a narrow fasciculus into modiolus. Often continuous below with Platysma.

Function:

Depresses lower lip and pulls down angle of mouth

Facial expression muscle (as in sadness)

Innervation:

Facial (VII) nerve (marginal mandibular branch)

24 DEPRESSOR LABII INFERIORIS

(Also called Quadratus labii inferioris)

Origin:

Mandible (oblique line between symphysis and mental foramen)

Insertion:

Skin and mucosa of lower lip

Modiolus

Description:

Passes upward and medially from a broad origin; then narrows and blends with Orbicularis oris and Depressor labii inferioris of opposite side

Function:

Draws lower lip down and laterally.

Facial expression muscle (sorrow, sadness)

Innervation:

Facial (VII) nerve (marginal mandibular branch)

25 ORBICULARIS ORIS

Origin:

No fascial attachments except the modiolus. This is a composite muscle with contributions from other muscles of the mouth, which form a complex sphincter-like structure, but it is not a true sphincter. Via its incisive components, the muscle attaches to the maxilla (Incisivus labii superioris) and mandible (Incisivus labii inferioris).

Insertion:

Modiolus

Labial connective tissue

Description[2]:

This muscle is not a complete ellipse of muscle surrounding the mouth. The fibers actually form four separate functional quadrants on each side that provide great diversity of oral movements. There is overlapping function among the quadrants (upper, lower, left, and right). The muscle is connected with the maxillae and septum of the nose by lateral and medial accessory muscles.

The Incisivus labii superioris is a lateral accessory muscle of the upper lip within the Orbicularis oris, and there is a similar accessory muscle, the Incisivus labii inferioris, for the lower lip. These muscles have bony attachments to the floor of the maxillary incisive (superior) fossa and the mandibular incisive (inferior) fossa. They arch laterally between the Orbicularis fibers on the respective lip and, after passing the buccal angle, insert into the modiolus. The modiolus acts as a force-transmission system to the lips from muscles attached to it.

The Orbicularis oris has another accessory muscle, the Nasolabialis, which lies medially and connects the upper lip to the nasal septum. (The interval between the contralateral Nasolabialis corresponds to the philtrum, the depression on the upper lip beneath the nasal septum.)

Function:

Closes lips

Protrudes lips

Holds lips tight against teeth

Shapes lips for whistling, kissing, sucking, drinking, etc.

Alters shape of lips for speech and musical sounds

Innervation:

Facial (VII) nerve (buccal and marginal mandibular branches)

This innervation is of interest because when one facial nerve is injured distal to the stylomastoid foramen, only half of the Orbicularis oris muscle is paralyzed. When this occurs, as in Bell's palsy, the mouth droops and may be drawn to the opposite side.

26 BUCCINATOR

Origin:
Maxilla and mandible (external surfaces of alveolar processes opposite molars)
Pterygomandibular raphe

Insertion:
Modiolus
Submucosa of cheek and lips

Description:
The principal muscle of the cheek is classified as a facial muscle (because of its innervation) despite its role in mastication. The Buccinator forms the lateral wall of the oral cavity, lying deep to the other facial muscles and filling the gap between the maxilla and the mandible.

Function:
Compresses cheek against the teeth
Expels air when cheeks are distended (in blowing)
Acts in mastication to control passage of food

Innervation:
Facial (VII) nerve (buccal branch)

EXTRINSIC MUSCLES OF THE EAR

Intrinsic muscles of the ear (6 in number) connect one part of the auricle to another and are not accessible or useful for manual testing. The three extrinsic muscles connect the auricle with the skull and scalp.

27 THE AURICULARES (Three Muscles)

Auricularis anterior

Origin:
Anterior fascia in temporal area (lateral edge of epicranial aponeurosis)

Insertion:
Spine of cartilaginous helix of ear

Auricularis superior

Origin:
Temporal fascia

Insertion:
Auricle (cranial surface)

Auricularis posterior

Origin:
Temporal bone (mastoid process) via a short aponeurosis

Insertion:
Auricle (cranial surface, concha)

Function (all):
Limited function in humans except at parties! The anterior muscle elevates the auricle and moves it forward; the superior muscle elevates the auricle slightly, and the posterior draws it back. Auditory stimuli may evoke minor responses from these muscles.

Innervation:
Facial (VII) nerve (temporal branch to anterior and superior Auriculares; posterior auricular branch to posterior auricular muscle)

MUSCLES OF JAW AND MASTICATION

28 Masseter

29 Temporalis

30 Lateral pterygoid

31 Medial pterygoid

28 MASSETER

Muscle has three parts

Superficial part:

Origin:
Maxilla (zygomatic process via an aponeurosis)
Zygomatic bone (maxillary process and inferior border of arch)

Insertion:
Mandible (ramus: angle and lower half of lateral surface)

Intermediate part:

Origin:
Zygomatic arch (inner surface of anterior 2/3)

Insertion:
Mandible (ramus, central part)

Deep part:

Origin:
Zygomatic arch (posterior 1/3 continuous with intermediate part)

Insertion:
Mandible (ramus [superior half] and lateral coronoid process)

Description:
A thick muscle connecting the upper and lower jaws and consisting of three layers that blend anteriorly. The superficial layer descends backward to the angle of the mandible and the lower mandibular ramus. (The middle and deep layers compose the deep part cited in *Nomina Anatomica*.) The muscle is easily palpable and lies under the parotid gland posteriorly; the anterior margin overlies the Buccinator.

Function:
Elevates the mandible (occlusion of the teeth in mastication)
Up-and-down biting motion

Innervation:
Trigeminal (V) nerve (mandibular division, masseteric branches)

29 TEMPORALIS

Origin:
Temporal bone (all of temporal fossa)
Temporal fascia (deep surface)

Insertion:
Mandible (coronoid process, medial surface, apex, and anterior border; anterior border of ramus almost to 3rd molar)

Description:
A broad muscle that radiates like a fan on the side of the head from most of the temporal fossa, converging downward to coronoid process of the mandible. The descending fibers converge into a tendon that passes between the zygomatic arch and the cranial wall. The more anterior fibers descend vertically, but the more posterior the fibers the more oblique their course until the most posterior fibers are almost horizontal. Difficult to palpate unless muscle is contracting as in clenching of teeth.

Function:
Elevates mandible to close mouth and approximate teeth (biting motion)
Retracts mandible (posterior fibers)
Participates in lateral grinding motions

Innervation:
Trigeminal (V) nerve (mandibular division, deep temporal branch)

30 LATERAL PTERYGOID

Has two heads

Origin:
Superior head: Sphenoid bone (greater wing, infratemporal crest and surface)
Inferior head: Sphenoid bone (lateral pterygoid plate, lateral surface)

Insertion:
Mandible (condylar neck, pterygoid fossa)
Temporomandibular joint (TMJ) (articular capsule and disc)

Description:
A short, thick muscle with two heads that runs posterolaterally to the mandibular condyle, neck, and disc of the TMJ. The fibers of the upper head are directed downward and laterally, while those of the lower head course horizontally. The muscle lies under the mandibular ramus.

Function:
Protracts mandibular condyle and disc of TMJ joint forward while the mandibular head rotates on disc (participates in opening of mouth).
The Lateral pterygoid, acting with the elevators of the mandible, protrudes the jaw, causing malocclusion of the teeth (i.e., the lower teeth project in front of the upper teeth).
When the Lateral and Medial pterygoids on the same side act jointly, the mandible and the jaw (chin) rotate to the opposite side (chewing motion).
Assists mouth closure: condyle retracts as muscle lengthens to assist Masseter and Temporalis.

Innervation:
Trigeminal (V) nerve (mandibular division, nerve to Lateral pterygoid)

31 MEDIAL PTERYGOID

Origin:
Sphenoid bone (lateral pterygoid plate)
Palatine bone (grooved surface of pyramidal process)
Maxilla (tuberosity)
Palatine bone (tubercle)

Insertion:
Mandible medial surface of ramus via a strong tendon, reaching as high as mandibular foramen

Description:
This short, thick muscle occupies the position on the inner side of the mandibular ramus, whereas the Masseter occupies the outer position. The Medial pterygoid is separated by the Lateral pterygoid from the mandibular ramus. The deep fibers arise from the palatine bone;

the more superficial fibers arise from the maxilla and lie superficial to the Lateral pterygoid. The fibers descend posterolaterally to the mandibular ramus.

Function:

Elevates mandible to close jaws (biting).

Protrudes mandible (with Lateral pterygoid).

Unilaterally the Medial and Lateral pterygoids together rotate the mandible forward and to the opposite side. This alternating motion is chewing.

The Medial pterygoid and Masseter are situated to form a sling that suspends the mandible. This sling is a functional articulation in which the TMJ acts as a guide. As the mouth opens and closes, the mandible moves on a center of rotation established by the sling and the spheno-mandibular ligament.

Innervation:

Trigeminal (V) nerve (mandibular division, nerve to Medial pterygoid)

MUSCLES OF THE TONGUE

Extrinsic Tongue Muscles

32 Genioglossus

33 Hyoglossus

34 Chondroglossus

35 Styloglossus

36 Palatoglossus

32 GENIOGLOSSUS

Origin:

Mandible (symphysis menti on inner surface of superior mental spine)

Insertion:

Hyoid bone via a thin aponeurosis

Middle pharyngeal constrictor muscle

Undersurface of tongue, whole length mingling with the intrinsic musculature of tongue

Description:

The tongue is separated into lateral halves by the lingual septum, which extends along its full length and inserts inferiorly into the hyoid bone. The extrinsics extend outside the tongue.

The Genioglossus is a thin, flat muscle that fans out backward from its mandibular origin, running parallel with and close to the midline. The lower fibers run downward to the hyoid; the median fibers run posteriorly and join the mid-

dle constrictor of the pharynx; the superior fibers run upward to insert on the whole length of the underside of the tongue. The muscles of the two sides are blended anteriorly and separated posteriorly by the medial lingual septum (see Fig. 7–51).

Function:

Protraction of tongue (tip protrudes beyond mouth)

Depression of central part of tongue

Innervation:

Hypoglossal (XII) nerve, muscular branch

33 HYOGLOSSUS

Origin:

Hyoid bone (side of body and whole length of greater horn)

Insertion:

Side of tongue

Description:

Thin, quadrilateral muscle whose fibers run almost vertically

Function:

Depression and retraction of tongue

Innervation:

Hypoglossal (XII) nerve, muscular branch

34 CHONDROGLOSSUS

Origin:

Hyoid bone (lesser horn, medial side)

Insertion:

Blends with intrinsic muscles on side of tongue

Description:

A very small muscle (about 2 cm long) that is sometimes considered part of the Hyoglossus

Function:

Assists in tongue depression

Innervation:

Hypoglossal (XII) nerve, muscular branch

35 STYLOGLOSSUS

Origin:

Temporal bone (styloid process, apex)

Stylomandibular ligament (styloid end)

Insertion:

Muscle divides into two portions before entering side of tongue

Side of tongue near dorsal surface to blend with intrinsics (longitudinal portion)

Overlaps Hyoglossus and blends with it (oblique portion)

Description:

Shortest and smallest of extrinsic tongue muscles. The muscle curves down anteriorly and divides into longitudinal and oblique portions. It lies between the internal and external carotid arteries.

Function:

Draws tongue up and backward

Innervation:

Hypoglossal (XII) nerve, muscular branch

36 PALATOGLOSSUS

Origin:

Soft palate (anterior surface)

Insertion:

Side of tongue intermingling with intrinsic muscles

Description:

Technically an extrinsic muscle of the tongue, this muscle is functionally closer to the palate muscles. It is a small fasciculus, narrower in the middle than at its ends. It passes anteroinferiorly and laterally in front of the tonsil to reach the side of the tongue. Along with the mucous membrane covering it, the Palatoglossus forms the palatoglossal arch or fold.

Function:

Elevates root of tongue

Closes palatoglossal arch (along with its opposite member) to close the oral cavity from the oropharynx

Innervation:

Vagus (X) nerve (pharyngeal plexus)

Intrinsic Tongue Muscles

37 Superior longitudinal

38 Inferior longitudinal

39 Transverse lingual

40 Vertical lingual

37 SUPERIOR LONGITUDINAL

Attachments and Description:

Oblique and longitudinal fibers run immediately under the mucous membrane on dorsum of tongue.

Arises from submucous fibrous layer near epiglottis and from the median lingual septum. Fibers run anteriorly to the edges of the tongue.

Function and innneration of intrinsics: See Vertical lingual (# 40).

38 INFERIOR LONGITUDINAL

Attachments and Description:

Narrow band of fibers close to the inferior lingual surface. Extends from the root to the apex of the tongue. Some fibers connect to hyoid body. Blends with Styloglossus anteriorly.

39 TRANSVERSE LINGUAL

Attachments and Description:

Passes laterally across tongue from the median lingual septum to the edges of the tongue. Blends with Palatopharyngeus.

40 VERTICAL LINGUAL

Attachments and Description:

Located only at the anterolateral regions and extends from the dorsal to the ventral surfaces of the tongue.

Function of intrinsics:

These muscles change the shape and contour of the tongue. The longitudinal muscles tend to shorten it. The Superior longitudinal also turns the apex and sides upward, making the dorsum concave. The Inferior longitudinal pulls the apex and sides downward to make the dorsum convex. The Transverse muscle narrows and elongates the tongue. The Vertical muscle flattens and widens it.

These almost limitless alterations give the tongue the incredible versatility and precision necessary for speech and swallowing functions.

Innervation of intrinsics:

Hypoglossal (XII) nerve

MUSCLES OF THE PHARYNX

41 Inferior pharyngeal constrictor

42 Middle pharyngeal constrictor

43 Superior pharyngeal constrictor

44 Stylopharyngeus

45 Salpingopharyngeus

49 Palatopharyngeus (see under *Muscles of the Palate*)

41 INFERIOR PHARYNGEAL CONSTRICTOR

Origin:
Cricoid cartilage (sides)
Thyroid cartilage (oblique line on the side as well as from inferior cornu)

Insertion:
Pharynx (posterior median fibrous raphe, along with its contralateral partner)

Description:
The thickest and largest of the pharyngeal constrictors, the muscle has two parts: the Cricopharyngeus and the Thyropharyngeus. Both parts spread to join the muscle of the opposite side at the fibrous median raphe. The lowest fibers run horizontally and circle the narrowest part of the pharynx. The other fibers course obliquely upward to overlap the Middle constrictor.
During swallowing the Cricopharyngeus acts like a sphincter; the Thyropharyngeus uses peristaltic action to propel food downward.

Function:
During swallowing all constrictors act as general sphincters and in peristaltic action during swallowing.

Innervation:
Pharyngeal plexus formed by components of vagus (X), accessory (XI), glossopharyngeal (IX), and external laryngeal nerves

42 MIDDLE PHARYNGEAL CONSTRICTOR

Origin (in two parts):
Hyoid bone (whole length of superior border of lesser cornu and stylohyoid ligament) [chondropharyngeal part]
Hyoid bone (whole border of greater cornu) [ceratopharyngeal part]
Stylohyoid ligament

Insertion:
Pharynx (posterior median fibrous raphe)

Description:
From their origin the fibers fan out in three directions: the lower ones descend to lie under the Inferior constrictor; the medial ones pass transversely, and the superior fibers ascend to overlap the Superior constrictor. At its insertion it joins with the muscle from the opposite side.

Function:
Serves as a sphincter and acts during peristaltic functions in deglutition

Innervation:
Pharyngeal plexus formed by components of vagus (X), accessory (XI), and glossopharyngeal (IX) nerves

43 SUPERIOR PHARYNGEAL CONSTRICTOR

Origin (in four parts):
Sphenoid bone (medial pterygoid plate and its hamulus [pterygopharyngeal part])
Pterygomandibular raphe (buccopharyngeal part)
Mandible (mylohyoid line) [mylopharyngeal part]
Side of tongue [glossopharyngeal part]

Insertion:
Median pharyngeal fibrous raphe
Occipital bone (pharyngeal tubercle on basilar part)

Description:
The smallest of the constrictors, the fibers of this muscle curve posteriorly and are elongated by an aponeurosis to reach the occiput. The attachments of this muscle are differentiated as pterygopharyngeal, buccopharyngeal, mylopharyngeal, and glossopharyngeal.
The interval between the superior border of this muscle and the base of the skull is closed by the pharyngobasilar fascia known as the sinus of Morgagni.
A small band of muscle blends with the Superior constrictor from the upper surface of the palatine aponeurosis and is called the palatopharyngeal sphincter. This band is visible when the soft palate is elevated; often it is hypertrophied in individuals with cleft palate.

Function:
Acts as a sphincter and has peristaltic functions in swallowing

Innervation:
Pharyngeal plexus (from Vagus and Accessory)

44 STYLOPHARYNGEUS

Origin:
Temporal bone (styloid process, medial side of base)

Insertion:
Blends with pharyngeal constrictors and Palatopharyngeus
Thyroid cartilage (posterior border)

Description:
A long thin muscle that passes downward along the side of the pharynx and between the

Superior and Middle constrictors to spread out beneath the mucous membrane

Function:
Elevation of upper lateral pharyngeal wall in swallowing

Innervation:
Glossopharyngeal (IX) nerve

45 SALPINGOPHARYNGEUS

Origin:
Auditory (pharyngotympanic) tube (inferior aspect of cartilage near orifice)

Insertion:
Blends with Palatopharyngeus

Description:
Small muscle whose fibers pass downward, lateral to the uvula, to blend with fibers of the Palatopharyngeus

Function:
Elevates pharynx to move a bolus of food

Innervation:
Pharyngeal plexus

MUSCLES OF THE PALATE

46 Levator veli palatini

47 Tensor veli palatini

48 Musculus uvulae

49 Palatopharyngeus

36 Palatoglossus (see under *Muscles of the Tongue*)

46 LEVATOR VELI PALATINI
(Levator Palati)

Origin:
Temporal bone (inferior surface of petrous bone)
Tympanic fascia
Auditory (pharyngotympanic) tube cartilage

Insertion:
Palatine aponeurosis (upper surface, where it blends with opposite muscle at the midline)

Description:
Fibers of this small muscle run downward and medially from the petrous temporal bone to pass above the margin of the Superior pharyngeal constrictor and anterior to the Salpingo-

pharyngeus. They form a sling for the palatine aponeurosis.

Function:
Elevates soft palate
Retracts soft palate

Innervation:
Pharyngeal plexus

47 TENSOR VELI PALATINI
(Tensor Palati)

Origin:
Sphenoid bone (pterygoid process, scaphoid fossa)
Auditory (pharyngotympanic) tube cartilage
Sphenoid spine (medial part)

Insertion:
Palatine aponeurosis
Palatine bone (horizontal plate)

Description:[13]
This small thin muscle lies lateral to the Levator veli palatini and the auditory tube. It descends vertically between the medial pterygoid plate and the Medial pterygoid muscle, converging into a delicate tendon, which turns medially around the pterygoid hamulus.

Function:
Draws soft palate to one side (unilateral)
Tightens soft palate, depressing it and flattening its arch (with its contralateral counterpart)
Opens auditory tube in yawning and swallowing and eases any buildup of air pressure between the nasopharynx and middle ear

Innervation:
Trigeminal (V) nerve (to medial pterygoid)[13]

48 MUSCULUS UVULAE
(Azygos Uvulae)

Origin:
Palatine bones (posterior nasal spine)
Palatine aponeurosis

Insertion:
Uvula (connective tissue and mucous membrane)

Description:
A bilateral muscle, its fibers descend into the uvular mucosa.

Function:
Elevates and retracts uvula to assist with palatopharyngeal closure
Seals nasopharynx (along with levators)

Innervation:
Pharyngeal plexus (X and XI)

49 PALATOPHARYNGEUS
(Pharyngopalatinus)

Origin (by two fasciculi):

Anterior fasciculus:
Soft palate (palatine aponeurosis)
Hard palate (posterior border)

Posterior fasciculus:
Pharyngeal aspect of soft palate (palatine aponeurosis)

Insertion:
Thyroid cartilage (posterior border)
Side of pharynx on an aponeurosis

Description:
Along with its overlying mucosa, it forms the palatopharyngeal arch. It arises by two fasciculi separated by the Levator veli palatini, all of which join in the midline with their opposite muscles. The two muscles unite and are joined by the Salpingopharyngeus to descend behind the tonsils. The muscle forms an incomplete longitudinal wall on the internal surface of the pharynx.

Function:
Elevates pharynx and pulls it forward, thus shortening it during swallowing. The muscles also narrow the palatopharyngeal arches (fauces). Depresses soft palate.

Innervation:
Pharyngeal plexus (X and XI)

36 PALATOGLOSSUS

See under *Muscles of the Tongue*

MUSCLES OF THE LARYNX
(Intrinsics)

These muscles are confined to the larynx:

50 Cricothyroid

51 Posterior cricoarytenoid

52 Lateral cricoarytenoid

53 Transverse arytenoid

54 Oblique arytenoid

55 Thyroarytenoid
Vocalis
Thyroepiglotticus

50 CRICOTHYROID

Origin:
Cricoid cartilage (front and lateral)

Insertion:
Thyroid cartilage (inferior cornu)
Thyroid lamina

Description:
The fibers of this paired muscle are arranged in two groups: a lower oblique group (pars obliqua), which slants posterolaterally to the inferior cornu, and a superior group (pars recta or vertical fibers), which ascends backward to the lamina.

Function:
Regulates tension of vocal folds
Stretches vocal ligaments by raising the cricoid arch, thus increasing tension in the vocal folds

Innervation:
Vagus (X) nerve (external laryngeal branch)

51 POSTERIOR CRICOARYTENOID

Origin:
Cricoid cartilage lamina (broad depression on corresponding half of posterior surface)

Insertion:
Arytenoid cartilage on same side (back of muscular process)

Description:
The fibers of this paired muscle pass cranially and laterally to converge on the back of the arytenoid cartilage on the same side. The lowest fibers are nearly vertical and become oblique and finally almost transverse at the superior border.

Function:
Regulates tension of vocal folds
Opens glottis by rotating arytenoid cartilages laterally and separating (abducting) the vocal folds
Retracts arytenoid cartilages, thereby helping to tense the vocal folds

Innervation:
Vagus (X) nerve (recurrent laryngeal nerve)

52 LATERAL CRICOARYTENOID

Origin:
Cricoid cartilage (cranial border of arch)

Insertion:

> Arytenoid cartilage on same side (front of muscular process)

Description:

> Fibers run obliquely upward and backward. The muscle is paired.

Function:

> Closes glottis by rotating arytenoid cartilages medially, approximating (adducting) the vocal folds for speech

Innervation:

> Vagus (X) nerve (recurrent laryngeal branch)

53 TRANSVERSE ARYTENOID

Attachments and Description:

> A single muscle (i.e., unpaired) that crosses transversely between the two arytenoid cartilages. Often considered a branch of an Arytenoid muscle. It attaches to the back of the muscular process and the adjacent lateral borders of both arytenoid cartilages.

Function:

> Approximates (adducts) the arytenoid cartilages, closing the glottis

Innervation:

> Vagus (X) nerve (recurrent laryngeal nerve)

54 OBLIQUE ARYTENOID

Origin:

> Arytenoid cartilage (back of muscular process)

Insertion:

> Arytenoid cartilage on opposite side (apex)

Description:

> A pair of muscles lying superficial to the Transverse arytenoid. Arrayed as two fasciculi that cross on the posterior midline. Often considered part of an Arytenoid muscle. Fibers that continue laterally around the apex of the Arytenoid are sometimes termed the Aryepiglottic muscle.

Function:

> Acts as a sphincter for the laryngeal inlet (by adducting the aryepiglottic folds and approximating the arytenoid cartilages)

Innervation:

> Vagus (X) nerve (recurrent laryngeal nerve)

55 THYROARYTENOID

Origin:

> Thyroid cartilage (caudal half of angle)
> Middle cricothyroid ligament

Insertion:

> Arytenoid cartilage (base and anterior surface)
> Vocal process (lateral surface)

Description:

> The paired muscles lie lateral to the vocal fold, ascending posterolaterally. Many fibers are carried to the aryepiglottic fold.
> The lower and deeper fibers, which lie medially, appear to be differentiated as a band inserted into the vocal process of the arytenoid cartilage. This band frequently is called the *Vocalis* muscle. It is adherent to the vocal ligament, to which it is lateral and parallel.
> Other fibers of this muscle continue as the *Thyroepiglotticus* muscle and insert into the epiglottic margin; other fibers that swing along the wall of the sinus to the side of the epiglottis are termed the *Superior thyroarytenoid* and relax the vocal folds.

Function:

> Regulates tension of vocal folds.
> Draws arytenoid cartilages toward thyroid cartilage, thus shortening and relaxing vocal ligaments.
> Rotates the arytenoid cartilages medially to approximate vocal folds.
> The Vocalis relaxes the posterior vocal folds while the anterior folds remain tense, thus raising the pitch of the voice.
> The Thyroepiglotticus widens the laryngeal inlet via action on the aryepiglottic folds.
> The Superior thyroarytenoids relax the vocal cords and aid in closure of the glottis.

Innervation:

> Vagus (X) nerve (recurrent laryngeal nerve)

MUSCLES OF THE NECK AND SUBOCCIPITAL TRIANGLE

Capital Extensor Muscles

This group of eight muscles consists of suboccipital muscles extending between the atlas, axis, and skull and large overlapping muscles from the 6th thoracic to the 3rd cervical vertebrae and rising to the skull.

56 Rectus capitis posterior major

57 Rectus capitis posterior minor

58 Obliquus capitis superior

59 Obliquus capitis inferior

60 Longissimus capitis

61 Splenius capitis

62 Semispinalis capitis

63 Spinalis capitis

The capital extensor muscles control the head as an entity separate from the cervical spine.[14] The muscles are paired.

83 Sternocleidomastoid (posterior) (see under cervical spine flexors)

124 Trapezius (upper) (see under shoulder muscles)

56 RECTUS CAPITIS POSTERIOR MAJOR

Origin:
Axis (spinous process)

Insertion:
Occiput (lateral part of inferior nuchal line; surface just inferior to nuchal line)

Description:
Starts as a small tendon and broadens as it rises upward and laterally (review suboccipital triangle in any anatomy text)

Function:
Capital extension
Rotation of head to same side
Lateral bending of head to same side

Innervation:
C1 spinal nerve (suboccipital nerve, dorsal rami)

57 RECTUS CAPITIS POSTERIOR MINOR

Origin:
Atlas (tubercle on posterior arch)

Insertion:
Occiput (medial portion of inferior nuchal line; surface between inferior nuchal line and foramen magnum)

Description:
Begins as a narrow tendon, which broadens into a wide band of muscle as it ascends

Function:
Capital extension

Innervation:
C1 spinal nerve (suboccipital nerve, dorsal rami)

58 OBLIQUUS CAPITIS SUPERIOR

Origin:
Atlas (transverse process, superior surface), where it joins insertion of Obliquus capitis inferior

Insertion:
Occiput (between superior and inferior nuchal lines; lies lateral to Semispinalis capitis)

Description:
Starts as a narrow muscle and then widens as it rises upward and medially. It is more a postural muscle than a muscle for major motion

Function:
Capital extension of head on atlas (muscle on both sides)
Lateral bending to same side (muscle on that side)

Innervation:
C1 spinal nerve (suboccipital nerve, dorsal rami)

59 OBLIQUUS CAPITIS INFERIOR

Origin:
Axis (apex of spinous process)

Insertion:
Atlas (transverse process, inferior and dorsal surface)

Description:
Passes laterally and slightly upward. This is the larger of the two obliquui.

Function:
Rotation of head to same side
Lateral bending (muscle on that side)

Innervation:
C1 spinal nerve (suboccipital nerve, dorsal rami)

60 LONGISSIMUS CAPITIS

Origin:
T1–T5 vertebrae (transverse processes)
C4–C7 vertebrae (articular processes)

Insertion:
Temporal bone (mastoid process [posterior margin])

Description:
A muscle with several tendons lying under the Splenius cervicis. Sweeps upward and laterally

and is considered a continuation of the Sacrospinalis.

Function:
Capital extension
Lateral bending and rotation of head to same side

Innervation:
C3–C8 cervical nerves with variations (dorsal rami)

61 SPLENIUS CAPITIS

Origin:
Ligamentum nuchae at C3–C7 vertebrae
C7–T4 vertebrae (spinous processes) with variations

Insertion:
Temporal bone (mastoid process)
Occiput (surface below lateral 1/3 of superior nuchal line)

Description:
Fibers directed upward and laterally as a broad band deep to the Rhomboids and Trapezius distally and the Sternocleidomastoid proximally. It forms the floor of the apex of the posterior triangle of the neck.

Function:
Capital extension
Rotation of head to same side (debated)
Lateral bending of head to same side

Innervation:
C3–C6 cervical nerves with variations (dorsal rami)
C1–C2 (suboccipital and greater occipital nerves off first two dorsal rami)

62 SEMISPINALIS CAPITIS

Origin:
C7 and T1–T6 vertebrae (variable) as series of tendons from tips of transverse processes
C4–C6 vertebrae (articular processes)

Insertion:
Occiput (between superior and inferior nuchal lines)

Description:
Tendons unite to form a broad muscle in the upper posterior neck, which passes vertically upward.

Function:
Capital extension (muscles on both sides)
Rotation of head to opposite side (debated)
Lateral bending of head to same side

Innervation:
C2–T1 spinal nerves (dorsal rami); greater occipital nerve (variable)

63 SPINALIS CAPITIS

Origin:
C5–C7 and T1–T3 vertebrae (variable) (spinous processes)

Insertion:
Occiput (between superior and inferior nuchal lines)

Description:
The smallest and thinnest of the Erector spinae, these muscles lie closest to the vertebral column. The Spinales are inconstant and are difficult to separate.

Function:
Capital extension

Innervation:
C3–T1 spinal nerves (dorsal rami) (variable)

Cervical Extensor Muscles

This group of eight overlapping cervical muscles arise from the thoracic vertebrae or ribs and insert into the cervical vertebrae. They are responsible for cervical spine extension in contrast to capital (head) extension.

64 Longissimus cervicis
65 Semispinalis cervicis
66 Iliocostalis cervicis
67 Splenius cervicis
68 Spinalis cervicis
69 Interspinales cervicis
70 Intertransversarii cervicis
71 Rotatores cervicis
94 Multifidi (see under Erector spinae)
124 Trapezius (see under Shoulder Girdle)
127 Levator scapulae (see under Shoulder Girdle)

64 LONGISSIMUS CERVICIS

Origin:
T1–T5 vertebrae (variable) (tips of transverse processes)

Insertion:
C2–C6 vertebrae (posterior tubercles of transverse processes)

Description:
A continuation of the Sacrospinalis group, the tendons are long and thin, and the muscle courses upward and slightly medially. The muscles are bilateral.

Function:
Extension of the cervical spine (both muscles)
Lateral bending of cervical spine to same side (one muscle)

Innervation:
C3–T3 spinal nerves (variable) (dorsal rami)

65 SEMISPINALIS CERVICIS

Origin:
T1–T5 vertebrae (variable) (transverse processes)

Insertion:
Axis (C2) to C5 vertebrae (spinous processes)

Description:
A narrow, thick muscle arising from a series of tendons and ascending vertically

Function:
Extension of the cervical spine (both muscles)
Rotation of cervical spine to opposite side (one muscle)
Lateral bending to same side

Innervation:
C2–T5 spinal nerves (dorsal rami) (variable)

66 ILIOCOSTALIS CERVICIS

Origin:
Ribs 3 to 6 (angles); sometimes ribs 1 and 2 also

Insertion:
C4–C6 vertebrae (transverse processes, posterior tubercles)

Description:
Flattened tendons arise from ribs on dorsum of back and become muscular as they rise and turn medially to insert on cervical vertebrae. The muscle lies lateral to the Longissimus cervicis. The Iliocostales form the lateral column of the Sacrospinalis group.

Function:
Extension of the cervical spine (both muscles)
Lateral bending to same side (one muscle)
Depression of ribs (accessory)

Innervation:
C4–T3 spinal nerves (variable) (dorsal rami)

67 SPLENIUS CERVICIS

Origin:
T3–T6 vertebrae (spinous processes)

Insertion:
C1–C3 vertebrae (variable) (transverse processes, posterior tubercles)

Description:
Narrow tendinous band arises from bone and intraspinous ligaments and forms a broad sheet along with the Splenius capitis. This muscle rises upward and laterally under the Trapezius and Rhomboids and medially to the Levator scapulae. The Splenii are often absent and are quite variable.

Function:
Extension of the cervical spine (both muscles)
Rotation of cervical spine to same side (one muscle)
Lateral bending to same side (one muscle)
Synergistic with opposite Sternocleidomastoid

Innervation:
C4–C8 spinal nerves (variable) (dorsal rami)

68 SPINALIS CERVICIS

Origin:
C6–C7 and sometimes T1–T2 vertebrae (spinous processes)
Ligamentum nuchae (lower part)

Insertion:
Axis (spine)
C2–C3 vertebrae (spinous processes)

Description:
The smallest and thinnest of the Erector spinae, it lies closest to the vertebral column. The Erector spinae are inconstant and difficult to separate. This muscle is often absent.

Function:
Extension of the cervical spine

Innervation:
C3–C8 spinal nerves (dorsal rami) (variable)

69 INTERSPINALES CERVICIS

Origin and Insertion:
Spinous processes of contiguous cervical vertebrae
Six pairs occur: The first pair runs between the axis and C3; the last pair between C7 and T1.

Description:
One of the smallest and least significant muscles but consists of short, narrow bundles more evident in cervical spine than at lower levels.

Function:
Extension of the cervical spine (weak)

Innervation:
C3–C8 spinal nerves (dorsal rami) (variable)

70 INTERTRANSVERSARII CERVICIS

Origin and Insertion:
Both anterior and posterior pairs occur at each segment. The anterior muscles interconnect the anterior tubercles of contiguous transverse processes and are innervated by the ventral primary rami. The posterior muscles interconnect the posterior tubercles of contiguous transverse processes and are innervated by the dorsal primary rami.

Description:
These muscles are small paired fasciculi which lie between the transverse processes of contiguous vertebrae. The cervicis is the most developed of this group which includes the following: the anterior Intertransversarii cervicis; the posterior Intertransversarii cervicis; a thoracic group; and a medial and lateral lumbar group.

Function:
Extension of spine (muscles on both sides)
Lateral bending to same side (muscles on one side)

Innervation:
Anterior cervicis: C3–C8 spinal nerves (ventral rami)
Posterior cervicis: C3–C8 spinal nerves (dorsal rami)

71 ROTATORES CERVICIS

(See comments under *Rotatores thoracis*)

Origin:
Transverse process of one cervical vertebra

Insertion:
Base of spine of next highest vertebra

Description:
The Rotatores cervicis lies deep to the Multifidus and cannot be readily separated from it. Both muscles are irregular and not functionally significant at the cervical level.

Function:
Extension of the cervical spine (assist)
Rotation of spine to opposite side

Innervation:
C3–C8 spinal nerves (dorsal rami)

Muscles of Capital Flexion

The primary capital flexors are the short recti that lie between the atlas and the skull and the Longus capitis. Reinforcing these muscles are the suprahyoid muscles from the mandibular area.

72 Rectus capitis anterior

73 Rectus capitis lateralis

74 Longus capitis

Suprahyoids:

75 Mylohyoid

76 Stylohyoid

77 Geniohyoid

78 Digastric

72 RECTUS CAPITIS ANTERIOR

Origin:
Atlas (C1) (transverse process and anterior surface of lateral mass)

Insertion:
Occiput (inferior surface of basilar part)

Description:
Short, flat muscle found immediately behind Longus capitis. Upward trajectory is vertical and slightly medial.

Function:
Capital flexion
Stabilization of atlanto-occipital joint

Innervation:
C1–C2 spinal nerves (ventral rami)

73 RECTUS CAPITIS LATERALIS

Origin:
Atlas (C1) (transverse process, upper surface)

Insertion:
Occiput (jugular process)

Description:
Short, flat muscle; courses upward and laterally

Function:
Lateral bending of head to same side (obliquity of muscle)
Assists head rotation
Stabilizes atlanto-occipital joint (assists)
Capital flexion

Innervation:
C1–C2 spinal nerves (ventral rami)

74 LONGUS CAPITIS

Origin:
C3–C6 vertebrae (transverse processes, anterior tubercles)

Insertion:
Occiput (inferior basilar part)

Description:
Starting as four tendinous slips, muscle merges and becomes broader and thicker as it rises, converging medially toward its contralateral counterpart.

Function:
Capital flexion
Rotation of head to same side (muscle of one side)

Innervation:
C1–C3 spinal nerves (ventral rami)

75 MYLOHYOID

Origin:
Mandible (whole length of mylohyoid line from symphysis in front to last molar behind)

Insertion:
Hyoid bone (body, superior surface)
Mylohyoid raphe (from symphysis menti of mandible to hyoid bone)

Description:
Flat triangular muscle; the muscles from the two sides form a floor for the cavity of the mouth.

Function:
Raises hyoid bone and tongue for swallowing
Depresses the mandible when hyoid bone fixed
Capital flexion (weak accessory)

Innervation:
Trigeminal (V) nerve (mylohyoid branch of inferior alveolar nerve off mandibular division)

76 STYLOHYOID

Origin:
Temporal bone, styloid process (posterolateral surface)

Insertion:
Hyoid bone (body at junction with greater horn)

Description:
Slim muscle passes downward and forward and is perforated by Digastric near its distal attachment. Muscle occasionally is absent.

Function:
Hyoid bone drawn upward and backward (in swallowing)
Capital flexion (weak accessory)
Assists in opening mouth (depression of mandible)
Participation in mastication and speech (roles not clear)

Innervation:
Facial (VII) nerve (posterior trunk, stylohyoid branch)

77 GENIOHYOID

Origin:
Mandible (symphysis menti, inferior mental spine)

Insertion:
Hyoid bone (body, anterior surface)

Description:
Narrow muscle lying superficial to the Mylohyoid, it runs backward and somewhat downward. It is in contact (or may fuse) with its contralateral counterpart at the midline.

Function:
Elevation and protraction of hyoid bone
Capital flexion (weak accessory)
Assists in depressing mandible

Innervation:
C1 spinal nerve via hypoglossal (XII) nerve

78 DIGASTRIC

Origin:
Posterior belly: temporal bone (mastoid notch)
Anterior belly: mandible (digastric fossa)

Insertion:
Intermediate tendon and from there to hyoid bone via a fibrous sling

Description:
Consists of two bellies united by a rounded intermediate tendon. Lies below the mandible and extends as a sling from the mastoid to the symphysis menti, perforating the Stylohyoid, where the two bellies are joined by the intermediate tendon.
EMG data show that the two bilateral muscles always work together.[15]

Function:
Mandibular depression (muscles on both sides)
Elevation of hyoid bone (in swallowing)
Anterior belly: draws hyoid forward
Posterior belly: draws hyoid backward
Capital flexion (weak synergist)

Innervation:
> *Anterior belly:* trigeminal (V) nerve (mylohyoid branch of inferior alveolar nerve)
> *Posterior belly:* facial (VII) nerve, digastric branch

Cervical Spine Flexors

The primary cervical spine flexors are the Longus colli (a prevertebral mass), the three scalene muscles, and the Sternocleidomastoid. Superficial accessory muscles are the infrahyoid muscles and the Platysma.

79 Longus colli

80 Scalenus anterior

81 Scalenus medius

82 Scalenus posterior

83 Sternocleidomastoid

88 Platysma

Infrahyoids:

84 Sternothyroid

85 Thyrohyoid

86 Sternohyoid

87 Omohyoid

79 LONGUS COLLI

Three heads

Superior oblique:

Origin:
> C3–C5 vertebrae (anterior tubercles of transverse processes)

Insertion:
> Atlas (tubercle on anterior arch)

Inferior oblique:

Origin:
> T1–T3 vertebrae (variable) (anterior bodies)

Insertion:
> C5–C6 vertebrae (anterior tubercles of transverse processes)

Vertical portion:

Origin:
> T1–T3 and C5–C7 vertebrae (anterolateral bodies) (variable)

Insertion:
> C2–C4 vertebrae (anterior bodies)

Description:
> Situated on the anterior surface of the vertebral column from the thoracic spine rising to the cervical vertebrae. It is cylindrical and tapers at each end.

Function:
> Cervical flexion (weak)
> Cervical rotation to opposite side (inferior oblique head)
> Lateral bending (superior and inferior oblique heads) (debatable)

Innervation:
> C2–C6 spinal nerves (ventral rami)

The Scalenes

These muscles are highly variable in their specific anatomy, and this possibly leads to disputes about minor functions. Though not described here, a fourth scalene muscle, the Scalenus minimus (of no functional significance), runs, when present, from C7 to the 1st rib.

80 SCALENUS ANTERIOR

Origin:
> C3–C6 vertebrae (anterior tubercles of transverse processes)

Insertion:
> 1st rib (scalene tubercle on inner border and ridge on upper surface)

Description:
> Lying deep at the side of the neck under the Sternocleidomastoid, it descends vertically. Attachments are highly variable.
> A fourth scalene (Scalenus minimus) is occasionally associated with the cervical pleura and runs from C7 to the 1st rib.

Function:
> Flexion of cervical spine (both muscles)
> Elevation of 1st rib in inspiration
> Rotation of cervical spine to opposite side
> Lateral bending of neck to same side

Innervation:
> C4–C6 cervical nerves (ventral rami)

81 SCALENUS MEDIUS

Origin:
> C2–C7 (posterior tubercles of transverse processes)
> Atlas (sometimes)

Insertion:
1st rib (widely over superior surface)

Description:
Longest and largest of the scalenes. Descends vertically alongside of vertebrae.

Function:
Cervical flexion (weak)
Lateral bending of cervical spine to same side
Elevation of 1st rib in inspiration
Cervical rotation to opposite side

Innervation:
C3–C8 cervical nerves (ventral rami)

82 SCALENUS POSTERIOR

Origin:
C4–C6 vertebrae (variable; posterior tubercles of transverse processes)

Insertion:
2nd rib (outer surface)

Description:
Smallest and deepest lying of the scalene muscles. Attachments are highly variable. Often not separable from Scalenus medius.

Function:
Cervical flexion (weak)
Elevation of 2nd rib in inspiration
Lateral bending of cervical spine to same side (accessory)
Cervical spine rotation to opposite side

Innervation:
C6–C8 cervical nerves (ventral rami)

83 STERNOCLEIDOMASTOID

Origin:
Sternal (medial) head: sternum (manubrium, ventral surface)
Clavicular (lateral) head: clavicle (superior and anterior surface of medial 1/3)

Insertion:
Temporal bone (mastoid process, lateral surface)
Occiput (lateral half of superior nuchal line)

Description:
The two heads of origin gradually merge in the neck as the muscle rises upward laterally and posteriorly. Their oblique (lateral to medial) course across the sides of the neck is a very prominent feature of surface anatomy.

Function:
Flexion of cervical spine (both muscles)
Lateral bending of cervical spine to same side
Rotation of head to opposite side
Capital extension (posterior fibers)
Raises sternum in forced inspiration

Innervation:
Accessory (XI) nerve (spinal part)
C2–C3 (sometimes C4) cervical nerves (ventral rami)

84 STERNOTHYROID

Origin:
Sternum (manubrium, posterior surface)
1st rib (cartilage)

Insertion:
Thyroid cartilage (oblique line)

Description:
A deep-lying, somewhat broad muscle rising vertically and slightly laterally just lateral to the thyroid gland.

Function:
Cervical flexion (weak)
Draws larynx down after swallowing or vocalization
Depression of hyoid, mandible, and tongue (after elevation)

Innervation:
C1–C3 cervical nerves (branch of ansa cervicalis)

85 THYROHYOID

Origin:
Thyroid cartilage (oblique line)

Insertion:
Hyoid bone (inferior border of greater horn)

Description:
Appears as an upward extension of Sternothyroid. It is a small rectangular muscle lateral to the thyroid cartilage.

Function:
Cervical flexion (This small muscle is attached to mobile structures and its role in cervical flexion seems unlikely as a functional entity.)
Draws hyoid bone downward
Elevates larynx and thyroid cartilage

Innervation:
Hypoglossal (XII) and branches of C1 spinal nerve (which run in hypoglossal nerve)

86 STERNOHYOID

Origin:
Clavicle (medial end, posterior surface)
Sternum (manubrium, posterior)
Sternoclavicular ligament

Insertion:
Hyoid bone (body, lower border)

Description:
Thin strap muscle that ascends slightly medially from clavicle to hyoid bone

Function:
Cervical flexion (weak)
Depresses hyoid bone after swallowing

Innervation:
Hypoglossal (XII) nerve
C1–C3 cervical nerves (branches of ansa cervicalis)

87 OMOHYOID

Has two bellies

Inferior Belly:

Origin:
Scapula (superior margin to variable extent; subscapular notch)
Superior transverse ligament

Insertion:
Intermediate tendon of Omohyoid under Sternocleidomastoid
Clavicle by fibrous expansion

Superior belly:

Origin:
Intermediate tendon of Omohyoid

Insertion:
Hyoid bone (lower border of body)

Description:
Muscle consists of two fleshy bellies united at an angle by a central tendon. The inferior belly is a narrow band that courses forward and slightly upward across the lower front of the neck. The superior belly rises vertically and lateral to the Sternohyoid.

Function:
Depression of hyoid after elevation
Cervical flexion
No EMG data to support function

Innervation:
Hypoglossal (XII) (ansa cervicalis) via C1 (branches from ansa cervicalis) and C2–C3 cervical nerves

88 PLATYSMA

Origin:
Fascia covering upper Pectoralis major and Deltoid

Insertion:
Mandible (below the oblique line)
Modiolus[10–12]
Skin and subcutaneous tissue of lower lip and face
Contralateral muscles join at midline

Description:
A broad sheet of muscle, it rises from the shoulder, crosses the clavicle, and rises obliquely upward and medially to the side of the neck.
The muscle is very variable.

Function:
Draws lower lip downward and backward (expression of surprise or horror) and assists with jaw opening.
Cervical flexion (weak). Electromyogram shows great activity in extreme effort and in sudden deep inspiration.[16]
Can pull skin up from clavicular region, increasing diameter of neck. Wrinkles skin of nuchal area obliquely, thereby decreasing concavity of neck.
Forced inspiration.
Platysma is not a very functional muscle.

Innervation:
Facial (VII) nerve (cervical branch)

MUSCLES OF THE TRUNK

Back
Thorax (respiration)
Abdomen
Perineum and anus

Deep Muscles of the Back

These muscles consist of groups of serially arranged muscles ranging from the occiput to the sacrum. There are four subgroups plus the Quadratus lumborum.

In this section readers will note that the cervical portions of each muscle group are not included. These muscles are described as part of the neck muscles because their functions involve capital and cervical motions. They are, however, mentioned in the identification of each group for a complete overview.

Splenius (in neck only)
Erector spinae
Transversospinalis group
Interspinal-intertransverse group
Quadratus lumborum

Erector spinae

The muscles of this group cover a large area of the back, extending laterally from the vertebral column to the angle of the ribs and vertically from the sacrum to the occiput. This large musculotendinous mass is covered by the Serratus posterior inferior and thoracodorsal fascia below the Rhomboid and Splenius muscles above. The Erector spinae vary in size and composition at different levels.

Sacral region: Strong, dense, tendinous sheet, narrow at base (common tendon)
Lumbar region: Expands into thick muscular mass (palpable); visible surface contour on lateral side
Thoracic region: Muscle mass much thinner than that found in lumbar region; surface groove along lateral border follows costal angles until covered by scapula

Common Tendon of Erector spinae:

This is the origin of the broad thick tendon as described in Grant:[7]
Sacrum (median and lateral crests, anterior surface of the tendon of Erector spinae; L1–L5 and T12 vertebrae (spinous processes); supraspinous, sacrotuberous, and sacroiliac ligaments; iliac crests (inner aspect of dorsal part).
From the common tendon the muscles rise to form a large mass that is divided in the upper lumbar region into three longitudinal columns based on their areas of attachment in the thoracic and cervical regions.

Lateral column of muscle

66 Iliocostalis cervicis (see *Muscles of the Neck*)

89 Iliocostalis thoracis

90 Iliocostalis lumborum

Intermediate column of muscle

60 Longissimus capitis (see *Muscles of the Neck*)

64 Longissimus cervicis (see *Muscles of the Neck*)

91 Longissimus thoracis

Medial column of muscle

63 Spinalis capitis (see *Muscles of the Neck*)

68 Spinalis cervicis (see *Muscles of the Neck*)

92 Spinalis thoracis

The Iliocostalis Column (Lateral)

66 Iliocostalis cervicis (see *Muscles of the Neck*)

89 ILIOCOSTALIS THORACIS

Origin:
Ribs 12 to 7 (upper borders at angles)

Insertion:
Ribs 1 to 6 (at angles)
C7 (transverse process, dorsum)

Innervation:
T1–T12 spinal nerves

90 ILIOCOSTALIS LUMBORUM

Origin:
Common tendon of Erector spinae (anterior surface)
Thoracolumbar fascia
Iliac crest (external lip)
Sacrum (posterior surface)

Insertion:
Lumbar vertebrae (all) (transverse processes)
Ribs 5 or 6 to 12 (angles on inferior border)

Description (All Iliocostales):
This is the most lateral column of the Erector spinae. The lumbar portion of this muscle is the largest, and it subdivides as it ascends.

Function:
Extension of spine
Lateral bending of spine (muscles on one side)
Depression of ribs (lumborum)
Elevation of pelvis

Innervation:
L1–L5 spinal nerves, dorsal rami (variable)

The Longissimus Column (Intermediate)

91 LONGISSIMUS THORACIS

Origin:
Thoracolumbar fascia
L1–L5 vertebrae (transverse and accessory processes)

Insertion:
T1–T12 vertebrae (transverse processes)
Ribs 2 to 12 (between tubercles and angles)

Description (All Longissimi):
These are the intermediate Erector spinae. They lie between the Iliocostales (laterally) and the Spinales (medially). The fibers of the Longis-

simus are inseparable from those of the Iliocostales until the upper lumbar region.

Function (Longissimus thoracis):
  Extension of the spine
  Lateral bending of spine to same side (muscles on one side)
  Depression of ribs

Innervation:
  T1–L1 spinal nerves (dorsal rami)

Spinalis Column (Medial)

92 SPINALIS THORACIS

Origin:
  T11–T12 and L1–L2 vertebrae (spinous processes)

Insertion:
  T1–T4 or through T8 vertebrae (spinous processes)

Description:
  The smallest and thinnest of the Erector spinae, they lie closest to the vertebral column. The Spinales are inconstant, and are difficult to separate.

Function:
  Extension of spine

Innervation:
  T1–T12 (variable) dorsal rami

Transversospinales Group
Muscles of this group lie deep to the Erector spinae, filling the concave region between the spinous and transverse processes of the vertebrae. They ascend obliquely and medially from the vertebral transverse processes to adjacent and sometimes more remote vertebrae. A span over four to six vertebrae is not uncommon.

  62 Semispinalis capitis (see Muscles of the Neck)
  65 Semispinalis cervicis (see Muscles of the Neck)
  93 Semispinalis thoracis
  94 Multifidi
  71 Rotatores cervicis (see Muscles of the Neck)
  95 Rotatores thoracis
  96 Rotatores lumborum

93 SEMISPINALIS THORACIS

Origin:
  T6–T10 vertebrae (transverse processes)

Insertion:
  C6–T4 vertebrae (spinous processes)

Description:
  This group is found only in the thoracic and cervical regions, extending to the head. They lie deep to the Spinalis and Longissimus columns of the Erector spinae.

Function:
  Extension of thoracic spine

Innervation:
  T1–T12 spinal nerves (dorsal rami) variable

94 MULTIFIDI

Origin:
  Sacrum (posterior, as low as the S4 foramen)
  Aponeurosis of Erector spinae
  Ilium (posterior superior iliac spine) and adjacent crest
  Sacroiliac ligaments (posterior)
  L1–L5 vertebrae (mamillary processes)
  T1–T12 vertebrae (transverse processes)
  C4–C7 vertebrae (articular processes)

Insertion:
  A higher vertebra (spinous process): Most superficial fibers run to the 3rd or 4th vertebra above; middle fibers run to the 2nd or 3rd above; deep fibers run between contiguous vertebrae.

Description:
  These muscles fill the grooves on both sides of the spinous processes of the vertebrae from the sacrum to the middle cervical vertebrae (or may rise as high as C1). They lie deep to the Erector spinae in the lumbar region and deep to the Semispinales above. Each fasciculus ascends obliquely, traversing over two to four vertebrae as it moves toward the midline to insert in the spinous process of a higher vertebra.

Function:
  Extension of spine
  Lateral bending of spine (muscle on one side)
  Rotation to opposite side

Innervation:
  Spinal nerves (whole length of spine), segmentally (dorsal rami)

The Rotatores

The Rotatores are the deepest muscles of the Transversospinales group, lying as 11 pairs of very short muscles beneath the Multifidi. The fibers run obliquely upward and and medially or almost horizontal. They may cross more than one vertebra on their ascending course, but most commonly they proceed to the next higher one. Found along the entire length of the vertebral column, they are distinguishable as developed muscles only in the thoracic area.

95 ROTATORES THORACIS

Origin:
T1 to T12 vertebrae (transverse processes)

Insertion:
Vertebra above (lamina)

Description:
There are 11 pairs of these small muscles. Adjacent muscles start from the posterior transverse process of one vertebra and rise to attach to the lower body and lamina of the next higher vertebra.

Function:
Extension of thoracic spine
Rotation to opposite side

Innervation:
T1–T12 spinal nerves (dorsal rami)

96 ROTATORES LUMBORUM

The Rotatores are highly variable and irregular in these regions.

Description:
This muscle lies deep to the Multifidi and cannot be readily separated from the deepest fibers of the multifidi. Pattern is similar to the thoracis.

Function:
Extension of spine
Rotation of spine to opposite side

Innervation:
L1–L5 spinal nerves (dorsal rami) (highly variable)

Interspinal-Intertransverse Group

69 Interspinalis cervicis (see under Muscles of the Neck)

70 Intertransversarii cervicis, anterior and posterior (see under Muscles of the Neck)

97 Interspinalis thoracis

98 Interspinalis lumborum

99 Intertransversarii thoracis

99 Intertransversarii lumborum, medial and lateral

The Interspinales and Intertransversarii

The short, paired muscles in the Interspinales group pass segmentally from the spinous processes (superior surface) of one vertebra to the inferior surface of the next on either side of the interspinous ligament. They are most highly developed in the cervical region, and quite irregular in distribution in the thoracic and lumbar spines.

The Intertransversarii are small fasciculi lying between the transverse processes of contiguous vertebrae. They are most developed in the cervical spine. The cervical muscles have both anterior and posterior parts; the lumbar muscles have medial and lateral fibers. The thoracic muscles are single without divisions as seen in the other spine areas and are not constant.

97 INTERSPINALES THORACIS

Origin and Insertion:
Between spinous processes of contiguous vertebrae
Three pairs are reasonably constant: (1) between the 1st and 2nd thoracic vertebrae; (2) between the 2nd and 3rd thoracic vertebrae (variable); (3) between the 11th and 12th thoracic vertebrae

Function:
Extension of spine

Innervation:
T1–T3; T11–T12 (irregular) spinal nerves (dorsal rami)

98 INTERSPINALES LUMBORUM

Origin:
There are four pairs lying between the five lumbar vertebrae. Fasciculi run from the spinous process (superior) of L2–L5.

Insertion:
To inferior surfaces of spinous processes of the vertebra above the vertebra of origin.

Function:
Extension of spine

Innervation:
L1–L4 spinal nerves (dorsal rami), variable

99 INTERTRANSVERSARII THORACIS AND LUMBORUM

Intertransversarii thoracis

Origin:
T11–L1 (transverse processes, superior surfaces)

Insertion:
T10–T12 (transverse processes, inferior surfaces)

Function:
Extension of spine (muscles on both sides)
Lateral bending to same side (muscles on one side)
Rotation to opposite side

Innervation:
T1–T12, L1–L5 spinal nerves (dorsal rami)

Intertransversarii lumborum—medial

Origin:
L2–S1 vertebrae (accessory processes)

Insertion:
Vertebra above the vertebra of origin (mamillary processes)

Function:
Lateral bending of lumbar spine
Most likely function is postural

Innervation:
Lumbar and sacral spinal nerves (dorsal rami)

**Intertransversarii lumborum—lateral
(two portions)**

Origin:
Ventral portion: L2–S1 vertebrae (costal processes, ventral part)
Dorsal portion: L2–S1 vertebrae (accessory processes, superior part)

Insertion:
Ventral portion: vertebra above the vertebra of origin (costal processes, inferior surfaces)
Dorsal portion: vertebra above the vertebra of origin (transverse processes, inferior surfaces)

Function:
Postural function and stabilization of adjacent vertebrae
Extension of the spine

Innervation:
Lateral muscles: lumbar and sacral spinal nerves (ventral rami)

100 QUADRATUS LUMBORUM

Origin:
Ilium (crest, inner lip)
Iliolumbar ligament

Insertion:
12th rib (lower border)

L1–L4 vertebrae (apices of transverse processes)
T12 vertebral body (occasionally)

Description:
An irregular quadrilateral muscle located against the posterior (dorsal) abdominal wall, this muscle is encased by layers of the thoracolumbar fascia. It fills the space between the 12th rib and the iliac crest. Its fibers run obliquely upward and medially from the iliac crest to the inferior border of the 12th rib and transverse processes of the lumbar vertebrae. The muscle is variable in size and occurrence.

Function:
Elevation of pelvis (weak in contrast to lateral abdominals)
Extension of lumbar spine (muscles on both sides)
Inspiration (via stabilization of lower attachments of diaphragm)
Fixation of lower portions of diaphragm for prolonged vocalization which needs sustained expiration.
Lateral bending of lumbar spine to same side (pelvis fixed)
Fixation and depression of 12th rib

Innervation:
T12–L3 spinal nerves (ventral rami)

Muscles of the Thorax for Respiration

101 Diaphragm

102 Intercostales externi

103 Intercostales interni

104 Intercostales intimi

105 Subcostales

106 Transversus thoracis

107 Levatores costarum

108 Serratus posterior superior

109 Serratus posterior inferior

101 DIAPHRAGM

Origin:
Muscle fibers take origin from the circumference of the thoracic outlet in three groups:
Sternal: Xiphoid (posterior surface)
Costal: Ribs 7 to 12 (bilaterally; inner surfaces of the cartilage and the deep surfaces on each side)
Lumbar: L1–L3 vertebrae (from the medial and lateral arcuate ligaments (also called lumbocostal arches) and from bodies of the vertebrae by two muscular crura)

Insertion:

Central tendon (trifoliate-shaped) of diaphragm immediately below the pericardium and blending with it. The central tendon has no bony attachments. It has three divisions called leaflets (because of its clover leaf pattern) in an otherwise continuous sheet of muscle, which affords the muscle great strength.

Description:

This half-dome–shaped muscle of contractile and fibrous structure forms the floor of the thorax (convex upper surface) and the roof of the abdomen (concave inferior surface) (Fig. 9–4).

The diaphragm is muscular on the periphery and its central area is tendinous. It closes the opening of the thoracic outlet and forms a convex floor for the thoracic cavity. The muscle is flatter centrally than at the periphery and higher on the right (reaching rib 5) than on the left (reaching rib 6). From the peak on each side, the diaphragm abruptly descends to its costal and vertebral attachments. This descending slope is much more precipitous and longer posteriorly.

Function:

Inspiration: Contraction of the diaphragm with the lower ribs fixed draws the central tendon downward and forward during inspiration. This increases the vertical thoracic dimensions and pushes the abdominal viscera downward. It also decreases the pressure within the thoracic cavity, forcing air into the lungs through the open glottis by the higher pressure of the atmospheric air.

These events occur along with intercostal muscle action, which elevates the ribs, sternum, and vertebrae, increasing the anteroposterior and transverse thoracic dimensions for the inspiratory effort.

The diaphragm adds power to expulsive efforts: lifting heavy loads, sneezing, coughing, laughing, parturition, evacuation of bladder and bowels. These activities are preceded by deep inspiration.

Expiration: Passive relaxation allows the half-dome to ascend, thus decreasing thoracic cavity volume and increasing its pressure.

Innervation:

Phrenic nerve, C4 (with contributions from C3 and C5)

The Intercostals

The intercostal muscles are slim layers of muscle and tendon occupying each of the intercostal spaces; the externals are the most superficial, the internals come next, and deepest are the intimi.

102 EXTERNAL INTERCOSTALS
(Intercostales Externi)

There are 11 pairs

Origin:

Ribs 1 to 11 (lower borders and costal tubercles)
Superior costotransverse ligaments

Insertion:

Ribs 2 to 12 (upper border of rib below)
Aponeurotic external intercostal membrane
Sternum (via aponeurosis)

Description:

There are 11 of these muscles on each side of the chest. Each arises from the inferior margin of one rib and inserts on the superior margin of the rib below. They extend in the intercostal spaces from the tubercles of the ribs dorsally to the cartilages of the ribs ventrally.

The muscle fibers run obliquely inferolaterally on the dorsal thorax; they run inferomedially and somewhat ventrally on the anterior thorax (down and toward the sternum).

The externi are the thickest of the three intercostal muscles. In appearance they may seem to be continuations of the external oblique abdominal muscles.

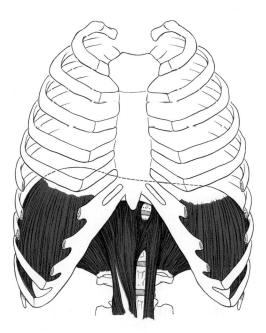

FIGURE 9–4
The diaphragm

Function:

The muscles of respiration are highly coordinated between abdominal and thoracic processes with the diaphragm being the major muscle of inspiration, accounting for about 2/3 of vital capacity. The External intercostals are more active in inspiration than expiration but work closely with the Internal intercostals to stiffen the chest wall, preventing paradoxical motion during descent of the diaphragm.

Elevation of ribs in inspiration. There are data to support this claim for the upper four or five muscles, but the more dorsal and lateral fibers of the same muscles also are active in early expiration. It is possible that the activity of the intercostals during respiration varies with the depth of breathing.[17]

Depression of the ribs in expiration (supporting data sparse).

Rotation of thoracic spine to opposite side (unilateral).

Stabilization of rib cage.

Innervation:

T1–T11 intercostal nerves (ventral rami)

These nerves are numbered sequentially according to interspace; e.g., the 5th intercostal nerve innervates muscle occupying the 5th intercostal space between the 5th and 6th ribs.

103 INTERNAL INTERCOSTALS
(Intercostales Interni)

Origin:

Ribs 1 to 11 (ridge on inner surface, then passing down and toward spine)

Costal cartilage of same rib

Sternum (anterior)

Upper border and costal cartilage of rib below

Internal intercostal membrane (aponeurosis)

Insertion:

Ribs 2 to 12 (upper border of next rib below)

Description:

There are 11 pairs of these muscles. They extend from the sternal end of the ribs anteriorly to the angle of the ribs posteriorly. The fibers run obliquely downward but at a 90° angle to the external intercostals.

Function:

Not as strong as the External intercostals.

Elevation of ribs in inspiration. This may be true at least for the 1st to 5th muscles. The more lateral muscle fibers run more obliquely inferior and posterior and are most active in expiration.[17]

Stabilization of rib cage.

Innervation:

T1–T11 intercostal nerves (ventral rami)

104 INTERCOSTALES INTIMI

Origin:

Costal groove of rib above the rib of insertion. Found in lower costal interspaces when present, but no consistent evidence in upper five to six interspaces

Insertion:

Upper margin of the rib below the rib of origin. Found in lower costal interspaces.

Description:

There is dispute about whether this is a separate muscle or just a part of the internal intercostals. It is a thin sheet lying deep to the internal intercostals, but arguments in favor of a separate muscle are not convincing. If they are separate, there may be five to six pairs, with no consistent presence in the upper costal interspaces. Considered insignificant.

Function:

Presumed to be identical to Intercostales interni.

Innervation:

T1–T11 intercostal nerves (ventral rami) (inconsistent)

105 SUBCOSTALES

Origin:

Lower ribs (variable) on inner surface near angle

Insertion:

Inner surface of two or three ribs below rib of origin

Description:

Lying on the dorsal thoracic wall, these muscles are discretely developed only in the lower thorax. Fibers run in the same direction as those of the Intercostales interni.

Function:

Draws adjacent ribs together or depresses ribs (no supporting data)

Innervation:

T7–T11 intercostal nerves (ventral rami)

106 TRANSVERSE THORACIS

Origin:

Sternum (caudal 1/3; xiphoid, posterior surface)

Ribs 3 to 6 (costal cartilages, inner side)

Insertion:
Ribs 2 to 5 (costal cartilages, caudal borders)

Description:
A thin plane on the inner surface of the anterior wall of the thorax. The fibers pass obliquely up and laterally, diverging more as they insert. The lowest fibers are horizontal and are continuous with the Transversus abdominis. The highest fibers are almost vertical. Attachments vary from side to side in the same person and among different persons.

Function:
Draws ribs downward; narrows chest
Active in forced expiration

Innervation:
T2–T11 intercostal nerves (ventral rami)

107 LEVATORES COSTARUM

12 pairs of muscles

Origin:
C7 and T1–T11 vertebrae (transverse processes)

Insertion:
Rib immediately below rib of origin (upper margin, outer edge between angle and tubercle)

Description:
There are 12 pairs of these muscles on either side of the thorax on its posterior wall. Fibers run obliquely inferolaterally, like those of the external intercostal muscles. The most inferior fibers divide into two fasciculi, one of which inserts as described; the other descends to the 2nd rib below its origin.

Function:
Elevation of ribs in inspiration (disputed)
Lateral bending of spine

Innervation:
T1–T11 intercostal nerves and sometimes C8 (dorsal rami)

108 SERRATUS POSTERIOR SUPERIOR

Origin:
C7 and T1–T3 vertebrae (spinous processes)
Ligamentum nuchae
Supraspinous ligaments

Insertion:
Ribs 2 to 5 (upper borders, lateral to angles)

Description:
Muscle lies on the upper dorsal thorax, over the

Erector spinae and under the Rhomboids. Fibers run inferolaterally.

Function:
Elevates upper ribs (debated)
Presumably increases thoracic volume (function uncertain)

Innervation:
T2–T5 spinal nerves (ventral rami)

109 SERRATUS POSTERIOR INFERIOR

Origin:
T11–T12 and L1–L2 vertebrae (spinous processes via thoracolumbar fascia)
Supraspinous ligaments

Insertion:
Ribs 9 to 12 (inferior borders, lateral to angles)

Description:
A thin muscle, composed of four digitations, lying at the border between the thoracic and lumbar regions. Fibers ascend laterally. It is much broader than the Serratus posterior superior and lies four ribs below it. It lies over the Erector spinae and under the Latissimus dorsi.[4] The muscle may have fewer than four digitations or may be absent.

Function:
Depresses lower ribs and moves them dorsally
Has an uncertain role in respiration

Innervation:
T9–T12 spinal nerves (ventral rami)

Muscles of the Abdomen
Anterolateral Walls

110 Obliquus externus abdominis

111 Obliquus internus abdominis

112 Transversus abdominis

113 Rectus abdominis

114 Pyramidalis

110 OBLIQUUS EXTERNUS ABDOMINIS

Origin:
Ribs 5 to 12 (by digitations that attach to the external and inferior surfaces and alternate with digitations of the Serratus anterior and Latissimus dorsi)

Insertion:
Iliac crest (anterior half of outer lip)
Iliac fascia
Aponeurosis from the prominence of 9th costal cartilage to anterior superior iliac spine (ASIS); aponeuroses from both sides meet at the linea alba

Description:
The largest and most superficial flat, thin muscle of the abdomen curves around the anterior and lateral walls. Its muscular fibers lie on the lateral wall while its aponeurosis traverses the anterior wall in front of the Rectus abdominis, meeting its opposite number to form the linea alba. The digitations form an oblique line that runs down and backward. The linea alba extends from the xiphoid process to the symphysis pubis.

The upper (superior) five digitations increase in size as they descend and alternate with the corresponding digitations of the Serratus anterior. The distal three digitations decrease in size as they descend and alternate with digitations of the Latissimus dorsi. The superior fibers travel inferomedially; the posterior fibers pass more vertically.

Function:
Flexion of trunk (bilateral muscles)
Tilts pelvis posteriorly
Elevates pelvis (unilateral)
Rotation of trunk to opposite side (unilateral)
Lateral bending of trunk (unilateral)
Support and compression of abdominal viscera, counteracting effect of gravity on abdominal contents
Assists defecation, micturition, emesis, and parturition (i.e., expulsion of contents of abdominal viscera and air from lungs)
Important accessory muscle of forced expiration (during expiration it forces the viscera upward to elevate the diaphragm)

Innervation:
T7–T12 spinal nerves (ventral rami)

111 OBLIQUUS INTERNUS ABDOMINIS

Origin:
Thoracolumbar fascia
Inguinal ligament (lateral 2/3 of upper aspect)
Iliac crest (anterior 2/3 of intermediate line)

Insertion:
Ribs 9 to 12 (inferior borders and cartilages by digitations that appear continuous with internal intercostals)

Aponeurosis that splits at the lateral border of the Rectus abdominis to encircle the muscle and reunite at the linea alba
Cartilages of ribs 7 to 9 (via an aponeurosis)
Pubis (crest and pecten pubis) from tendinous sheath of Transverse abdominis

Description:
This muscle is smaller and thinner than the external oblique under which it lies in the lateral and ventral abdominal wall. The fibers from the iliac crest pass upward and medially to ribs 9 to 12 and the aponeurosis; the more lateral the fibers, the more they run toward the vertical. The lowest fibers pass almost horizontally on the lower abdomen.

Function:
Flexion of spine (bilateral)
Lateral bending of spine (unilateral)
Rotation of trunk to same side (unilateral)
Increases abdominal pressure to assist in defecation and other expulsive actions
Forces viscera upward during expiration to elevate diaphragm
Elevation of pelvis

Innervation:
T7–T12 spinal nerves (ventral rami)
L1 spinal nerve (iliohypogastric and ilioinguinal branches) (ventral rami)

112 TRANSVERSE ABDOMINIS

Origin:
Inguinal ligament (lateral 1/3)
Iliac crest (anterior 2/3 of inner lip)
Thoracolumbar fascia (between iliac crest and 12th rib)
Ribs 7 to 12 (costal cartilages)

Insertion:
Pubis (crest and pecten pubis) via aponeurosis along with aponeurosis of the internal oblique to form the falx inguinalis
Linea alba (upper and middle fibers pass medially to blend with the posterior layer of the broad aponeurosis encircling the Rectus abdominis)

Description:
The innermost of the flat abdominal muscles, the Transversus abdominis lies under the internal oblique. Its name derives from the direction of its fibers, which pass horizontally across the lateral abdomen to an aponeurosis and the linea alba. The length of the fibers varies considerably depending on the insertion site, the most inferior to the pubis being the longest. At its origin on ribs 7 to 12, the muscle interdigitates

with similar diaphragmatic digitations separated by a narrow raphe.

Function:
> Constricts (flattens) abdomen, compressing the abdominal viscera and assisting in expelling their contents
> Forced expiration

Innervation:
> T7–T12 spinal nerves (ventral rami)
> L1 spinal nerve (iliohypogastric and ilioinguinal branches) (ventral rami)

113 RECTUS ABDOMINIS

Origin:
> By two tendons inferiorly:
> *Lateral:* pubis (tubercle on crest and pecten pubis)
> *Medial:* ligaments covering front of symphysis pubis

Insertion:
> Ribs 5 to 7 (costal cartilages by three fascicles of differing size)
> Sternum (xiphoid process, costoxiphoid ligaments)

Description:
> A long muscular strap extending from the ventral lower sternum to the pubis. Its vertical fibers lie centrally along the abdomen, each separated from its contralateral partner by the linea alba. The muscle is interrupted (but not all the way through) by three (or more) fibrous bands called the *tendinous intersections,* which pass transversely across the muscle in a zigzag fashion. The most superior intersection generally is at the level of the xiphoid; the lowest is at the level of the umbilicus, and the second intersection is midway between the two. These are readily visible on bodybuilders or others with well-developed musculature.

Function:
> Flexion of spine (draws symphysis and sternum toward each other)
> Posterior tilt of pelvis
> With other abdominal muscles, compresses abdominal contents

Innervation:
> T7–T12 spinal nerves (ventral rami)
> T7 innervates fibers above the superior tendinous intersection; T8 innervates fibers between the superior and middle intersections; T9 innervates fibers between the middle and distal intersections.

114 PYRAMIDALIS

Origin:
> Pubis (front of body and symphysis via ligamentous fibers)

Insertion:
> Linea alba (midway between umbilicus and pubis)

Description:
> A small triangular muscle located in the extreme distal portion of the abdominal wall and lying anterior to the lower Rectus abdominis. Its origin on the pubis is wide, and it narrows as it rises to a pointed insertion. The muscle varies considerably from side to side, and may be present or absent.

Function:
> Tenses the linea alba

Innervation:
> T12 spinal nerve (subcostal nerve) (ventral ramus)

Muscles of the Perineum

115 Levator ani

116 Coccygeus

117 Cremaster

118 Transversus perinei superficialis

119 Transversus perinei profundus

120 Bulbospongiosus

121 Ischiocavernosus

122 Sphincter urethrae

123 Sphincter ani externus

> Corrugator cutis ani (involuntary muscle, not described)

> Internal anal sphincter (involuntary muscle, not described)

115 LEVATOR ANI

Origin:
> *Pubococcygeus part:* Pubis (inner surface of superior ramus)
> Coccyx (anterior)
> Blends with longitudinal rectus muscle and fascia
> *Puborectal part:* Same origin as pubococcygeus but splits off to join its opposite member, along with Sphincter externus, to form an anorectal sling
> *Iliococcygeus part:* Ischium (inner surface of spine)
> *Iliosacralis part:* Accessory slip
> Obturator fascia

Insertion:
Coccyx (last two segments)
Anococcygeal raphe
Sphincter ani externus

Description:
A part of the pelvic diaphragm, this broad, thin sheet of muscle unites with its contralateral partner to form a complete pelvic floor. Anteriorly it is attached to the pubis lateral to the symphysis, posteriorly to the ischial spine, and between these to the obturator fascia. The fibers course medially with varying obliquity.

There are links to the Sphincter urethrae, to the prostate as the Levator prostatae, to the Pubovaginalis walls of the vagina in the female, and to the perineal body and rectum in both men and women. In animals these parts are attached to caudal vertebrae and control tail motions. Loss of a tail in humans leaves these muscles to form a stronger pelvic floor.

Function:
Constriction of rectum and vagina contributing to continence; they must relax to permit expulsion.

Along with the coccygei, the levator forms a muscular pelvic diaphragm that supports the pelvic viscera and opposes sudden increases in intra-abdominal pressure, as in forced expiration, or the Valsalva maneuver.

Innervation:
S2–S3 spinal nerves (pudendal nerve) (ventral rami) and nerves from sacral plexus

116 COCCYGEUS

Origin:
Ischium (spine and pelvic surface)
Sacrospinous ligament

Insertion:
Coccyx (lateral margins)
Sacrum (last or 5th segment, side)

Description:
The paired muscle lies posterior and superior to the Levator ani and contiguous with it in the same plane. The muscle occasionally is absent. It is considered the pelvic aspect of the sacrospinous ligament.

Function:
The coccygei pull the coccyx forward and support it after it has been pushed back for defecation or parturition.

With the Levatores ani and Piriformis, compresses the posterior pelvic cavity and outlet in women ("the birth canal").

Innervation:
S3–S4 spinal nerves (pudendal plexus) (ventral rami)

117 CREMASTER

Origin:
Lateral part: Inguinal ligament (continuous with internal oblique and occasionally from Transverse abdominis). Technically this is an abdominal muscle.
Medial part: Pubis (crest, tubercle, and falx inguinalis) This part is inconstant.

Insertion:
Pubis (tubercle and crest)
Sheath of Rectus abdominis and Transversus abdominis

Description:
Consists of loose fasciculi lying along the spermatic cord and held together by areolar tissue to form the cremasteric fascia around the cord and testis. Often said to be continuous with the Internal oblique abdominal muscle or with the Transversus abdominis. After passage through the superficial inguinal ring, the muscle spreads into loops of varying lengths over the spermatic cord.

Although the muscle fibers are striated, this is not usually a voluntary muscle. Stimulation of the skin on the medial thigh evokes a reflex response, the cremasteric reflex.

Found as a vestige in women.

Function:
Elevation of testis toward superficial inguinal ring
Thermoregulation of testes by adjusting position

Innervation:
L1–L2 spinal nerves (genitofemoral nerve) (ventral rami)

118 TRANSVERSUS PERINEI SUPERFICIALIS

Origin:
Ischial tuberosity (inner and anterior part)

Insertion:
Perineal body (a centrally placed, modiolar-like structure on which perineal muscles and fascia converge)
Tendon of perineum

Description:
A narrow slip of muscle in both the male and female perineum, it courses almost transversely across the perineal area in front of the anus. It

is joined on the perineal body by the muscle from the opposite side. The muscle is sometimes absent, poorly developed, or may be doubled.

Function:
Bilateral action serves to fix the centrally located perineal body.
Support of pelvic viscera.

Innervation:
S2–S4 spinal nerves (pudendal nerve) (ventral rami)

119 TRANSVERSUS PERINEI PROFUNDUS

Origin:
Ischium (ramus, medial aspect)

Insertion:
Male: Perineal body
Female: Vagina (side); perineal body

Description:
Small deep muscle with similar structure and function in both male and female. The bilateral muscles meet at the midline on the perineal body. This muscle is in the same plane as the Sphincter urethrae, and together they form most of the bulk of the urogenital diaphragm. (Together they used to be called the Constrictor urethrae.) Together, the two muscles "tether" the perineal body.

Function:
Fixation of perineal body
Supports pelvic viscera

Innervation:
S2–S4 spinal nerves (pudendal nerve) (ventral rami)

120 BULBOSPONGIOSUS

Formerly called:
Male: Bulbocavernosus; Accelerator urinae
Female: Sphincter vaginae

In the Female:

Origin:
Perineal body
Blending with Sphincter ani externus and median raphe
Fascia of urogenital diaphragm

Insertion:
Corpora cavernosus clitoridis

Description:
Surrounds the orifice of the vagina and covers the lateral parts of the vestibular bulb. The fibers run anteriorly on each side of the vagina and send a slip to cover the clitoral body.

Function:
Arrests micturition; helps to empty urethra after bladder empties
Constriction of vaginal orifice
Constriction of deep dorsal vein of clitoris by anterior fibers, contributing to erection of clitoris

Innervation:
S2–S4 spinal nerves (pudendal nerve) (ventral rami)

In the Male:

Origin:
Perineal body
Median raphe over bulb of penis

Insertion:
Urogenital diaphragm (inferior fascia)
Aponeurosis over corpus spongiosum penis
Body of penis anterior to Ischiocavernosus
Tendinous expansion over dorsal vessels of penis

Description:
Located in the midline of the perineum anterior to the anus and consisting of two symmetrical parts united by a tendinous raphe. Its fibers divide like the halves of a feather. The posterior fibers disperse on the inferior fascia of the urogenital diaphragm; the middle fibers encircle the penile bulb and the corpus spongiosum and form a strong aponeurosis with fibers from the opposite side; and the anterior fibers spread out over the corpora cavernosa.

Function:
Empties urethra at end of micturition (is capable of arresting urination).
Middle fibers assist in penis erection by compressing the bulbar erectile tissue; anterior fibers assist by constricting the deep dorsal vein.
Contracts repeatedly in ejaculation.

Innervation:
S2–S4 spinal nerves (pudendal nerve) (ventral rami)

121 ISCHIOCAVERNOSUS

In the Female:

Origin:
Ischium (tuberosity [inner surface] and ramus)
Crus clitoridis (surface)

Insertion:
Aponeurosis inserting into sides and inferior surface of crus clitoridis

Description:
Covers the unattached surface of crus clitoridis. Muscle is smaller than the male counterpart.

Function:
Compresses crus clitoridis, retarding venous return and thus assisting erection

Innervation:
S2–S4 spinal nerves (pudendal)

In the Male:

Origin:
Ischium (tuberosity, medial aspect dorsal to crus penis and ischial rami)

Insertion:
Aponeurosis into the sides and undersurface of the body of the penis

Description:
The muscle is paired and covers the crus of the penis.

Function:
Compression of crus penis, maintaining erection by retarding return of blood through the veins

Innervation:
S2–S4 spinal nerves (pudendal nerve, perineal branch) (ventral rami)

122 SPHINCTER URETHRAE

In the Female:

Origin:
Pubis (inferior ramus on each side)
Transverse perineal ligament and fascia

Insertion:
Surrounds lower urethra, neck of bladder; sends fibers to wall of vagina.
Blends with fibers from opposite muscle posterior to urethra.
Peroneal membrane (posterior edge)

Description:
Has both superior and inferior fibers. The inferior fibers arise on the pubis and course across the pubic arch in front of the urethra to circle around it. The superior fibers merge into the smooth muscle of the bladder.

Function:
Constricts urethra, particularly when the bladder contains fluid.
It is relaxed during micturition but contracts to expel remaining urine after micturition.

Innervation:
Pudendal nucleus (Onuf's nucleus)
S2–S4 spinal nerves (pudendal nerve) (ventral rami)

In the Male:

Origin:
Ischiopubic ramus (superior fibers)
Transverse perineal ligament (inferior fibers)

Insertion:
Perineal body (converges with muscles from other side)

Description:
Surrounds entire length of membranous portion of urethra and is enclosed in the urogenital diaphragm fascia

Function:
Compression of urethra (bilateral action)
Active in ejaculation
Relaxes during micturition but contracts to expel last of urine

Innervation:
Pudendal nerve nucleus (Onuf's nucleus)
S2–S4 spinal nerves (ventral rami)

123 SPHINCTER ANI EXTERNUS

Origin:
Skin surrounding margin of anus
Coccyx (via anococcygeal ligament)

Insertion:
Perineal body
Blends with other muscles in area

Description:
Surrounds entire anal canal and is adherent to skin. Consists of three parts, all skeletal muscle:

1. *Subcutaneous:* Around lower anal canal; fibers course horizontally beneath the skin at the anal orifice. Some fibers join perineal body and others the anococcygeal ligament.
2. *Superficial:* Surrounds the lower part of the internal sphincter; attaches to both the perineal body and coccyx (via the terminal coccygeal ligament, the only bony attachment of the muscle).
3. *Deep part:* Thick band around the upper internal sphincter with fibers blending with the Puborectalis of the Levator ani and fascia.

Function:

Keeps anal orifice closed. It is always in a state of tonic contraction and has no antagonist. Muscle relaxes during defecation, allowing orifice to open. The muscle can be voluntarily contracted to close the orifice more tightly as in forced expiration or the Valsalva maneuver.

Innervation:

S2–S3 spinal nerves (pudendal nerve, inferior rectal branch) (ventral rami)

S4 spinal nerve (perineal branch)

MUSCLES OF THE UPPER EXTREMITY
(Shoulder Girdle, Elbow, Forearm, Wrist, Fingers, Thumb)

Muscles of the Shoulder Girdle Acting on the Scapula

124 Trapezius

125 Rhomboid major

126 Rhomboid minor

127 Levator scapulae

128 Serratus anterior

129 Pectoralis minor

124 TRAPEZIUS

A paired muscle

Origin:

Upper:
Occiput (external protuberance and medial 1/3 of superior nuchal line)
Ligamentum nuchae
C7 vertebra (spinous process)

Middle:
T1–T5 vertebrae (spinous processes)
Supraspinous ligaments

Lower:
T6–T12 vertebrae (spinous processes)
Supraspinous ligaments

Insertion:

Upper:
Clavicle (posterior surface, lateral 1/3)

Middle:
Scapula (medial margin of acromion; spine of scapula and crest of its superior lip)

Lower:
Scapula (spine: tubercle at lateral apex and aponeurosis at root of spine)

Description:

A flat, triangular muscle lying over the posterior neck, shoulder, and upper thorax. The upper trapezius fibers course down and laterally from the occiput; the middle fibers are horizontal; and the lower fibers move upward and laterally from the vertebrae to the scapular spine. The name of the muscle is derived from the shape of the muscle with its contralateral partner: a diamond-shaped quadrilateral figure, or trapezoid.

Function:

All: Stabilizes scapula during movements of the arm.

Upper and Lower:
Rotation of the scapula so glenoid faces up (inferior angle moves laterally and forward)

Upper:
Elevation of scapula and shoulder ("shrugging") (with Levator scapulae)
Rotation of head to opposite side (one)
Capital extension (both)
Cervical extension (both)

Middle:
Scapular adduction (retraction) (with Rhomboids)

Lower:
Scapular adduction, depression, and upward rotation

Innervation:

Accessory (XI) nerve (upper and middle)

While the accessory nerve provides the major motor supply to the Trapezius, there also is some supply from the cervical plexus (C3–C4) and this may be the primary supply of the lower fibers with contributions from the accessory nerve.[18]

125 RHOMBOID MAJOR
(Rhomboideus Major)

Origin:

T2–T5 vertebrae (spinous processes)
Supraspinous ligaments

Insertion:

Scapula (medial [vertebral] border between root of spine above and inferior angle below)

Description:

Fibers of the muscle run slightly inferolaterally between the thoracic spine and the vertebral border of the scapula.

Function:

Scapular adduction

Downward rotation of scapula (glenoid faces down)
Scapular elevation

Innervation:
C5 Dorsal scapular nerve

126 RHOMBOID MINOR

Origin:
C7–T1 vertebrae (spinous processes)
Ligamentum nuchae (lower)

Insertion:
Scapula (root of spine on medial [vertebral] border)

Description:
Lies just superior to Rhomboid major, and its fibers run parallel with the larger muscle.

Function:
Scapular adduction
Scapular downward rotation (glenoid faces down)
Scapular elevation

Innervation:
C5 Dorsal scapular nerve

127 LEVATOR SCAPULAE

Origin:
C1–C4 vertebrae (transverse processes and posterior tubercles)

Insertion:
Scapula (vertebral border between superior angle and root of scapular spine)

Description:
Lies on the dorsolateral neck and descends deep to the Sternocleidomastoid on the floor of the posterior triangle of the neck. Its vertebral attachments vary considerably.

Function:
Elevates and adducts scapula
Scapular downward rotation (glenoid faces down)
Lateral bending of cervical spine to same side (one)
Cervical rotation to same side (one)
Cervical extension (both assist)

Innervation:
C3–C4 spinal nerves (ventral rami)
C5 Dorsal scapular nerve (to lower fibers) (ventral rami)

128 SERRATUS ANTERIOR

Origin:
Ribs 1 to 8 (often 9 and 10 also) by digitations (superior and outer surfaces). Each digitation (except first) arises from a single rib. The 1st digitation arises from the 1st and 2nd ribs. All others arise from a single rib and fascia covering the intervening intercostals.
Aponeurosis of intercostal muscles.

Insertion:
Scapula (ventral surface of whole vertebral border)
First digitation: Superior angle of scapula on anterior aspect
Second and third digitations: Anterior (costal) surface of whole vertebral border
Fourth to eighth digitations: Inferior angle of scapula (costal surface)

Description:
This large sheet of muscle curves posteriorly around the thorax from its origin on the lateral side of the ribs, passing under the scapula to attach to its vertebral border.

Function:
Scapular abduction
Upward rotation of the scapula (glenoid faces up)
Medial border of scapula drawn anteriorly close to the thoracic wall (preventing "winging")

Functional Relationships:
The Serratus works with the Trapezius in a force couple to rotate the scapula upward (glenoid up), allowing the arm to be elevated fully (150° to 180°). Three component forces act around a center of rotation located in the center of the scapula: (1) upward pull on the acromial end of the spine of the scapula by the upper Trapezius; (2) downward pull on the base of the spine of the scapula by the lower Trapezius; (3) lateral and anterior pull on the inferior angle by the inferior fibers of the Serratus.[19-21]
The reader is referred to comprehensive texts on kinesiology for further detail.

Innervation:
C5–C7 Long thoracic nerve

129 PECTORALIS MINOR

Origin:
Ribs 3 to 5 and sometimes 2 to 4 (upper and outer surfaces near the costal cartilages)
Aponeurosis of intercostal muscles

Insertion:
Scapula (coracoid process, medial border, and superior surface)

Description:

This muscle, broader at its origins, lies on the upper thorax directly under the Pectoralis major. It forms part of the anterior wall of the axilla (along with the Pectoralis major). The fibers pass upward and laterally and converge in a flat tendon.

Function:

Scapular protraction (abduction): scapula moves forward around the chest wall. Works here with Serratus anterior.

Elevation of ribs in forced inspiration when scapula is fixed by the Levator scapulae

Innervation:

C5–T1 Medial and lateral pectoral nerves

Vertebrohumeral Muscles

130 Latissimus dorsi

131 Pectoralis major

130 LATISSIMUS DORSI

Origin:

T6–T12 vertebrae (spinous processes)

L1–L5 and sacral vertebrae (spinous processes by way of the thoracolumbar fascia)

Ribs 9 to 12 (interdigitates with the external abdominal oblique)

Ilium (posterior 1/3 of iliac crest)

Supraspinous ligament

Insertion:

Humerus (intertubercular groove, floor, distal)

Deep fascia of arm

Description:

A broad sheet of muscle that covers the lumbar and lower portion of the posterior thorax. From this wide origin, the muscle fibers converge on the proximal humerus. The superior fibers are almost horizontal, passing over the inferior angle of the scapula, whereas the lowest fibers are almost vertical. As the muscle approaches its tendinous insertion, the fibers from the upper and lower portions fold on themselves so that the superior fibers are attached inferiorly in the intertubercular groove; similarly, the sacral and lumbar fibers become more superior.

Function:

Extension, adduction, and internal rotation of shoulder.

Hyperextension of spine (muscles on both sides), as in lifting.

The muscle is most powerful in overhead activities (such as swimming [downstroke] and climb-

ing), crutch walking (elevation of trunk to arms, i.e., shoulder depression), or swinging.[22]

Adducts raised arm against resistance (with Pectoralis major and Teres major).

It is very active in strong expiration, as in coughing and sneezing, and in deep inspiration.

Elevation of pelvis with arms fixed.

Innervation:

C6–C8 Thoracodorsal nerve (ventral rami)

131 PECTORALIS MAJOR

Origin:

Clavicular (upper) portion:

Clavicle (sternal half of anterior surface)

Sternocostal portion:

Sternum (half of the anterior surface down to level of 6th rib)

Ribs (cartilage of all true ribs except rib 1 and sometimes rib 7)

Aponeurosis of Obliquus externus abdominis

Insertion:

Humerus (intertubercular sulcus, lateral border via a bilaminar tendon)

Description:

This muscle is a large, thick, fan-shaped muscle covering the anterior and superior surfaces of the thorax. The Pectoralis major forms part of the anterior wall of the axilla (the anterior axillary fold, conspicuous in abduction). The muscle is divided into two portions that converge toward the axilla.

The clavicular fibers pass downward and laterally toward the humeral insertion. The sternocostal fibers pass horizontally from midsternum and upward and laterally from the rib attachments. The lower fibers rise almost vertically toward the axilla. Both parts unite in a common tendon of insertion to the humerus.

Function:

Adduction of shoulder (glenohumeral) joint (whole muscle, proximal attachment fixed)

Internal rotation of shoulder

Elevation of thorax in forced inspiration (with both upper extremities fixed)

Clavicular fibers:

Internal rotation of shoulder

Flexion of shoulder

Horizontal shoulder adduction

Sternocostal fibers:

Horizontal shoulder adduction

Extension of shoulder

Draws trunk upward and forward in climbing

Innervation:

Clavicular fibers: C5–C7 Lateral pectoral nerve

Sternocostal fibers: C6–T1 medial and lateral pectoral nerves

Scapulohumeral Muscles

There are six shoulder muscles, which extend from the scapula to the humerus. Also included here are the Subclavius and the Coracobrachialis.

132 Subclavius

133 Deltoid

135 Supraspinatus

136 Infraspinatus

134 Subscapularis

138 Teres major

137 Teres minor

139 Coracobrachialis

All act on the shoulder (glenohumeral) joint. The largest of the muscles (Deltoid) also attaches to the clavicle and overlies the remaining muscles.

132 SUBCLAVIUS

Origin:
Rib 1 and its cartilage (at their junction)

Insertion:
Clavicle (inferior surface, groove in middle 1/3)

Description:
A small elongated muscle lying under the clavicle between it and the 1st rib. The fibers run upward and laterally following the contour of the clavicle.

Function:
Shoulder depression (assist)
Depresses and moves clavicle forward, thus stabilizing it during shoulder motion

Innervation:
C5–C6 (nerve to Subclavius off brachial plexus) (ventral rami)

133 DELTOID

Origin:
Anterior fibers: Clavicle (shaft: anterior border and superior surface of lateral 1/3)
Middle fibers: Scapula (acromion, lateral margin, and superior surface)
Posterior fibers: Scapula (spine on lower lip of posterior border)

Insertion:
Humerus (deltoid tuberosity on lateral midshaft via humeral tendon)

Description:
This large multipennate, triangular muscle covers the shoulder anteriorly, posteriorly, and laterally. From a wide origin on the scapula and clavicle, all fibers converge on the humeral insertion, where it gives off an expansion to the deep fascia of the arm. The anterior fibers descend obliquely backward and laterally; the middle fibers descend vertically; the posterior fibers descend obliquely forward and laterally.

Function:
Abduction of shoulder (glenohumeral joint): primarily the acromial middle fibers. The anterior and posterior fibers in this motion stabilize the limb in its cantilever position.
Flexion and internal rotation of shoulder (anterior fibers).
Extension and external rotation: posterior fibers.
The Deltoid tends to displace the humeral head upward.
Shoulder horizontal abduction (posterior fibers).
Shoulder horizontal adduction (anterior fibers).

Innervation:
C5–C6 Axillary nerve (ventral rami)

134 SUBSCAPULARIS

Origin:
Scapula (subscapular fossa and groove along axillary margin)
Aponeurosis separating this muscle from the Teres major and Triceps brachii (long head)
Tendinous laminae

Insertion:
Humerus (lesser tubercle)
Capsule of glenohumeral joint (anterior)

Description:
This is one of the rotator cuff muscles. It is a large triangular muscle that fills the subscapular fossa of the scapula. The tendon of insertion is separated from the scapular neck by a large bursa, which is really a protrusion of the synovial lining of the joint. Variations are rare.

Function:
Internal rotation of shoulder joint
Stabilization of glenohumeral joint by humeral depression (keeps humeral head in glenoid fossa)

Innervation:
C5–C6 Subscapular nerves (upper and lower)

135 SUPRASPINATUS

Origin:
Scapula (supraspinous fossa, medial 2/3)
Supraspinatus fascia

Insertion:
Humerus (greater tubercle, highest facet)
Articular capsule of glenohumeral joint

Description:
This is one of the four rotator cuff muscles. Occupying all of the supraspinous fossa, the muscle fibers converge to form a flat tendon that crosses above the glenohumeral joint (beneath the acromion) on its way to a humeral insertion. This tendon is the most commonly ruptured element of the rotator cuff mechanism around the joint.

Function:
Maintains humeral head in glenoid fossa (with other rotator cuff muscles)
Abduction of shoulder
External rotation of shoulder

Innervation:
C5–C6 Suprascapular nerve

136 INFRASPINATUS

Origin:
Scapula (fills most of infraspinous fossa, rises from medial 2/3)
Infraspinous fascia

Insertion:
Humerus (greater tubercle, middle facet)

Description:
Occupies most of the infraspinous fossa. The muscle fibers converge to form the tendon of insertion, which glides over the lateral border of the scapular spine and then passes across the posterior aspect of the articular capsule to insert on the humerus. This is the third of the rotator cuff muscles.

Function:
Stabilizes shoulder joint by depressing humeral head in glenoid fossa
External rotation of shoulder

Innervation:
C5–C6 Suprascapular nerve

137 TERES MINOR

Origin:
Scapula (proximal 2/3 of flat surface on dorsal aspect of axillary border)
Aponeurotic laminae (two such), one of which separates it from the Teres major, the other from the Infraspinatus

Insertion:
Humerus (greater tubercle, most inferior facet, upper fibers)

Humerus (shaft: below the lowest facet, lower fibers)
Capsule of glenohumeral joint (posterior)

Description:
A somewhat cylindrical and elongated muscle, the Teres minor ascends laterally and upward from its origin to form a tendon that inserts on the greater tubercle of the humerus. It lies inferior to the Infraspinatus, and its fibers lie in parallel with that muscle. It is one of the rotator cuff muscles.

Function:
Maintains humeral head in glenoid fossa, thus stabilizing the shoulder joint
External rotation of shoulder
Adduction of shoulder (weak)

Innervation:
C5–C6 Axillary nerve

138 TERES MAJOR

Origin:
Scapula (dorsal surface near the inferior scapular angle on its lateral margin)
Fibrous septa between this muscle and the Teres minor and Infraspinatus

Insertion:
Humerus (intertubercular sulcus, medial lip)

Description:
The Teres major is a flattened but thick muscle that ascends laterally and upward to the humerus. Its tendon lies behind that of the Latissimus dorsi, and they generally unite for a short distance.

Function:
Internal rotation of shoulder
Adduction and extension of shoulder
Extension of shoulder from a flexed position

Innervation:
C5–C6 Subscapular nerve (lower)

139 CORACOBRACHIALIS

Origin:
Scapula, coracoid process (apex)
Intermuscular septum

Insertion:
Humerus (midway along medial border of shaft)

Description:
The smallest of the muscles of the arm, it lies along the upper medial portion of the arm, appearing as a small rounded ridge. The muscle

fibers lie along the axis of the humerus. The origin on the coracoid process is in common with the tendon of the Biceps brachii (short head).

Function:
Flexion of arm
Adduction of shoulder

Innervation:
C5–C7 Musculocutaneous nerve

Muscles Acting on the Elbow

140 Biceps brachii

141 Brachialis

142 Triceps brachii

143 Brachioradialis

144 Anconeus

140 BICEPS BRACHII

Origin:
Short head:
Scapula (apex of coracoid process)
Long head:
Capsule of glenohumeral joint and glenoid labrum
Scapula (supraglenoid tubercle at apex of glenoid cavity)

Insertion:
Radius (radial tuberosity on posterior rough surface)
Broad bicipital aponeurosis fusing with deep fascia over forearm flexors

Description:
Long muscle on the anterior surface of the arm consisting of two heads. The tendon of origin of the short head is thick and flat; the tendon of the long head is long and narrow, curving up, over and down the humeral head before giving way to the muscle belly. The muscle fibers of both heads lie fairly parallel to the axis of the humerus. The heads can be readily separated except for the distal portion near the elbow joint, where they join before ending in a flat tendon.
The distal tendon spirals so that its anterior surface becomes lateral at the point of insertion.
Both the short head and the Coracobrachialis arise from the coracoid apex. The muscle flexes the elbow most forcefully when the forearm is in supination. It is attached, via the bicipital aponeurosis, to the posterior border of the ulna, the distal end of which is drawn medially in supination.

Function:
Both heads:
Flexion of elbow
Supination of forearm (powerful)
Long head: Stabilizes and depresses humeral head in glenoid fossa during Deltoid activity.

Innervation:
C5–C6 Musculocutaneous nerve

141 BRACHIALIS

Origin:
Humerus (shaft: distal 1/2 of anterior surface)
Intermuscular septa (medial 1/2)

Insertion:
Ulna (ulnar tuberosity and rough surface of coronoid process, anterior aspect)
Anterior ligament of elbow joint
Bicipital aponeurosis (occasionally)

Description:
Positioned over the distal half of the front of the humerus and the anterior aspect of the elbow joint. It may be divided into several parts or may be fused with nearby muscles.
The C7 innervation by the radial nerve is to the lateral part of the muscle and is not large.

Function:
Flexion of elbow, forearm supinated or pronated.

Innervation:
C5–C6 Musculocutaneous nerve
C7 Radial nerve[23]

142 TRICEPS BRACHII

Has three heads

Origin:
Long head:
Scapula (infraglenoid tuberosity)
Blends above with capsule of glenohumeral joint
Lateral head:
Humerus (shaft: oblique ridge on posterior surface)
Lateral intermuscular septum
Medial head:
Humerus (shaft: entire posterior surface distal to radial groove down almost to trochlea)
Medial and lateral intermuscular septa
Humerus (medial border)

Insertion:
Three heads join in a common tendon
Ulna (olecranon process, proximal posterior surface)
Antebrachial fascia
Capsule of elbow joint

Description:

Located along the entire dorsal aspect of the arm in the extensor compartment. It is a large muscle arising in three heads: long, lateral, and medial. All heads join in a common tendon of insertion, which begins at the midpoint of the muscle. A fourth head is not uncommon.

Function:

Extension of elbow

Long and lateral heads: Especially active in resisted extension, otherwise minimally active[24]

Long head: Extension and adduction of shoulder (assist)

Medial head: Active in all forms of extension

Innervation:

C6–C8 Radial nerve (ventral rami)

143 BRACHIORADIALIS

Origin:

Humerus (lateral supracondylar ridge, proximal 2/3)

Lateral intermuscular septum (anterior)

Insertion:

Radius (lateral side of shaft just proximal to styloid process)

Description:

The most superficial muscle on the radial side of the forearm, it forms the lateral side of the cubital fossa. It has a rather thin belly, which descends to the midforearm, where its long flat tendon begins and continues to the distal radius. The Brachioradialis often is fused proximally with the Brachialis. Its tendon may be divided and the muscle may be absent (rarely).

This is a flexor muscle despite its innervation by an "extensor" nerve.

Function:

Flexion of elbow

Note: This muscle evolved with the extensor muscles and is innervated by the radial nerve, but its action is that of a forearm flexor. Muscle is less active when the forearm is fully supinated because it crosses the joint laterally rather than anteriorly. It works most efficiently when the forearm is in some pronation.

Innervation:

C5–C6 Radial nerve (C7 innervation sometimes cited)

144 ANCONEUS

Origin:

Humerus (lateral epicondyle, posterior surface)

Capsule of elbow joint

Insertion:

Ulna (olecranon, lateral aspect, and posterior surface of upper 1/4 of shaft)

Description:

A small triangular muscle on the dorsum of the elbow whose fibers descend medially a short distance to their ulnar insertion. Considered a continuation of the Triceps and often blended with it.

Function:

Elbow extension (assist)

Innervation:

C6–C8 Radial nerve

Muscles Acting on the Forearm

145 Supinator

140 Biceps brachii (see under *Muscles Acting on the Elbow*)

146 Pronator teres

147 Pronator quadratus

145 SUPINATOR

Origin:

Humerus (lateral epicondyle)

Radial collateral ligament of elbow joint

Annular ligament of radioulnar joint

Ulna (dorsal surface of shaft, supinator crest)

Aponeurosis of supinator

Insertion:

Radius (tuberosity and oblique line; shaft: lateral surface of proximal 1/3)

Description:

Broad muscle whose fibers form two planes that curve around the upper radius. The two planes arise together from the epicondyle: the superficial plane from the tendon and the deep plane from the muscle fibers. This muscle is subject to considerable variation.

Function:

Supination of forearm

Innervation:

C6–C7 Radial nerve (posterior interosseous branch)

146 PRONATOR TERES

Has two heads

Origin:

Humeral head (superficial and larger head): Shaft proximal to medial epicondyle

Common tendon of origin of forearm flexor muscles
    Intermuscular septum
    Antebrachial fascia
Ulnar head (deep head):
    Coronoid process, medial side
    Joins tendon of humeral head

Insertion:
    Radius (shaft: lateral surface of middle)

Description:
    The humeral head is much larger; the thin ulnar head joins its companion at an acute angle, and together they pass obliquely across the forearm to end in a flat tendon of insertion near the radius. The lateral border of the ulnar head is the medial limit of the cubital fossa, which lies just anterior to the elbow joint. The Pronator teres is less active than the Pronator quadratus.[25]

Function:
    Pronation of forearm
    Elbow flexion (accessory)

Innervation:
    C6–C7 Median nerve

147 PRONATOR QUADRATUS

Origin:
    Ulna (shaft: oblique ridge, anterior and medial surfaces of distal 1/4)
    Aponeurosis over middle 1/3 of the muscle

Insertion:
    Radius (shaft: anterior surface of distal 1/4; deeper fibers to a narrow triangular area above ulnar notch)

Description:
    This small, flat quadrilateral muscle passes across the anterior aspect of the distal ulna to the distal radius. Its fibers are quite horizontal. The Pronator quadratus is the main pronator of the forearm, being joined by the Pronator teres only in rapid or strong motions.[25]

Function:
    Pronation of forearm

Innervation:
    C7–C8 Median nerve (anterior interosseous branch)

Muscles Acting at the Wrist

148 Extensor carpi radialis longus

149 Extensor carpi radialis brevis

150 Extensor carpi ulnaris

151 Flexor carpi radialis

152 Palmaris longus

153 Flexor carpi ulnaris

148 EXTENSOR CARPI RADIALIS LONGUS

Origin:
    Humerus (distal 1/3 of lateral supracondylar ridge)
    Lateral intermuscular septum
    Common extensor tendon

Insertion:
    2nd metacarpal (dorsal surface of base on radial side). Occasionally slips to 1st and 3rd metacarpals.

Description:
    Descends lateral to Brachioradialis. Muscle fibers end at midforearm in a flat tendon, which descends along the lateral radius.

Function:
    Extension and radial deviation of wrist
    Synergist for finger flexion by stabilization of wrist
    Elbow flexion (accessory)

Innervation:
    C6–C7 Radial nerve (lateral muscular branch)

149 EXTENSOR CARPI RADIALIS BREVIS

Origin:
    Humerus (lateral epicondyle via common extensor tendon)
    Radial collateral ligament of elbow joint
    Aponeurotic sheath and intermuscular septa

Insertion:
    3rd metacarpal (dorsal surface of base on radial side distal to styloid process)
    Slips sent to 2nd metacarpal base

Description:
    This short, thick muscle lies partially under the Extensor carpi radialis longus in the upper forearm. Its muscle fibers end well above the wrist in a flattened tendon, which descends alongside the Extensor carpi radialis longus tendon to the wrist.

Function:
    Extension of wrist
    Radial deviation of wrist (weak)
    Finger flexion synergist (by stabilizing the wrist)

Innervation:
    C7–C8 Radial nerve (posterior interosseous branch)

150 EXTENSOR CARPI ULNARIS

Origin:
    Humerus (lateral epicondyle via common extensor tendon)
    Ulna (posterior border by an aponeurosis common to Flexor carpi ulnaris and Flexor digitorum profundus)
    Overlying fascia

Insertion:
    5th metacarpal (tubercle on ulnar side of base)

Description:
    Muscle fibers descend on the dorsal ulnar side of the forearm and join a tendon located in the distal 1/3 of the forearm that is the most medial tendon on the dorsum of the hand. This tendon can be palpated lateral to the groove found just over the ulna's posterior border.

Function:
    Extension of wrist
    Ulnar deviation (adduction) of wrist

Innervation:
    C7–C8 Radial nerve (posterior interosscous branch)

151 FLEXOR CARPI RADIALIS

Origin:
    Humerus (medial epicondyle by common flexor tendon)
    Intermuscular septa
    Antebrachial fascia

Insertion:
    2nd and 3rd metacarpals (base, palmar surface)

Description:
    A slender aponeurotic muscle at its origin, it descends in the forearm between the Pronator teres and the Palmaris longus. It increases in size as it descends to end in a tendon about halfway down the forearm.

Function:
    Flexion of wrist
    Radial deviation (abduction) of wrist
    Extends fingers (tenodesis action)
    Flexion of elbow (weak assist)
    Pronation of forearm (weak assist)

Innervation:
    C6–C7 Median nerve

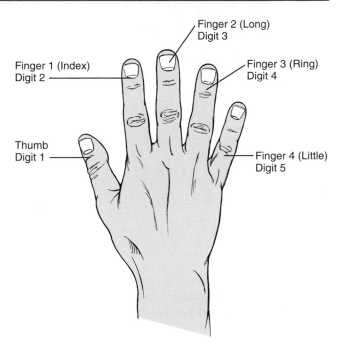

FIGURE 9-5
Fingers and digits of the hand

152 PALMARIS LONGUS

Origin:
    Humerus (medial epicondyle via common flexor tendon)
    Intermuscular septa and deep fascia

Insertion:
    Flexor retinaculum
    Palmar aponeurosis
    Slip sent frequently to the short thumb muscles

Description:
    A slim fusiform muscle, it ends in a long tendon midway in the forearm. Muscle is quite variable and frequently is absent.

Function:
    Tension of palmar fascia (anchor for palmar fascia and skin)
    Flexion of wrist (weak or questionable)
    Flexion of elbow (weak or questionable)
    Abduction of thumb

Innervation:
    C7–C8 Median nerve

153 FLEXOR CARPI ULNARIS

Has two heads

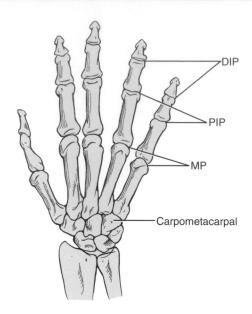

FIGURE 9–6
The bones and joints of the hand

Muscles Acting on the Fingers
(see Figs. 9–5 and 9–6)

154 Extensor digitorum

155 Extensor indicis

156 Flexor digitorum superficialis

157 Flexor digitorum profundus

154 EXTENSOR DIGITORUM

Origin:
Humerus (lateral epicondyle via common extensor tendon)
Intermuscular septa
Antebrachial fascia

Insertion:
Digits 2 to 5: Divides distally into four tendons that insert into the digital expansion over the proximal and middle phalanges.
Intermediate slips: To middle phalanges
Lateral slips: Distal phalanges (dorsum of base of digits 2 to 5)

Description:
The Extensor digitorum is the only extensor of the metacarpophalangeal (MP) joints. The muscle divides above the wrist into four distinct tendons, which traverse (with the Extensor indicis) a tunnel under the extensor retinaculum in a common sheath. Over the dorsum of the hand the four tendons diverge, one to each finger. The tendon to the index finger is accompanied by the Extensor indicis tendon.
The digital attachments are achieved by a fibrous expansion dorsal to the proximal phalanges. All of the digital extensors, as well as the lumbricales and interossei, are integral to this mechanism.

Function:
Extension of MP and proximal (PIP) and distal interphalangeal (DIP) joints, digits 2 to 5.
Extensor digitorum can extend any and all joints over which it passes via the dorsal expansion
Independent action of the Extensor digitorum:
Hyperextends MP joint (proximal phalanges) by displacing dorsal expansion proximally
Extends IP joints (middle and distal phalanges) when MP joints are slightly flexed by intrinsics
Wrist extension (accessory)
Abduction of ring, index, and little fingers with extension but no such action on the middle finger

Innervation:
C7–C8 Radial nerve, posterior interosseous branch

Origin:
Humeral head:
Humerus (medial epicondyle via common flexor tendon)
Ulnar head:
Ulna (olecranon, medial border and shaft: upper 2/3 of posterior border via an aponeurosis)
Intermuscular septum

Insertion:
Pisiform bone
Hamate bone
5th metacarpal (occasionally 4th)
Flexor retinaculum

Description:
This is the most ulnar-lying of the flexors in the forearm. The humeral head is small in contrast to the extensive origin of the ulnar head. The two heads are connected by a tendinous arch under which the ulnar nerve descends. The muscle fibers end in a tendon that forms along the anterolateral border of the muscle's distal half.

Function:
Flexion of wrist
Ulnar deviation (adduction) of wrist
Flexion of elbow (assist)

Innervation:
C7–T1 Ulnar nerve

155 EXTENSOR INDICIS

Origin:
> Ulna (posterior surface of shaft below origin of Extensor pollicis longus)
> Interosseous membrane

Insertion:
> Index finger (2nd digit) (extensor hood)

Description:
> Arises just below the Extensor pollicis longus and travels adjacent with it down to the level of the wrist. After passing under the extensor retinaculum near the head of the 2nd metacarpal, it joins with the index tendon of the Extensor digitorum on its ulnar side and then inserts into the extensor hood of the 2nd digit.

Function:
> Extension of MP joint of index finger
> Extension of IP joints (with intrinsics)
> Adduction of index finger (accessory)
> Wrist extension (accessory)

Innervation:
> C7–C8 Radial nerve, posterior interosseous branch

156 FLEXOR DIGITORUM SUPERFICIALIS

Has two heads

Origin:
> *Humeral-ulnar head:*
>> Humerus (medial epicondyle via the common flexor tendon)
>> Ulnar collateral ligament of elbow joint
>> Ulna (coronoid process, medial side)
>> Intermuscular septa
> *Radial head:*
>> Radius (oblique line on anterior surface of shaft)

Insertion:
From four tendons arranged in two pairs:
> *Superficial pair:* Long and ring fingers (sides of middle phalanges)
> *Deep pair:* Index and little fingers (sides of middle phalanges)

Description:
> Lies deep to the other forearm flexors but is the largest superficial flexor. The muscle separates into two planes of fibers, superficial and deep. The superficial plane (joined by radial head) divides into two tendons for digits 3 and 5. The deep plane fibers divide and join the tendons to digits 2 and 5. This can be remembered by touching the tips of the little and index fingers (deep) together underneath the ring and middle fingers (superficial).
> The four tendons sweep under the flexor retinaculum arranged in pairs (for the long and ring fingers, and for the index and little fingers). The tendons diverge again in the palm, and at the base of the proximal phalanges each divides into two slips to permit passage of the Flexor digitorum profundus to each finger. The slips reunite and then divide again for a final time to insert on both sides of each middle phalanx.
> The radial head may be absent.

Function:
> Flexion of PIP joints of digits 2 to 5
> Flexion of MP joints of digits 2 to 5 (assist)
> Flexion of wrist (accessory, especially in forceful grasp)

Innervation:
> C8–T1 Median nerve

157 FLEXOR DIGITORUM PROFUNDUS

Origin:
> Ulna (shaft: upper 3/4 of anterior and medial surfaces; also coronoid process, medial side via an aponeurosis)
> Interosseous membrane (ulnar half)

Insertion:
Ends in four tendons:
> Digits 2 to 5 (distal phalanges, palmar surface and base). Index finger tendon is distinct in its course.

Description:
> Lying deep to the superficial flexors, the profundus is located on the ulnar side of the forearm. The muscle fibers end in four tendons below the midforearm; the tendons pass into the hand under the transverse carpal ligament. The tendon for the index finger remains distinct, but the tendons for the other fingers are intertwined and connected to tendinous slips down into the palm.
> After passing through the tendons of the Flexor digitorum superficialis they move to their insertions on each distal phalanx. The four lumbrical muscles arise from the profundus tendons in the palm.
> The profundus, like the superficialis, can flex any or all joints over which it passes, but it is the only muscle that can flex the DIP joints.

Function:
Flexion of DIP joints of digits 2 to 5
Flexion of MP and PIP joints of digits 2 to 5 (assist)
Flexion of wrist (accessory)

Innervation:
C8–T1 Median nerve (anterior interosseous nerve) for digits 2 and 3
C8–T1 Ulnar nerve for digits 4 and 5

Muscles Acting on the Little Finger (and Hypothenar Muscles)

158 Extensor digiti minimi

159 Abductor digiti minimi

160 Flexor digiti minimi brevis

161 Opponens digiti minimi

162 Palmaris brevis

158 EXTENSOR DIGITI MINIMI

Origin:
Common extensor tendon
Intermuscular septa
Antebrachial fascia

Insertion:
Digit 5 via extensor hood on the radial side, as a separate long tendon to the little finger. From its origin in the forearm the long tendon passes under the extensor retinaculum at the wrist. The tendon divides into two slips: one joining the Extensor digitorum to the 5th digit. All three tendons then join the extensor hood, which covers the dorsum of the proximal phalanx.

Description:
A slim extensor muscle that lies medial to the Extensor digitorum and usually is associated with that muscle. It descends in the forearm (between the Extensor digitorum and the Extensor carpi ulnaris), passes under the extensor retinaculum at the wrist in its own compartment, and then divides into two tendons. The lateral tendon joins directly with the tendon of the Extensor digitorum; all three join the extensor expansion, and all insert on the middle phalanx of digit 5. The Extensor digiti minimi can extend any of the joints of digit 5 via the dorsal digital expansion.

Function:
Extension of MP, IP, and DIP joints of digit 5 (little finger)
Wrist extension (accessory)
Abduction of digit 5 (accessory)

Innervation:
C7–C8 Radial nerve (posterior interosseous branch)

159 ABDUCTOR DIGITI MINIMI

Origin:
Pisiform bone (often passes a slip to 5th metacarpal)
Tendon of Flexor carpi ulnaris
Pisohamate ligament

Insertion:
5th digit (proximal phalanx, base on ulnar side)
Into dorsal digital expansion of Extensor digiti minimi

Description:
Located on the ulnar border of the palm

Function:
Abduction of 5th digit away from ring finger
Flexion of proximal phalanx of 5th digit at the MP joint
Opposition of 5th digit (assist)

Innervation:
C8–T1 Ulnar nerve (deep branch)

160 FLEXOR DIGITI MINIMI BREVIS

Origin:
Hamate bone (hamulus or "hook")
Flexor retinaculum (palmar surface along with Abductor digiti minimi)

Insertion:
5th digit (proximal phalanx, base on ulnar side along with Abductor digiti minimi)

Description:
This short flexor of the little finger lies in the same plane as the Abductor digiti minimi on its radial side. The muscle may be absent or fused with the Abductor.

Function:
Flexion of little finger at the MP joint
Opposition of 5th digit (assist)

Innervation:
C8–T1 Ulnar nerve (deep branch)

161 OPPONENS DIGITI MINIMI

Origin:
Hamate (hamulus, often called "hook")
Flexor retinaculum

Insertion:
5th metacarpal (entire length of ulnar margin)

Description:

A triangular muscle lying deep to the abductor and the flexor. It commonly is blended with its neighbors.

Function:

Opposition of little finger to thumb (abduction, flexion, and lateral rotation, deepening the palmar hollow)

Innervation:

C8–T1 Ulnar nerve (deep branch)

162 PALMARIS BREVIS

Origin:

Flexor retinaculum and palmar aponeurosis

Insertion:

Skin on ulnar border of palm (hypothenar eminence)

Description:

A thin superficial muscle whose fibers run directly laterally across the hypothenar eminence

Function:

Draws the skin of the ulnar side of the hand toward the palm. This deepens the hollow of the hand and seems to increase the height of the hypothenar eminence, possibly assisting in grasp.

Innervation:

C8–T1 Ulnar nerve (superficial branch)

Intrinsic Muscles of the Hand

163 Lumbricales

164 Interossei, dorsal

165 Interossei, palmar

163 LUMBRICALES (Fig. 9-7)

Origin:

Flexor digitorum profundus tendons:

1st Lumbrical: Index finger (digit 2) Arises by single head from the radial side, palmar surface

2nd Lumbrical: Long (middle) finger (digit 3), radial side, palmar surface

3rd Lumbrical: Long and ring fingers (digits 3 and 4) by double heads from adjacent sides of tendons of Flexor digitorum profundus

4th Lumbrical: Ring and little fingers (digits 4 and 5), adjacent sides of tendon

Insertion:

Extensor digitorum expansion.

Each muscle extends distally to the radial side of

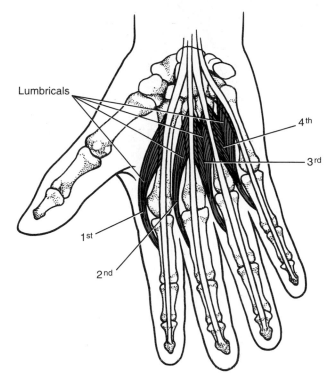

FIGURE 9-7
The lumbricales, palmar view

its corresponding digit and attaches to the dorsal digital expansion:

1st Lumbrical: To index finger (digit 2)

2nd Lumbrical: To long (middle) finger (digit 3)

3rd Lumbrical: To ring finger (digit 4)

4th Lumbrical: To little finger (digit 5)

Description:

These four small muscles arise from the tendon of the Flexor digitorum profundus over the metacarpals. They may be unipennate or bipennate. They extend to the middle phalanges of digits 2 to 5 (fingers 1 to 4), where they join the dorsal extensor hood on the radial side of each digit (see Fig. 9–7). Essentially, they link the flexor to the extension tendon systems in the hand. The exact attachments are quite variable. This gives rise to complexity of movement and differences in description.[26]

Function:

Flexion of MP joints (proximal phalanges) of digits 2 to 5 and simultaneous extension of the PIP and DIP joints

Opposition of digit 5 (4th Lumbrical)

Innervation:

1st and 2nd Lumbricales: C8–T1 Median nerve

3rd and 4th Lumbricales: C8–T1 Ulnar nerve

Note: The 3rd Lumbrical may receive innervation from both the ulnar and median nerves or all from the median.

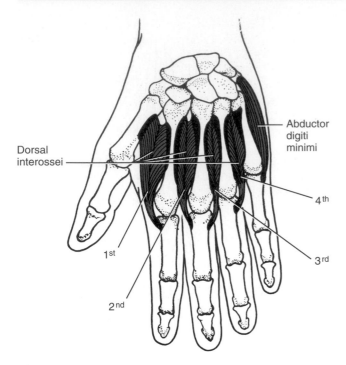

FIGURE 9-8
The dorsal interossei

164 DORSAL INTEROSSEI (Fig. 9-8)

These are four bipennate muscles

Origin:
Each muscle arises by two heads from adjacent sides of the metacarpals between which each lies.

> *1st Dorsal:* (also called Abductor indicis): Between thumb and index fingers
> *2nd Dorsal:* Between index and long fingers
> *3rd Dorsal:* Between long and ring fingers
> *4th Dorsal:* Between ring and little fingers

Insertion:
All: Dorsal extensor expansion.

> Proximal phalanges (bases)
> *1st Dorsal:* Index finger (radial side)
> *2nd Dorsal:* Long finger (radial side)
> *3rd Dorsal:* Long finger (ulnar side)
> *4th Dorsal:* Ring finger (ulnar side)

Description:
> This group comprises four bipennate muscles (see Fig. 9-8). In general, they originate via two heads from the adjacent metacarpal but more so from the metacarpal of the digit where they will insert distally. They insert into the bases of the proximal phalanges and dorsal expansions.

Function:
> Abduction of fingers away from an axis drawn through the center of the long (middle) finger

Flexion of fingers at MP joints (assist)
Extension of fingers at IP joints (assist)
Thumb adduction (assist)

Innervation:
C8-T1 ulnar nerve (deep branch)

165 PALMAR (VOLAR) INTEROSSEI (Fig. 9-9)

There are three palmar Interossei muscles (a 4th muscle is described)

Origin:
Metacarpal bones 2, 4, and 5. These muscles lie on the palmar surface of the metacarpals rather than between them. There is no palmar interosseous on the long finger.

> *1st Palmar:* 2nd metacarpal (ulnar side)
> *2nd Palmar:* 4th metacarpal (radial side)
> *3rd Palmar:* 5th metacarpal (radial side)

Insertion:
All: Dorsal expansion

> Proximal phalanges
> *1st Palmar:* Index finger (ulnar side)
> *2nd Palmar:* Ring finger (radial side)
> *3rd Palmar:* Little finger (radial side)

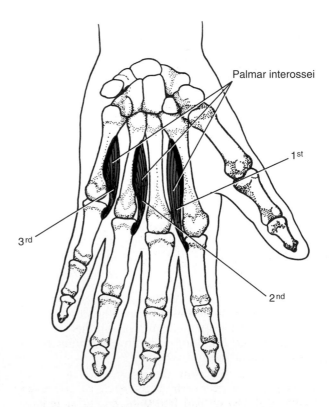

FIGURE 9-9
The palmar (volar) interossei

Description:

The palmar Interossei are smaller than their dorsal counterparts. They are found on the palmar surface of the hand at the metacarpal bones. There are three very distinct volar Interossei (see Fig. 9–9), and some authors describe a 4th Interosseus, to which they give the number 1 for its attachment on the thumb. When this is found as a discrete muscle, the other palmar Interossei become numbers 2, 3, and 4, respectively. When the thumb Interosseus exists it is on the ulnar side of the metacarpal and proximal phalanx. Some authors (including us) consider the Interosseus of the thumb part of the Adductor pollicis.

The middle finger has no Interosseous muscle.

Function:

Adduction of fingers (index, ring, and little) toward an axis drawn through the center of the long finger

Flexion of MP joints (assist)

Extension of IP joints (assist)

Opposition of digit 5 (3rd Interroseus)

Innervation:

C8–T1 Ulnar nerve (deep branch)

Muscles Acting on the Thumb

166 Abductor pollicis longus

167 Extensor pollicis longus

168 Extensor pollicis brevis

169 Flexor pollicis longus

171 Abductor pollicis brevis

172 Opponens pollicis

170 Flexor pollicis brevis

173 Adductor pollicis

166 ABDUCTOR POLLICIS LONGUS

Origin:

Ulna (posterior surface of shaft)

Radius (middle 1/3 of posterior surface of shaft)

Interosseous membrane

Insertion:

1st metacarpal bone (radial side of base)

Trapezium bone

Description:

Lies immediately below the Supinator and sometimes is fused with that muscle. Traverses obliquely down and lateral to end in a tendon at the wrist. The tendon passes through a groove on the lateral side of the distal radius along with the tendon of the Extensor pollicis brevis. Its tendon is commonly split; one slip attaches to the radial side of the 1st metacarpal and the other to the trapezium.[27]

Function:

Abduction and extension of thumb at carpometacarpal (CMC) joint

Extension of thumb at CMC joint (in concert with thumb extensors)

Radial deviation of wrist (assist)

Wrist flexion (weak)

Innervation:

C7–C8 Radial nerve (posterior interosseous branch)

167 EXTENSOR POLLICIS LONGUS

Origin:

Ulna (posterolateral surface of middle shaft)

Interosseous membrane

Insertion:

Thumb (base of distal phalanx, dorsal side)

Description:

The muscle rises distal to the Abductor pollicis longus and courses down and lateral into a tendon over the distal radius, which lies in a narrow oblique groove on the dorsal radius. It descends obliquely over the tendons of the carpal extensors. It separates from the Extensor pollicis brevis and can be seen during thumb extension as the ulnar margin of a triangular depression called the *anatomical snuff box*. This is a larger muscle than the Extensor pollicis brevis.

Function:

Extension of the thumb at all joints:

Distal phalanx (alone)

MP and CMC joints (along with Extensor pollicis brevis and Abductor pollicis longus)

Radial deviation of wrist (accessory)

Innervation:

C7–C8 Radial nerve (posterior interosseous branch)

168 EXTENSOR POLLICIS BREVIS

Origin:

Radius (posterior surface of shaft)

Interosseous membrane

Insertion:

Thumb (proximal phalanx base on dorsal surface)

Attachment to distal phalanx via tendon of Extensor pollicis longus is common.[27]

Description:

Arises distal and lies medial to the Abductor pollicis longus and descends with it so that the tendons of the two muscles pass through the same groove on the lateral side of the distal radius. During its descent it wraps itself around a bony fulcrum (Lister's tubercle), which alters the line of pull from forearm to thumb.

The muscle often is connected with the abductor or may be absent. Its tendon forms the radial margin of the "snuff box."

Function:

Extension of MP joint of thumb

Extension and abduction of 1st CMC joint of thumb

Radial deviation of wrist (accessory)

Innervation:

C7–C8 Radial nerve (posterior interosseous branch)

169 FLEXOR POLLICIS LONGUS

Origin:

Radius (grooved anterior surface of middle of shaft)

Interosseous membrane

Ulna (coronoid process), variable

Humerus (medial epicondyle), variable[28]

Insertion:

Thumb (base of distal phalanx, palmar surface)

Description:

Descends on the radial side of the forearm in the same plane as, but lateral to, the Flexor digitorum profundus

Function:

Flexion of IP joint of thumb

Flexion of the MP and CMC joints of thumb (accessory)

Flexion of wrist (accessory)

Innervation:

C7–C8 Median nerve (anterior interosseous branch)

170 FLEXOR POLLICIS BREVIS

Has two heads

Origin:

Superficial head:

Flexor retinaculum (distal border)

Trapezium bone (tubercle)

Deep head:

Trapezoid bone

Capitate bone

Palmar ligaments of distal row of carpal bones

Insertion:

Pollex (both heads: proximal phalanx, base on radial side)

Description:

The superficial head runs more laterally and accompanies the Flexor pollicis longus. Its tendon of insertion contains the radial sesamoid bone at a point where it unites with the tendon of the deep head. The deep head is sometimes absent. Of the thenar muscles, only the Abductor pollicis brevis consistently joins the dorsal extensor expansion of the thumb.

Function:

Flexion of the MP and CMC joints of the thumb

Opposition of thumb (assist)

Innervation:

Superficial head: C8–T1 Median nerve (lateral branch)

Deep head: C8–T1 Ulnar nerve (deep branch)

171 ABDUCTOR POLLICIS BREVIS

Origin:

Flexor retinaculum

Scaphoid bone (tubercle)

Trapezium bone (tubercle)

Tendon of Abductor pollicis longus

Insertion:

Thumb (proximal phalanx, radial side of base)

Dorsal extensor expansion of thumb

Description:

The most superficial muscle on the radial side of the thenar eminence

Function:

Abduction at CMC and MP joints (in a plane 90° from the palm)

Opposition of thumb (assist)

Extension of IP joint (assist)

Innervation:

C8–T1 Median nerve

172 OPPONENS POLLICIS

Origin:

Trapezium bone (tubercle)

Flexor retinaculum

Insertion:

1st metacarpal bone (along entire length of radial [lateral] side of shaft)

Description:

A small triangular muscle lying deep to the abductor

Function:
    Flexion of CMC joint medially across the palm
    Abduction of CMC joint
    Medial rotation of CMC joint

These motions occur simultaneously in the motion called opposition, which brings the thumb into contact with any of the other fingers on their palmar digital aspect (pads)

Innervation:
    C8–T1 Median nerve
    C8–T1 Ulnar nerve[29–31] (terminal branch)

173 ADDUCTOR POLLICIS

Rises from two heads

Origin:
    Oblique head:
        Capitate bone
        2nd and 3rd metacarpal bones (bases)
        Palmar carpal ligaments
        Tendon sheath of Flexor carpi radialis
        Flexor retinaculum (small slip)
        Unites with tendon of transverse head
    Transverse head:
        3rd metacarpal bone (distal 2/3 of palmar surface)
        Converges with oblique head and with 1st palmar Interosseous

Insertion (both heads):
    Thumb (base, proximal phalanx on ulnar side)
    Extensor retinaculum (on its medial side) of the thumb

Description:
    The muscle lies deep on the palmar side of the hand and has two heads, which vary in their comparative sizes. Both heads arise from the 3rd metacarpal and insert into both sides of the proximal phalanx,[7] or, as more frequently cited, the medial side of the proximal phalanx. The two heads are divided by the radial artery and the extent of their convergence also is variable.

Function:
    Adduction of CMC joint of thumb (approximates the thumb to the palm)
    Adduction and flexion of MP joint (assist)

Innervation:
    C8–T1 Ulnar nerve (deep branch)

MUSCLES OF THE LOWER EXTREMITY
(Knee, Ankle, Toes, Hallux)

Muscles of the Hip

174 Psoas major

175 Psoas minor

176 Iliacus

177 Pectineus

178 Gracilis

179 Adductor longus

180 Adductor brevis

181 Adductor magnus

182 Gluteus maximus

183 Gluteus medius

184 Gluteus minimus

185 Tensor fasciae latae

186 Piriformis

187 Obturator internus

188 Obturator externus

189 Gemellus superior

190 Gemellus inferior

191 Quadratus femoris

192 Biceps femoris (long head)

193 Semitendinosus

194 Semimembranosus

195 Sartorius

174 PSOAS MAJOR

Origin:
    L1–L5 vertebrae (transverse processes, inferior border)
    T12–L5 vertebral bodies and intervertebral discs between them (by five digitations)
    Tendinous arches across the lumbar vertebral bodies

Insertion:
    Femur (lesser trochanter)

Description:
    A long muscle lying next to the lumbar spine, its fibers descend downward and laterally. It decreases in size as it descends along the pelvic brim. It passes anterior to the hip joint and joins in a tendon with the Iliacus to insert on the lesser trochanter.
    The Iliopsoas muscle is a compound muscle consisting of the Iliacus and the Psoas major, which join in a common tendon of insertion on the lesser trochanter of the femur.
    The roots from the lumbar plexus enter the muscle directly and are contained within the muscle, its branches move out and away from its borders.

Function:
Hip flexion with origin fixed[32]
Trunk flexion (sit-up) with insertion fixed
(These two functions occur in conjunction with the Iliacus)
Hip external (lateral) rotation
Flexion of lumbar spine (muscles on both sides)
Lateral bending of lumbar spine to same side (muscle on one side)

Innervation:
L2–L4 (lumbar plexus) spinal nerves (ventral rami)
L1 also cited

175 PSOAS MINOR

Origin:
T12–L1 vertebral bodies (sides) and the intervertebral disc between them

Insertion:
Pecten pubis (i.e., pectineal line)
Ilium (iliopectineal eminence and linea terminalis of inner surface of the pelvis)
Iliac fascia

Description:
Lying anterior to the Psoas major, this is a long thin muscle whose belly lies entirely within the abdomen along its posterior wall, but its long flat tendon descends to the ilium. The muscle frequently is absent.
The pecten pubis, or pectineal line, is the distal end of the iliopectineal line, which in turn is a segment of the linea terminalis. These three segments together form the anterior part of the pelvic brim.

Function:
Flexion of trunk and lumbar spine (both; weak)

Innervation:
L1 spinal nerve

176 ILIACUS

Origin:
Ilium (superior 2/3 of iliac fossa)
Iliac crest (inner lip)
Anterior sacroiliac and iliolumbar ligaments
Sacrum (lateral)

Insertion:
Femur (lesser trochanter via insertion on tendon of the Psoas major and shaft below lesser trochanter)

Description:
A broad flat muscle, it fills the iliac fossa and descends along the fossa, converging laterally with

the tendon of the Psoas major. The Iliacus, acting alone in contraction on a fixed femur, results in flexion of the pelvis on the femur (an anterior tilt termed "symphysis down") of the pelvis. This leads to increased lumbar extension (lordosis).

Function:
Hip flexion
Flexes pelvis on femur

Innervation:
L2–L3 Femoral nerve

177 PECTINEUS

Origin:
Pecten pubis (between iliopectineal eminence and pubic tubercle)
Anterior fascia

Insertion:
Femur (shaft: on a line from lesser trochanter to linea aspera)

Description:
A flat muscle forming part of the wall of the femoral triangle in the upper medial aspect of the thigh. It descends posteriorly and laterally on the medial thigh.

Function:
Hip adduction
Hip flexion (accessory)

Innervation:
L2–L3 Femoral nerve
L3 Accessory obturator nerve (when present)

178 GRACILIS

Origin:
Pubis (inferior ramus near symphysis via aponeurosis)
Ischial ramus

Insertion:
Tibia (medial surface of shaft below tibial condyle)
Pes anserina
Deep fascia of leg

Description:
Lies most superficially on the medial thigh as a thin and broad muscle that tapers and narrows distally. The fibers are directed vertically and join a tendon that curves around the medial condyle of the femur and then around the medial condyle of the tibia. Its tendon is one of three (along with those of the Sartorius and

Semitendinosus) that unite to form the pes anserinus.

Function:
    Hip adduction
    Knee flexion
    Internal (medial) rotation of knee (accessory)

Innervation:
    L2–L3 Obturator nerve (anterior division) (ventral rami)

179 ADDUCTOR LONGUS

Origin:
    Pubis (anterior at the angle where the crest meets the symphysis)

Insertion:
    Femur (by an aponeurosis on the middle 1/3 of the linea aspera on its medial lip)

Description:
    The most anterior of the adductor muscles arises in a narrow tendon and widens into a broad muscle belly as it descends backward and laterally to insert on the femur.
    As part of their function, the hip adductors are not frequently called upon for strenuous activity, but they are capable of such. They play a major synergistic role in the complexity of gait and in some postural activities, but are relatively quiescent in quiet standing.

Function:
    Hip adduction
    Hip flexion (accessory)
    Hip rotation (depends on position of thigh)[29]
    Hip external (lateral) rotation (when hip is in extension; accessory)

Innervation:
    L2 or L3–L4 Obturator nerve (anterior division)

180 ADDUCTOR BREVIS

Origin:
    Pubis (inferior ramus and body, external aspect)

Insertion:
    Femur (along a line from the lesser trochanter to the proximal 1/3 of medial lip of the linea aspera via an aponeurosis)

Description:
    The muscle lies under the Pectineus and Adductor longus with its fibers coursing laterally and posteriorly as it broadens and descends

Function:
    Hip adduction
    Hip flexion

Innervation:
    L2–L3 or L4 Obturator nerve (posterior division)

181 ADDUCTOR MAGNUS

Origin:
    Pubis (inferior ramus)
    Ischium (inferior ramus; ischial tuberosity, inferior and lateral aspect)

Insertion:
    Femur (whole length of linea aspera and medial supracondylar line by an aponeurosis; adductor tubercle on medial condyle via a rounded tendon; the rounded tendon attaches to the medial supracondylar line by a fibrous expansion)

Description:
    The largest of the adductor group, this muscle is located on the medial thigh and appears as three distinct bundles. The superior fibers from the pubic ramus are short and horizontal. The medial fibers move down and laterally. The most distal bundle descends almost vertically to a tendon on the distal 1/3 of the thigh.
    Occasionally the fibers that arise from the ramus of the pubis are inserted into a line from the greater trochanter to the linea aspera and seem to form a distinct separate muscle. When this occurs the muscle is called the *Adductor minimus.*
    The innervation of the Adductor magnus comes from the anterior divisions of the lumbar plexus suggesting a primitive flexor action for the muscle.

Function:
    Hip adduction
    Hip extension (inferior fibers)
    Hip flexion (superior fibers; weak)
    The role of the Adductor magnus in rotation of the hip is dependent on the position of the thigh.[33]

Innervation:
    Superior and middle fibers: L2–L4 Obturator nerve (posterior division)
    Inferior fibers: L2–L4 Sciatic nerve (tibial division)

182 GLUTEUS MAXIMUS

Origin:
    Ilium (posterior gluteal line and crest)
    Sacrum (dorsal surface)
    Coccyx (lateral surface)
    Erector spinae aponeurosis
    Sacrotuberous ligament
    Aponeurosis of Gluteus medius

Insertion:
    Iliotibial tract of fascia lata
    Femur (gluteal tuberosity)

Description:

The maximus is the largest and most superficial of the gluteal muscles, forming the prominence of the buttocks. The fibers descend laterally, inserting widely on the thick tendinous iliotibial tract.

Function:

Hip extension (powerful)
Hip external (lateral) rotation
Hip abduction (upper fibers)
Hip adduction (lower fibers)
Through its insertion into the iliotibial band it stabilizes the knee

Innervation:

L5–S2 Inferior gluteal nerve

183 GLUTEUS MEDIUS

Origin:

Ilium (outer surface between the iliac crest and the posterior gluteal line)
Gluteal aponeurosis

Insertion:

Femur (greater trochanter, oblique ridge on lateral surface)

Description:

The posterior fibers of the medius lie deep to the maximus; its anterior 2/3 is covered by fascia (gluteal aponeurosis). It lies on the outer surface of the pelvis.

The Gluteus medius helps to maintain erect posture in walking. During single-limb stance when the swing limb is raised from the ground, all body weight is placed on the opposite (stance) limb, which should result in a noted sagging of the pelvis of the swing limb. The action of the Gluteus medius on the stance limb prevents such a tilt or sag. When the Gluteus medius is weak, the trunk tilts (lateral lean) to the weak side with each step in an attempt to maintain balance (this is the deliberate compensation for the positive Trendelenburg sign). It is called a *Gluteus medius sign* or gait.

The uncompensated positive Trendelenburg results in a pelvic drop of the contralateral side. This is the so-called Trendelenburg gait.

Function:

Hip abduction (in all positions)
Hip internal rotation (anterior fibers)
Hip external (lateral) rotation (posterior fibers)
Hip flexion (anterior fibers) and hip extension (posterior fibers) as accessory functions

Innervation:

L4–S1 Superior gluteal nerve (inferior branch)

184 GLUTEUS MINIMUS

Origin:

Ilium (outer surface between the anterior and inferior gluteal lines; also from margin of the greater sciatic notch).

Insertion:

Femur (greater trochanter, anterior border)
Expansion to capsule of hip joint

Description:

The minimus is the smallest of the gluteal muscles and lies immediately under the medius. Its fibers pass obliquely lateral and down, forming a fan-shaped muscle that converges on the great femoral trochanter.

Function:

Hip abduction
Hip internal (medial) rotation

Innervation:

L4–S1 Superior gluteal nerve (superior branch)

185 TENSOR FASCIAE LATAE

Origin:

Ilium (iliac crest; anterior part of outer lip; anterior superior iliac spine [ASIS])
Fascia lata (deep surface)

Insertion:

Iliotibial tract (both layers)

Description:

The Tensor descends between and is attached to the deep and superficial layers of the iliotibial band.

The smallish muscle belly is highly variable in length. The muscle lies superficially on the border between the anterior and lateral thigh. Functions at the knee that have been attributed to the Tensor could not be confirmed in EMG studies; indeed, there was no electrical activity in the Tensor during knee motions.[34–36]

Function:

Hip flexion
Hip internal (medial) rotation
Knee flexion (accessory via iliotibial band) once the knee is flexed beyond 30° (no confirmation)
Knee extension with external rotation (no confirmation)
Knee external (lateral) rotation (assist) (no confirmation)

Innervation:

L4–S1 Superior gluteal nerve (inferior branch)

186 PIRIFORMIS

Origin:

Sacrum (via three digitations attached between the 1st and 4th anterior sacral foramina)

Ilium (gluteal surface near posterior inferior iliac spine (PIIS)

Capsule of sacroiliac joint

Sacrotuberous ligament (pelvic surface)

Insertion:

Femur (greater trochanter, superior border of medial aspect)

Description:

Runs parallel to the posterior margin of the Gluteus medius posterior to the hip joint. It lies against the posterior wall on the interior of the pelvis. The broad muscle belly narrows to exit through the greater sciatic foramen and converge on the greater trochanter. The insertion tendon often is partly blended with the common tendon of the Obturator internus and Gemelli.

Function:

Hip external (lateral) rotation

Abducts the flexed hip (assist) (muscle probably too small to do much of this)

Innervation:

S1–S2 spinal nerves (nerve to Piriformis)

187 OBTURATOR INTERNUS

Origin:

Pelvis (obturator foramen, around most of its margin; from pelvic brim to greater sciatic foramen above and obturator foramen below)

Ischium (ramus)

Pubis (inferior ramus)

Obturator membrane (pelvic surface)

Obturator fascia

Insertion:

Femur (greater trochanter, medial surface proximal to the trochanteric fossa)

Tendon fuses with Gemelli

Description:

Muscle lies internal in the osteoligamentous pelvis and also external behind the hip joint. The fibers converge toward the lesser sciatic foramen and hook around the body of the ischium, which acts as a pulley; it exits the pelvis via the lesser sciatic foramen, crosses the capsule of the hip joint, and proceeds to the greater trochanter.

Function:

Hip external (lateral) rotation

Abduction of flexed hip (assist)

Innervation:

L5–S1 Nerve to Obturator internus off lumbosacral plexus

188 OBTURATOR EXTERNUS

Origin:

Pubic ramus

Ischial ramus

Obturator foramen (margin)

Obturator membrane (medial 2/3 of outer surface)

Insertion:

Femur (trochanteric fossa)

Description:

This flat, triangular muscle covers the external aspect of the anterior pelvic wall from a very broad origin on the medial margin of the obturator foramen. Its fibers pass posteriorly and laterally in a spiral to a tendon that passes behind the femoral neck to insert in the trochanteric fossa.

This muscle, along with the other small lateral rotators, may serve more postural functions (such as stability) than prime movement. They maintain the integrity of hip joint actions.

Function:

Hip external (lateral) rotation

Hip adduction (assist)

Innervation:

L3–L4 Obturator nerve (posterior branch)

189 GEMELLUS SUPERIOR

Origin:

Ischial spine (gluteal surface)

Insertion:

Femur (greater trochanter, medial surface)

Description:

Muscle lies in parallel with and superior to the tendon of Obturator internus, which it joins. This is the smaller of the two Gemelli and may be absent.

Function:

Hip external (lateral) rotation

Hip abduction with hip flexed (accessory)

Innervation:

L5–S1 Nerve to Obturator internus (off lumbar plexus)

190 GEMELLUS INFERIOR

Origin:

Ischium (tuberosity, superior surface)

Insertion:
Femur (greater trochanter, medial surface)

Description:
This small muscle parallels and joins the tendon of the Obturator internus on its inferior side. The two Gemelli may be considered adjunct to the Obturator internus.

Function:
Hip external (lateral) rotation
Hip abduction with hip flexed (weak assist)

Innervation:
L5–S1 Nerve to Quadratus femoris (off lumbar plexus)

191 QUADRATUS FEMORIS

Origin:
Ischium (tuberosity, upper external border)

Insertion:
Femur (quadrate tubercle on posterior aspect)

Description:
This flat quadrilateral muscle lies between the Gemellus inferior and the Adductor magnus. Its fibers pass almost horizontally, posterior to the hip joint and femoral neck.

Function:
Hip external (lateral) rotation

Innervation:
L5–S1 Nerve to Quadratus femoris (off lumbar plexus)

192 BICEPS FEMORIS

Origin:
Long head:
Ischium (tuberosity, inferior and medial aspects, in common with tendon of Semitendinosus)
Sacrotuberous ligament
Short head:
Femur (linea aspera, entire length of lateral lip; lateral supracondylar line)
Lateral intermuscular septum

Insertion:
Aponeurosis of long head distally. The short head inserts into the deep surface of this aponeurosis to form the "lateral hamstring tendon."
Fibula (head, lateral aspect via main portion of lateral hamstring tendon).
Tibia (lateral condyle via lamina from lateral hamstring tendon).[37]
Fascia on lateral leg.

Description:
This lateral hamstring muscle is a two-head muscle on the posterolateral thigh. Its long head is a two-joint muscle. The muscle fibers of the long head descend laterally, ending in an aponeurosis that covers the posterior surface of the muscle. Fibers from the short head also converge into the same aponeurosis, which narrows into the lateral hamstring tendon of insertion. At the insertion the tendon divides into two slips to embrace the fibular collateral ligament. The short head is sometimes absent.
The different nerve supply, tibial division for the long head and common peroneal division for the short head, reflects both flexor and extensor muscle derivations.
The Biceps femoris as a posterior femoral muscle flexes the knee and extends the hip (from a stooped posture) against gravity. When the hip is extended, this muscle is an external rotator of the hip. When the knee is flexed, the Biceps is an external rotator of the knee. When at any time the body's center of gravity moves forward of the transverse axis of the hip joint, the Biceps femoris contracts.

Function:
Knee flexion (only the short head is a pure knee flexor)
Knee external rotation
Hip extension and external rotation (long head)

Innervation:
Long head: L5–S2 Sciatic nerve (tibial division)
Short head: L5–S2 Sciatic nerve (common peroneal division)

193 SEMITENDINOSUS

Origin:
Ischium (tuberosity, inferior medial aspect)
Aponeurosis to share tendon with Biceps femoris (long head)
Pes anserina

Insertion:
Tibia (shaft on proximal medial side)
Deep fascia of leg

Description:
A muscle on the posteromedial thigh known for its long, round tendon, which extends from midthigh to the tibia. The Semitendinosus unites with the tendons of the Sartorius and the Gracilis to form a flattened aponeurosis called the *pes anserinus.*

Function:
Knee flexion
Knee internal rotation
Hip extension
Hip internal rotation (accessory)

Innervation:
L5–S2 Sciatic nerve (tibial division)

194 SEMIMEMBRANOSUS

Origin:
Ischium (tuberosity, superior and lateral facets)
Complex proximal tendon along with fibers from Biceps femoris and Semitendinosus

Insertion:
Tibia (tubercle on medial condyle)
Oblique popliteal ligament of knee joint
Aponeurosis over distal part of muscle to form tendon of insertion

Description:
The Semimembranosus is the larger of the two medial hamstrings. Its name derives from its flat, membranous tendon of origin that partially envelops the anterior surface of the upper portion of the Biceps femoris and Semitendinosus. Its fibers descend from midthigh to a distal aponeurosis, which narrows into a short, thick tendon before inserting on the tibia. The Semitendinosus is superficial to the Semimembranosus throughout its extent.

Function:
Knee flexion
Knee internal rotation
Hip extension
Hip internal rotation (accessory)

Innervation:
L5–S2 Sciatic nerve (tibial division)

195 SARTORIUS

Origin:
Ilium (ASIS; notch below ASIS)

Insertion:
Tibia (proximal medial surface of the shaft distal to the tibial condyle)
Aponeurosis
Capsule of knee joint

Description:
The longest muscle in the body, its parallel fibers form a narrow, thin muscle. It descends obliquely from lateral to medial to just above the knee, where it turns abruptly downward and passes posterior to the medial condyle of the femur. It expands into a broad aponeurosis before inserting on the medial surface of the tibia. The Sartorius is the most superficial of the anterior thigh muscles and occasionally is absent. It forms the lateral border of the femoral triangle.

Function:
Hip external rotation, abduction, and flexion
Knee flexion
Knee internal rotation
Assists in "tailor sitting"

Innervation:
L2–L3 Femoral nerve (two branches usually)

Muscles of the Knee

196-200 Quadriceps femoris

201 Articularis genus

192 Biceps femoris (see *Muscles Acting on the Hip*)

193 Semitendinosus (see *Muscles Acting on the Hip*)

194 Semimembranosus (see *Muscles Acting on the Hip*)

202 Popliteus

196-200 QUADRICEPS FEMORIS

This muscular mass on the anterior thigh has five component muscles (or heads), which together make this the most powerful muscle group in the human body. The five components are the great extensors of the knee.

196 Rectus femoris

197 Vastus lateralis

198 Vastus intermedius

199 Vastus medialis longus

200 Vastus medialis oblique

196 RECTUS FEMORIS

Origin:
Arises by two tendons, which conjoin to form an aponeurosis from which the muscle fibers arise:
Ilium (anterior inferior iliac spine)
Acetabulum (groove above posterior rim and superior margin of labrum)
Capsule of hip joint

Insertion:
Patella (base; from an aponeurosis which gradually narrows into a tendon which inserts into the center portion of the Quadriceps tendon, thence into the ligamentum patellae to a final insertion on the tibial tuberosity)

Description:

This most anterior of the Quadriceps lies 6° medial to the axis of the femur. Its superficial fibers are bipennate, but the deep fibers are parallel. It traverses a vertical course down the thigh. It is a two-joint muscle, crossing both the hip and knee, whereas the vasti are one-joint muscles crossing only the knee.

197 VASTUS LATERALIS

Origin:

Femur (linea aspera, lateral lip; greater trochanter, anterior and inferior borders; proximal intertrochanteric line; gluteal tuberosity)
Lateral intermuscular septum

Insertion:

Patella, into an underlying aponeurosis over the deep surface of the muscle, which narrows and attaches to the lateral border of the quadriceps tendon; to a lateral expansion, which blends with the capsule of the knee and the iliotibial tract.
The quadriceps tendon joins the ligamentum patellae to insert into the tibial tuberosity.

Description:

The lateralis is the largest of the Quadriceps group and, as its name suggests, it forms the bulk of the lateral thigh musculature. It arises via a broad aponeurosis lateral to the femur. Its fibers run at an angle of 17° to the axis of the femur. It descends to the thigh under the iliotibial band. It is the muscle of choice for biopsy in the lower extremity.

198 VASTUS INTERMEDIUS

Origin:

Femur (anterior and lateral surfaces of upper 2/3 of shaft)
Lateral intermuscular septum (lower part)

Insertion:

Patella (base: into an anterior aponeurosis of muscle which attaches to the middle part of the deep layer of the Quadriceps tendon, and then into the ligamentum patellae to insert into the tibial tuberosity)

Description:

The deepest of the Quadriceps muscles, this muscle lies under the Rectus femoris, the Vastus medialis, and the Vastus lateralis. It often appears inseparable from the medialis. It almost completely surrounds the proximal 2/3 of the shaft of the femur. A small muscle, the Articularis genus, occasionally is distinguishable from the intermedius, but more commonly it is part of the intermedius.

199 VASTUS MEDIALIS LONGUS[38, 39]

Origin:

Femur (intertrochanteric line, lower half; linea aspera, medial lip, proximal portion)
Tendons of Adductors longus and magnus
Medial intermuscular septum

Insertion:

Patella, via an aponeurosis into the superior medial margin of the Quadriceps tendon, thence to the ligamentum patellae and insertion into the tibial tuberosity

Description:

The fibers of this muscle course upward at an angle of 15° to 18° to the longitudinal axis of the femur.

200 VASTUS MEDIALIS OBLIQUE[38, 39]

Origin:

Femur (linea aspera, medial lip, distal portion; medial supracondylar line, proximal portion)
Tendon of Adductor magnus
Medial intermuscular septum

Insertion:

Patella:
Into the medial Quadriceps tendon and along medial margin of the patella
Expansion aponeurosis to the capsule of the knee joint
Tibial tuberosity via ligamentum patellae

Description:

The fibers of this muscle run at an angle of 50° to 55° to the longitudinal axis of the femur. The muscle appears to bulge quickly with training and to atrophy with disuse before the other Quadriceps show changes. This is deceiving because the Medialis oblique has the most sparse and thinnest fascial investment, making changes in it more obvious to observation.

Insertion (all):

The tendons of the five heads unite at the distal thigh to form a common strong tendon (Quadriceps tendon) that inserts into the proximal margin of the patella. Fibers continue across the anterior surface to become the patellar tendon (ligamentum patellae), which inserts into the tuberosity of the tibia.

Function (all):

Knee extension (none of the heads functions independently)
Hip flexion (by Rectus femoris, which crosses the hip joint)

Innervation (all):

L2–L4 Femoral nerve

201 ARTICULARIS GENUS

Origin:
Femur (shaft, lower anterior surface)

Insertion:
Knee joint (synovial membrane, upper part)

Description:
This small muscle is mostly distinct but also it may be inseparable from the Vastus intermedius

Function:
Retracts the synovial membrane during knee extension, purportedly preventing this membrane from being entrapped between the patella and the femur

Innervation:
L2–L4 Femoral nerve

202 POPLITEUS

Origin:
Capsule of knee joint (by a strong tendon to lateral condyle of the femur)
Femur (lateral condyle, popliteal groove on anterior surface)
Arcuate popliteal ligament
Lateral meniscus of knee joint[40]

Insertion:
Tibia (posterior triangular surface above soleal line)
Tendinous expansion of muscle

Description:
Sweeps across the upper leg from lateral to medial just below the knee. Forms the lower floor of the popliteal fossa. It is believed to protect the lateral meniscus from a crush injury during external rotation of the femur and flexion of the knee.[40]

Function:
Knee flexion
Knee internal rotation (proximal attachment fixed)
Hip external rotation (tibia fixed)

Innervation:
L4–S1 Tibial nerve (high branch)

Muscles of the Ankle

203 Tibialis anterior
204 Tibialis posterior
205 Gastrocnemius
206 Soleus
207 Plantaris

208 Peroneus longus
209 Peroneus brevis
210 Peroneus tertius

203 TIBIALIS ANTERIOR

Origin:
Tibia (lateral condyle and proximal 2/3 of lateral surface)
Interosseous membrane
Deep surface of crural fascia
Intermuscular septum

Insertion:
1st (medial) cuneiform bone (on medial and plantar surfaces)
1st metatarsal bone (base)

Description:
Located on the lateral aspect of the tibia, the muscle has a thick belly proximally but is tendinous distally. The fibers drop vertically and end in a prominent tendon on the anterior surface of the lower leg. Muscle is contained in the most medial compartments of the extensor retinacula.

Function:
Ankle dorsiflexion (talocrural joint)
Foot inversion and adduction (supination) at subtalar and midtarsal joints
Supports medial-longitudinal arch of foot in walking

Innervation:
L4–L5 (often S1) Deep peroneal nerve

204 TIBIALIS POSTERIOR

Origin:
Tibia (proximal 2/3 of posterior lateral shaft)
Fibula (proximal 2/3 of posterior medial shaft and head)
Interosseous membrane (entire posterior surface except lower portion where Flexor hallucis longus originates)
Deep transverse fascia and intermuscular septa

Insertion:
Navicular bone (tuberosity)
Cuneiform bones (media, intermediate, lateral)
Cuboid (slip)
2nd, 3rd, and 4th metatarsals (bases) (variable)

Description:
Most deeply placed of the flexor group, high on the posterior leg, this muscle is overlapped by both the Flexor hallucis longus and the Flexor digitorum longus. It rises by two narrow heads and descends centrally on the leg, forming its

distal tendon in the distal 1/4. This tendon passes behind the medial malleolus (with the Flexor digitorum longus), enters the foot on the plantar surface (where it contains a sesamoid bone), and then divides to its several insertions.

During weight bearing the Tibialis posterior assists in arch support and distribution of weight on the foot to maintain balance.

Function:
Foot inversion
Ankle plantar flexion (accessory)

Innervation:
L4–L5 (sometimes S1) Tibial nerve (low branches)

205 GASTROCNEMIUS

Rises via two heads

Origin:
Medial head:
Femur (medial condyle, depression on upper posterior part; popliteal surface adjacent to medial condyle)
Capsule of knee joint
Aponeurosis
Lateral head:
Femur (lateral condyle and posterior surface of shaft above lateral condyle; lower supracondylar line)
Capsule of knee joint
Aponeurosis

Insertion:
Calcaneus (via tendo calcaneus into middle posterior surface). Fibers of tendon rotate 90° such that those associated with Gastrocnemius are attached more laterally on the calcaneus.

Description:
The most superficial of the calf muscles, it gives the characteristic contour to the calf. It is a two-joint muscle with two heads arising from the condyles of the femur and descending to the calcaneus. The medial head is the larger, and its fibers extend further distally before spreading into a tendinous expansion, as does the lateral head. The two heads join as the aponeurosis narrows and form the tendo calcaneus. The belly of the muscle extends to about midcalf (the medial head is the longer) before inserting into the aponeurosis.

Function:
Ankle plantar flexion
Knee flexion (accessory)
Foot eversion

Innervation:
S1–S2 Tibial nerve

206 SOLEUS

Origin:
Fibula (head, posterior surface; shaft: proximal 1/3 on posterior surface)
Tibia (soleal line and middle 1/3 of medial side of shaft)
Fibrous arch between tibia and fibula
Aponeurosis (anterior aspect)

Insertion:
Aponeurosis over posterior surface of muscle, which, with tendon of Gastrocnemius, thickens to become the tendo calcaneus
Calcaneus (posterior surface via tendo calcaneus along with Gastrocnemius)[41]
Tendinous raphe in midline of muscle

Description:
This is a one-joint muscle, the largest of the Triceps surae. It is broad and flat and lies just under the Gastrocnemius. Its anterior attachment is a wide aponeurosis, and most of its fibers course obliquely to the descending tendon on its posterior side. Below midcalf the Soleus is wider than the tendon of the Gastrocnemius and on both sides. It is, thereby, accessible for biopsy and electrophysiological studies.

The Soleus is constantly active in quiet stance. It responds to the forward center of mass to prevent the body from falling forward.

Function:
Ankle plantar flexion
Foot inversion

Innervation:
S1–S2 Tibial nerve

207 PLANTARIS

Origin:
Femur (supracondylar line, lateral)
Oblique popliteal ligament of knee joint

Insertion:
Tendo calcaneus (medial border) to calcaneum
Plantar aponeurosis

Description:
This small fusiform muscle lies between the Gastrocnemius and the Soleus. It is sometimes absent; at other times it is doubled. Its short belly is followed by a long slender tendon of insertion along the medial border of the tendo calcaneus and inserts with it on the posterior calcaneum.

Plantaris is somewhat like Palmaris longus in the hand and is of little function in humans.[41]

Function:
Ankle plantar flexion (assist)
Knee flexion (weak accessory)

Innervation:
S1–S2 Tibial nerve (high branches)

208 PERONEUS LONGUS

Origin:
Fibula (head and upper 2/3 of lateral shaft)
Tibia (lateral condyle, occasionally)
Deep crural fascia and intermuscular septa

Insertion:
1st metatarsal (lateral plantar side of base)
1st (medial) cuneiform (lateral plantar aspect)
2nd metatarsal (occasionally by a slip)

Description:
Muscle is found proximally on the fibular side of the leg where it is superficial to the Peroneus brevis. The belly ends in a long tendon that passes behind the lateral malleolus (with the brevis) and then runs obliquely forward lateral to the calcaneus and crosses the plantar aspect of the foot to reach the 1st metatarsal and medial cuneiform.
It maintains concavity of foot (along with brevis) during toe-off and tiptoeing.

Function:
Foot eversion
Ankle plantar flexion (assist)
Depression of 1st metatarsal
Support of longitudinal and transverse arches

Innervation:
L5–S1 Superficial peroneal nerve

209 PERONEUS BREVIS

Origin:
Fibula (shaft: distal 2/3 of lateral surface)
Intermuscular septa

Insertion:
5th metatarsal (tuberosity on lateral surface of base)

Description:
The Peroneus brevis lies deep to the longus and is the shorter and smaller muscle of the two. The belly fibers descend vertically to end in a tendon, which courses (with the longus) behind the lateral malleolus (the pair of muscles share a synovial sheath). It bends forward on the lateral

side of the calcaneus, passing forward to the 5th metatarsal.

Function:
Foot eversion
Ankle plantar flexion (accessory)

Innervation:
L5–S1 Superficial peroneal nerve

210 PERONEUS TERTIUS

Origin:
Fibula (distal 1/3 of medial surface)
Interosseous membrane (anterior)
Intermuscular septum

Insertion:
5th metatarsal (dorsal surface of base; shaft: medial aspect)

Description:
This muscle is considered part of the Extensor digitorum longus (i.e., the 5th tendon). The muscle descends on the lateral leg, diving under the extensor retinaculum in the same passage as the Extensor digitorum longus, to insert on the 5th metatarsal. Muscle varies greatly.

Function:
Ankle dorsiflexion
Foot eversion (accessory)

Innervation:
L5–S1 Deep peroneal nerve

Muscles Acting on the Toes

211 Extensor digitorum longus

212 Extensor digitorum brevis

213 Flexor digitorum longus

214 Flexor digitorum brevis

215 Abductor digiti minimi

216 Flexor digiti minimi brevis

217 Quadratus plantae (Flexor digitorum accessorius)

218 Lumbricales

219 Interossei, dorsal (foot)

220 Interossei, plantar

211 EXTENSOR DIGITORUM LONGUS

Origin:
Tibia (lateral condyle on lateral side)
Fibula (shaft: upper 3/4 of medial surface)

Interosseous membrane (anterior surface)
Deep crural fascia and intermuscular septum

Insertion:
Tendon of insertion divides into four tendon slips
to dorsum of foot that form an expansion over
each toe:
Toes 2 to 5:
Middle phalanges (PIP joints) of the four lesser
toes (intermediate slip to dorsum of base of
each)
Distal phalanges (two lateral slips to dorsum of
base of each)

Description:
Muscle lies in the lateral aspect of the anterior leg.
It descends lateral to the Tibialis anterior, and
its distal tendon accompanies the tendon of the
Peroneus tertius before dividing. It is attached
in the manner of the Extensor digitorum of the
hand.

Function:
MP extension of four lesser toes
PIP and DIP extension (assist) of four lesser toes
Ankle dorsiflexion (accessory)
Foot eversion (accessory)

Innervation:
L5–S1 Deep peroneal nerve

212 EXTENSOR DIGITORUM BREVIS

Origin:
Calcaneus (superior proximal surface anterolateral
to the calcaneal sulcus)
Lateral talocalcaneal ligament
Extensor retinaculum (inferior)

Insertion:
Ends in four tendons:
(1) Hallux (proximal phalanx). This tendon is the
largest and most medial. It frequently is described as a separate muscle, the Extensor hallucis brevis.
(2, 3, 4) Three tendons join the tendon of
Extensor digitorum longus (lateral surfaces).

Description:
The muscle passes medially and distally across the
dorsum of the foot to end in four tendons, one
to the hallux and three to toes 2, 3, and 4.
Varies considerably.

Function:
Hallux (great toe): MP extension
Toes 2 to 4: MP extension
Toes 2 to 4: IP extension (assist)

Innervation:
L5–S1 Deep peroneal nerve, lateral terminal
branch

213 FLEXOR DIGITORUM LONGUS

Origin:
Tibia (shaft: posterior surface of middle 2/3)
Fascia covering Tibialis posterior

Insertion:
Toes 2 to 5 (distal phalanges: base, plantar surface)

Description:
Muscle lies deep on the tibial side of the leg and
increases in size as it descends. The tendon of
insertion extends almost the entire length of
the muscle and is joined in the sole of the foot
by the tendon of the Quadratus plantae. It finally divides into four slips, which insert into
the four lateral toes.

Function:
Toes 2 to 5: MP, PIP, and DIP flexion
Ankle plantar flexion (accessory)
Foot inversion (accessory)

Innervation:
L5–S2 Tibial nerve

214 FLEXOR DIGITORUM BREVIS

Origin:
Calcaneus (tuberosity, medial process)
Intermuscular septa (adjacent)
Plantar aponeurosis (central part)

Insertion:
Toes 2 to 5 (by four tendons to middle phalanges,
both sides)

Description:
This muscle is located in the middle of the sole of
the foot immediately above the plantar aponeurosis. It divides into four tendons, one for each
of the four lesser toes. At the base of the proximal phalanx each is divided into two slips,
which encircle the tendon of the Flexor digitorum longus. The tendons divide a second time
and insert onto both sides of the middle phalanges. The pattern of insertion is the same as
the tendons of the Flexor digitorum superficialis in the hand

Function:
Toes 2 to 5 MP and PIP flexion

Innervation:
S1–S2 Medial plantar nerve

215 ABDUCTOR DIGITI MINIMI (Foot)

Origin:
Calcaneus (tuberosity, medial and lateral processes)
Plantar aponeurosis and intermuscular septum

Insertion:
Toe 5 (base of proximal phalanx, lateral aspect)
Insertion is in common with Flexor digiti minimi brevis

Description:
Lies along the lateral border of the foot and inserts in common with the Flexor digiti minimi brevis. Its insertion on the lateral side of the base of the 5th toe makes it as much a flexor as an abductor.

Function:
Toe 5 abduction
Toe 5 MP flexion

Innervation:
S1–S3 Lateral plantar nerve

216 FLEXOR DIGITI MINIMI BREVIS

Origin:
5th metatarsal (base, plantar surface)
Sheath of Peroneus longus

Insertion:
Toe 5 (proximal phalanx, lateral aspect of base)

Description:
Muscle lies superficial to the 5th metatarsal and looks like an Interosseous muscle. Sometimes fibers are inserted into the lateral distal half of the 5th metatarsal, and these have been described as a distinct muscle called the *Opponens digiti minimi.*

Function:
Toe 5 MP flexion

Innervation:
S2–S3 Lateral plantar nerve (superficial branch)

217 QUADRATUS PLANTAE (Flexor Digitorum Accessorius)

Rises via two heads

Origin:
Lateral head:
Calcaneus (lateral border distal to lateral process of tuberosity)
Long plantar ligament

Medial head:
Calcaneus (medial concave surface)
Long plantar ligament (medial border)

Insertion:
Tendon of Flexor digitorum longus (lateral margin) may fuse with long flexor tendon.[42]

Description:
This muscle is sometimes known as the Flexor digitorum accessorius, or just Flexor accessorius.
The medial head is larger, whereas the lateral head is more tendinous. They rise from either side of the calcaneus, pass medially, and join in an acute angle at midfoot, to end in the lateral margin of the tendon of the Flexor digitorum longus. Muscle may be absent.

Function:
Toes 2 to 5 DIP flexion (in synergy with the Flexor digitorum longus)

Innervation:
S1–S3 Lateral plantar nerve

218 LUMBRICALES (Foot)

These are four small muscles considered accessories to the Flexor digitorum longus.

Origin:
1st Lumbrical: Originates by a single head from the medial side of the tendon of the Flexor digitorum longus bound for toe 2.
2nd, 3rd, and 4th Lumbricales: Originate by double heads from adjacent sides of tendons of the Flexor digitorum longus bound for toes 3, 4, and 5.

Insertion (all):
Toes 2 to 5 (proximal phalanges and dorsal expansions of the tendons of Extensor digitorum longus)

Description:
The Lumbricales are four small muscles intrinsic to the foot. They are numbered from the medial (hallux) side of the foot so that the 1st Lumbrical goes to toe 2 and the 4th Lumbrical goes to toe 5.

Function:
Toes 2 to 5: MP flexion
Toes 2 to 5: PIP and DIP extension (assist)

Innervation:
1st Lumbrical: L5–S1 Medial plantar nerve
2nd, 3rd, and 4th Lumbricales: S2–S3 Lateral plantar nerve, deep branch

219 DORSAL INTEROSSEI (Foot)

There are four dorsal Interossei

Origin:
Metatarsal bones (each head arises from the adjacent sides of the metatarsal bones between which it lies)

Insertion:
1st Dorsal: Toe 2 proximal phalanx, medial side of base
2nd Dorsal: Toe 2 proximal phalanx, lateral side of base
3rd Dorsal: Toe 3 proximal phalanx, lateral side of base
4th Dorsal: Toe 4 proximal phalanx, lateral side of base
All: Tendons of Extensor digitorum longus via dorsal digital expansion

Description:
The dorsal Interossei are four bipennate muscles, each arising by two heads. They are similar to the interossei of the hand except that their action is considered relative to the midline of the 2nd digit (the longitudinal axis of the foot). The muscles are innervated by the lateral plantar nerve, deep branch, except for the 4th dorsal muscle which lies in the 4th interosseous space; it is supplied by the superficial branch of the same nerve.

Function:
Toes 2 to 4: abduction from longitudinal axis of foot, which lines up through toe 2
Toes 2 to 4: MP flexion (accessory)
Toes 2 to 4: IP extension (possibly)

Innervation:
1st, 2nd, and 3rd Dorsals: S2–S3 Lateral plantar nerve, deep branch
4th Dorsal: S2–S3 Lateral plantar nerve, superficial branch (1st dorsal also may receive a slip from the deep peroneal, medial branch; the 2nd dorsal may receive a slip from the deep peroneal, lateral branch)

220 PLANTAR INTEROSSEI

Origin:
3rd, 4th, and 5th metatarsal bones (bases and medial sides)

Insertion:
Proximal phalanges of same toe (bases and medial sides)
Dorsal digital expansion

Description:
These are three muscles that lie along the plantar surface of the metatarsals rather than between them. Each connects with only one metatarsal. As with the dorsal Interossei, the muscles are innervated by the deep branch of the lateral plantar nerve except for the 3rd plantar muscle, which lies in the 4th interosseous space and is innervated by the superficial branch of the same nerve.

Function:
Toes 3, 4, and 5: Adduction (toward the axis of toe 2)
MP flexion
IP extension (assist)

Innervation:
1st and 2nd Plantars: S2–S3 Lateral plantar nerve (deep branch)
3rd plantar: S2–S3 Lateral plantar nerve (superficial branch)

Muscles Acting on the Great Toe

221 Extensor hallucis longus

222 Flexor hallucis longus

223 Flexor hallucis brevis

224 Abductor hallucis

225 Adductor hallucis

221 EXTENSOR HALLUCIS LONGUS

Origin:
Fibula (shaft: medial aspect of middle half)
Interosseous membrane

Insertion:
Hallux (base of distal phalanx, dorsal surface)
Expansion to base of proximal phalanx of hallux

Description:
This thin muscle travels lateral to medial as it descends in the leg between and largely covered by the Tibialis anterior and the Extensor digitorum longus. Its tendon does not emerge superficially until it reaches the distal 1/3 of the leg. It may be joined with the Extensor digitorum longus.

Function:
Hallux: MP and IP extension
Ankle dorsiflexion (accessory)
Foot inversion (accessory)

Innervation:
L5 Deep peroneal nerve
L4–S1 also cited

222 FLEXOR HALLUCIS LONGUS

Origin:
Fibula (shaft: inferior 2/3 of posterior surface)

Interosseous membrane
Posterior crural intermuscular septum
Fascia over Tibialis posterior

Insertion:
Hallux (distal phalanx at base on plantar surface)
Slip to tendon of flexor digitorum longus

Description:
This muscle lies deep in the lateral side of the leg. Its fibers pass obliquely down via a long tendon that runs along the whole length of its posterior surface and then crosses over the distal end of the tibia, talus, and the inferior surface of the calcaneus. It then runs forward on the sole of the foot to the distal phalanx of the hallux.

Function:
Hallux IP flexion
Hallux MP flexion (accessory)
Ankle plantar flexion and foot inversion (accessory)

Innervation:
L5–S2 Tibial nerve (low branches)

223 FLEXOR HALLUCIS BREVIS

Origin:
Lateral part:
Cuboid (medial part of plantar surface)
Cuneiform (lateral)

Medial part:
Tendon of Tibialis posterior
Medial intermuscular septum

Insertion:
Hallux: sides of base of proximal phalanx
The medial part blends with the Abductor hallucis
The lateral part blends with Adductor hallucis

Description:
One of the muscles of the third layer (of four layers) of plantar muscles. It is located adjacent to the plantar surface of the 1st metatarsal.

Function:
Hallux abduction (away from toe 2)
Hallux MP flexion

Innervation:
S1–S2 Medial plantar nerve

224 ABDUCTOR HALLUCIS

Origin:
Flexor retinaculum
Calcaneus (tuberosity, medial process)
Plantar aponeurosis and intermuscular septum

Insertion:
Hallux (base of proximal phalanx, medial side)
Medial sesamoid of hallux
Joins tendon of Flexor hallucis brevis

Description:
This muscle lies along the medial border of the foot. Its tendon attaches distally to the medial tendon of the Flexor hallucis brevis and they insert together on the hallux.
When fibers from the muscle are attached to the first metatarsal, it can be considered an Opponens hallucis

Function:
Hallux abduction (away from toe 2)
Hallux MP flexion (accessory)

Innervation:
S1–S2 Medial plantar nerve

225 ADDUCTOR HALLUCIS

Arises from two heads

Origin:
Oblique head:
2nd, 3rd, and 4th metatarsals (bases)
Sheath of Peroneus longus tendon
Transverse head:
Toes 3 to 5: Plantar metatarsophalangeal ligaments
Deep transverse metatarsal ligaments between toes

Insertion:
Oblique:
Hallux (base of proximal phalanx, lateral aspect)
Lateral sesamoid bone of hallux
Blends with Flexor hallucis brevis
Transverse:
Proximal phalanx of hallux (debated)
Lateral sesamoid of hallux

Description:
The two heads are unequal in size, the oblique being the larger and more muscular. It is located in the third layer of plantar muscles. The oblique head crosses the foot from center to medial on a long oblique axis; the transverse head courses transversely across the metatarsophalangeal joints.

Function:
Hallux adduction (toward toe 2)
Hallux MP flexion (accessory)
Support of transverse metatarsal arch

Innervation:
S2–S3 Lateral plantar nerve, deep branch

PART 4. MOTIONS AND THEIR PARTICIPATING MUSCLES
(MOTIONS OF THE NECK, TRUNK, AND LIMBS)

In this part of the ready reference chapter, each motion of the axial skeleton and trunk is listed along with the muscles that participate in that motion regardless of the extent of their contribution.

As with all aspects of human anatomy, widely different opinions about functional anatomy are cited in the literature. We have used the American and British (primarily) versions of *Gray's Anatomy* as the principal references, but occasionally kinesiologic imperatives have caused us to deviate from orthodoxy for some muscles.

MOTIONS OF THE CERVICAL SPINE AND HEAD

Note: The small muscles of the neck are variably innervated.

Capital Extension (All muscles act bilaterally)

56.	Rectus capitis posterior major	C1 (suboccipital)
57.	Rectus capitis posterior minor	C1 (suboccipital)
58.	Obliquus capitis superior	C1 (suboccipital)
59.	Obliquus capitis inferior (extension doubtful)	C1 (suboccipital)
60.	Longissimus capitis	C3–C8 (greater occipital)
61.	Splenius capitis	C3–C6
62.	Semispinalis capitis	C2–T1
63.	Spinalis capitis	C3–T1
83.	Sternocleidomastoid (posterior)	Accessory (XI) and C2–C3
124.	Trapezius (upper)	Accessory (XI) and C3–C4

Capital Flexion (All muscles act bilaterally)

72.	Rectus capitis anterior	C1–C2
73.	Rectus capitis lateralis	C1–C2
74.	Longus capitis	C1–C3
75.	Mylohyoid	Trigeminal (V)
76.	Stylohyoid	Facial (VII)
77.	Geniohyoid	Hypoglossal (XII) with fibers from C1
78.	Digastric	
	Anterior belly	Trigeminal (V)
	Posterior belly	Facial (VII)

Cervical Extension (All muscles act bilaterally)

64.	Longissimus cervicis	C3–T3
65.	Semispinalis cervicis	C2–T5
66.	Iliocostalis cervicis	C4–T3
67.	Splenius cervicis	C4–C8
69.	Interspinales cervicis	C3–C8
68.	Spinalis cervicis	C4–C8
124.	Trapezius (upper)	Accessory (XI) and C3–C4
70.	Intertransversarii cervicis	C3–C8
71.	Rotatores cervicis	C3–C8
94.	Multifidus	Segmental spinal nerves (axis to sacrum)
127.	Levator scapulae	C3–C4 spinal nerves (ventral rami) C5 dorsal scapular nerve

Cervical Flexion (All muscles act bilaterally and are variable)

79.	Longus colli	C2–C6
80.	Scalenus anterior	C4–C6
81.	Scalenus medius	C3–C8
82.	Scalenus posterior	C6–C8
83.	Sternocleidomastoid	Accessory (XI), C2–C3
84.	Sternothyroid	C1–C3
85.	Thyrohyoid	Hypoglossal (XII) and C1
86.	Sternohyoid	Hypoglossal (XII) and C1–C3
87.	Omohyoid	C1–C3
88.	Platysma	Facial (VII)

Lateral Bending (Ear to shoulder)

The muscles used in this movement are the capital extensors and flexors on that side, and the cervical flexors and extensors on that side.

Rotation to Same Side (Turn face to same side; all variable)

56.	Rectus capitis posterior major	C1 (suboccipital)
59.	Obliquus capitis inferior	C1 (suboccipital)
60.	Longissimus capitis	C3–C8
61.	Splenius capitis (debated)	C3–C6
67.	Splenius cervicis	C4–C8
74.	Longus capitis	C1–C3
127.	Levator scapulae	C5 (dorsal scapular) and C3–C4

Rotation to Opposite Side (All innervations variable)

124.	Trapezius (upper)	Accessory (XI) and C3–C4
62.	Semispinalis capitis	C2–T1
65.	Semispinalis cervicis	C2–T5
71.	Rotatores cervicis	C3–C8
79.	Longus colli	C2–C6
80.	Scalenus anterior	C4–C6
81.	Scalenus medius	C3–C8
82.	Scalenus posterior	C6–C8
83.	Sternocleidomastoid	Accessory (XI) and C2–C3
94.	Multifidus	Segmental spinal nerves

MOTIONS OF THE THORACIC SPINE

Thoracic Extension

89.	Iliocostalis thoracis	T1–T12 (variable)
91.	Longissimus thoracis	T1–L1
92.	Spinalis thoracis	T1–T12 (variable)
93.	Semispinalis thoracis	T1–T12
94.	Multifidus	T1–T12 spinal nerves; whole spine
95.	Rotatores thoracis	T1–T12 (variable)
97.	Interspinales thoracis	T1–T3, T11–T12 (variable)
99.	Intertransversarii thoracis	Thoracic spinal nerves (very variable)

MOTIONS OF THE LUMBAR SPINE AND PELVIS

Lumbar Forward Flexion

110.	Obliquus externus abdominis (both)	T7–T12
111.	Obliquus internus abdominis (both)	T7–L1
113.	Rectus abdominis (both)	T7–T12
174.	Psoas major	L2–L4
175.	Psoas minor	L1

Lumbar Extension

90.	Iliocostalis lumborum (both)	L1–L5
94.	Multifidus	Spinal nerves: axis to sacrum
96.	Rotatores lumborum (both)	Lumbar spinal nerves (variable)
98.	Interspinales lumborum	Lumbar spinal nerves (variable)
99.	Intertransversarii thoracis and lumborum	Thoracic and lumbar spinal nerves (dorsal rami)
100.	Quadratus lumborum (both)	T12–L3 (ventral rami)
182.	Gluteus maximus	L5–S2 inferior gluteal nerve

Lumbar Lateral Bending

90.	Iliocostalis lumborum	Lumbar spinal nerves (variable)
99.	Intertransversarii lumborum	Lumbar spinal nerves (variable)
100.	Quadratus lumborum	T12–L3
110.	Obliquus externus abdominis	T7–T12
111.	Obliquus internus abdominis	T7–L1
174.	Psoas major	L2–L4

Lumbar Rotation to Same Side

111.	Obliquus internus abdominis	T7–L1

Lumbar Rotation to Opposite Side

94.	Multifidi	Spinal nerves, axis to sacrum
96.	Rotatores lumborum	Lumbar spinal nerves (variable)
110.	Obliquus externus abdominis	T7–T12

MOTIONS OF RESPIRATION

Quiet Inspiration

101.	Diaphragm	C4 (phrenic)
102.	Intercostales externi	T1–T11 (intercostal)
103.	Intercostales interni	T1–T11 (intercostal)
104.	Intercostales intimi	T1–T11 (intercostal)
107.	Levatores costarum	T1–T11 (intercostal)
80.	Scalenus anterior	C4–C6
81.	Scalenus medius	C3–C8
82.	Scalenus posterior	C6–C8
108.	Serratus posterior superior	T2–T5 (intercostal)
	Deep back extensors	Segmental spinal nerves

Expiration (During exertion, coughing, Valsalva maneuver, etc.)

110.	Obliquus externus abdominis	T7–T12
111.	Obliquus internus abdominis	T7–L1
113.	Rectus abdominis	T7–T12
112.	Transversus abdominis	T7–L1 (intercostal)
102.	Intercostales externi (supporting data scarce)	T1–T11 (intercostal)
103.	Intercostales interni	T1–T11 (intercostal)
106.	Transversus thoracis	T2–T11 (intercostal)
130.	Latissimus dorsi	C6–C8 (thoracodorsal)

Forced Inspiration

All muscles of quiet inspiration plus:

83.	Sternocleidomastoid	Accessory (XI); C2–C3
88.	Platysma	Facial (VII)
131.	Pectoralis major	C5–T1 (medial and lateral pectorals)
129.	Pectoralis minor	C5–T1 (medial and lateral pectorals)
130.	Latissimus dorsi	C6–C8 (thoracodorsal)

Elevation of Pelvis

100.	Quadratus lumborum	T12–L3 spinal nerves
130.	Latissimus dorsi	C6–C8 (thoracodorsal)
110.	Obliquus externus abdominis	T7–T12 spinal nerves
111.	Obliquus internus abdominis	T7–T12 spinal nerves
90.	Iliocostalis lumborum	L1–L5 spinal nerves

UPPER EXTREMITY MOTIONS

The Scapula

Scapular Elevation (Shrugging)

124.	Trapezius (upper)	Accessory (XI) and C3–C4
127.	Levator scapulae	C3–C4; C5 (dorsal scapular)
125.	Rhomboid major	C5 (dorsal scapular)
126.	Rhomboid minor	C5 (dorsal scapular)

Scapular Depression

124.	Trapezius (lower)	Accessory (XI) and C3–C4
132.	Subclavius	C5–C6 (nerve to Subclavius)

Scapular Abduction (Protraction)

128. Serratus anterior	C5–C7 (long thoracic)
129. Pectoralis minor	C5–T1 (medial pectoral)

Scapular Adduction (Retraction)

124. Trapezius (middle and lower)	Accessory (XI) and C3–C4
125. Rhomboid major	C5 (dorsal scapular)
126. Rhomboid minor	C5 (dorsal scapular)
127. Levator scapulae	C3–C4; C5 (dorsal scapular)

Scapular Upward Rotation (Glenoid fossa up)

124. Trapezius (upper and lower)	Accessory (XI) and C3–C4
128. Serratus anterior	C5–C7 (long thoracic)

Scapular Downward Rotation (Glenoid fossa down)

125. Rhomboid major	C5 (dorsal scapular)
126. Rhomboid minor	C5 (dorsal scapular)
127. Levator scapulae	C3–C4; C5 (dorsal scapular)

The Shoulder (Glenohumeral Motions)

Shoulder Flexion (Musculocutaneous)

139. Coracobrachialis	C5–C7 (musculocutaneous)
133. Deltoid (anterior and middle)	C5–C6 (axillary)
131. Pectoralis major (clavicular part)	C5–C6 (lateral pectoral)

Shoulder Abduction

133. Deltoid (middle)	C5–C6 (axillary)
135. Supraspinatus	C5–C6 (suprascapular)

Shoulder Adduction

130. Latissimus dorsi	C6–C8 (thoracodorsal)
131. Pectoralis major	C5–T1 (medial and lateral pectorals)
137. Teres minor	C5–C6 (axillary)
138. Teres major	C5–C6 (subscapular)
139. Coracobrachialis	C5–C7 (musculocutaneous)

Shoulder Internal Rotation (Medial rotation)

130. Latissimus dorsi	C6–C8 (thoracodorsal)
131. Pectoralis major	C5–T1 (medial and lateral pectorals)
134. Subscapularis	C5–C6 (subscapular)
138. Teres major	C5–C6 (subscapular)
133. Deltoid (anterior)	C5–C6 (axillary)

Shoulder Horizontal Adduction

131. Pectoralis major	C5–T1 (medial and lateral pectorals)
133. Deltoid (anterior)	C5–C6 (axillary)

Shoulder Horizontal Abduction

133. Deltoid (posterior)	C5–C6 (axillary)

Shoulder External Rotation (Lateral rotation)

133. Deltoid (posterior)	C5–C6 (axillary)
136. Infraspinatus	C5–C6 (suprascapular)
137. Teres minor	C5–C6 (axillary)

Shoulder Extension

130. Latissimus dorsi	C6–C8 (thoracodorsal)
133. Deltoid (posterior)	C5–C6 (axillary)

138. Teres major	C5–C7 (subscapular)	
142. Triceps brachii (long head)	C6–C8 (radial)	

Elbow and Forearm Motions

Elbow Flexion

140. Biceps brachii	C5–C6 (musculocutaneous)
141. Brachialis	C5–C6 (musculocutaneous)
143. Brachioradialis	C5–C6 (radial)
146. Pronator teres	C6–C7 (median)
148. Extensor carpi radialis longus	C6–C7 (radial)
151. Flexor carpi radialis	C6–C7 (median)
152. Palmaris longus	C7–C8 (median)
153. Flexor carpi ulnaris	C7–T1 (ulnar)

Elbow Extension

142. Triceps brachii	C6–C8 (radial)
144. Anconeus	C6–C8 (radial)

Forearm Pronation

146. Pronator teres	C6–C7 (median)
147. Pronator quadratus	C7–C8 (median)
151. Flexor carpi radialis	C6–C7 (median)

Forearm Supination

145. Supinator	C6–C7 (radial)
140. Biceps brachii	C5–C6 (musculocutaneous)

Wrist and Hand Motions

Wrist Flexion

151. Flexor carpi radialis	C6–C7 (median)
153. Flexor carpi ulnaris	C7–T1 (ulnar)
156. Flexor digitorum superficialis	C8–T1 (median)
157. Flexor digitorum profundus Digits 2 and 3 Digits 4 and 5	C8–T1 (median) C8–T1 (ulnar)

166. Abductor pollicis longus	C7–C8 (radial)
169. Flexor pollicis longus	C7–C8 (median)
152. Palmaris longus	C7–C8 (median)

Wrist Extension

148. Extensor carpi radialis longus	C6–C7 (radial)
149. Extensor carpi radialis brevis	C7–C8 (radial)
150. Extensor carpi ulnaris	C7–C8 (radial)
154. Extensor digitorum	C7–C8 (radial)
158. Extensor digiti minimi	C7–C8 (radial)
155. Extensor indicis	C7–C8 (radial)

Wrist Radial Deviation (Abduction)

148. Extensor carpi radialis longus	C6–C7 (radial)
149. Extensor carpi radialis brevis	C7–C8 (radial)
151. Flexor carpi radialis	C6–C7 (median)
167. Extensor pollicis longus	C7–C8 (radial)
168. Extensor pollicis brevis	C7–C8 (radial)
166. Abductor pollicis longus	C7–C8 (radial)

Wrist Ulnar Deviation (Adduction)

150. Extensor carpi ulnaris	C7–C8 (radial)
153. Flexor carpi ulnaris	C7–T1 (ulnar)

Thumb Motions

Thumb Flexion

Carpometacarpal (CMC)

169. Flexor pollicis longus	C7–C8 (median)
172. Opponens pollicis	C8–T1 (median)
170. Flexor pollicis brevis: Superficial head Deep head	C8–T1 (median) C8–T1 (ulnar)

Metacarpophalangeal (MP)

170. Flexor pollicis brevis: Superficial head Deep head	C8–T1 (median) C8–T1 (ulnar)
169. Flexor pollicis longus	C7–C8 (median)
173. Adductor pollicis	C8–T1 (ulnar)

Interphalangeal (IP)

169. Flexor pollicis longus   C7–C8 (median)

Thumb Extension

Carpometacarpal (CMC)

168. Extensor pollicis brevis   C7–C8 (radial)

167. Extensor pollicis longus   C7–C8 (radial)

166. Abductor pollicis longus   C7–C8 (radial)

Metacarpophalangeal (MP)

168. Extensor pollicis brevis   C7–C8 (radial)

167. Extensor pollicis longus   C7–C8 (radial)

Interphalangeal (IP)

167. Extensor pollicis longus   C7–C8 (radial)

171. Abductor pollicis brevis   C8–T1 (median)

Thumb Abduction *(Away from digit 2 [index finger])*

Carpometacarpal (CMC)

166. Abductor pollicis longus   C7–C8 (radial)

168. Extensor pollicis brevis   C7–C8 (radial)

171. Abductor pollicis brevis   C8–T1 (median)

172. Opponens pollicis   C8–T1 (median)

152. Palmaris longus   C7–C8 (median)

Metacarpophalangeal (MP)

171. Abductor pollicis brevis   C8–T1 (median)

Thumb Adduction *(Toward digit 2)*

Carpometacarpal (CMC)

173. Adductor pollicis   C8–T1 (ulnar)

164. 1st dorsal Interosseous   C8 T1 (ulnar)

Metacarpophalangeal (MP)

173. Adductor pollicis   C8–T1 (ulnar)

Thumb Opposition *(Combination of internal rotation, abduction, and flexion)*

172. Opponens pollicis   C8–T1 (median)
                      C8–T1 (ulnar) frequently

171. Abductor pollicis brevis   C8–T1 (median)

170. Flexor pollicis brevis:
     Superficial head   C8–T1 (median)
     Deep head   C8–T1 (ulnar)

Finger Motions: Digit 2, 3, and 4 Motions (Index, Long, and Ring Fingers)

Finger Flexion

Metacarpophalangeal (MP)

163. Lumbricales, 1st and 2nd, for digits 2 and 3   C8–T1 (median)

163. Lumbricales, 3rd and 4th, for digits 4 and 5   C8–T1 (median)

165. Palmar Interossei for digits 2, 4, and 5   C8–T1 (ulnar)

164. Dorsal Interossei for digits 2, 3, and 4   C8–T1 (ulnar)

156. Flexor digitorum superficialis for digits 2 to 5   C8–T1 (median)

157. Flexor digitorum profundus for digits 2 and 3   C8–T1 (median)

157. Flexor digitorum profundus for digits 4 and 5   C8–T1 (ulnar)

Proximal Interphalangeal (PIP)

156. Flexor digitorum superficialis   C8–T1 (median)

157. Flexor digitorum profundus:
     For digits 2 and 3   C8–T1 (median)
     For digits 4 and 5   C8–T1 (ulnar)

Distal Interphalangeal (DIP)

157. Flexor digitorum profundus:
     For digits 2 and 3   C8–T1 (median)
     For digits 4 and 5   C8–T1 (ulnar)

Finger Extension

Metacarpophalangeal (MP)

154. Extensor digitorum (digits 2 to 5)   C7–C8 (radial)

155. Extensor indicis (digit 2)   C7–C8 (radial)

Proximal and Distal Interphalangeal (PIP and DIP)

154. Extensor digitorum (digits 2 to 5)   C7–C8 (radial)

155. Extensor indicis (digit 2)   C7–C8 (radial)

163. Lumbricales:
    1st and 2nd, for digits C8–T1 (median)
    2 and 3
    3rd and 4th, for digits C8–T1 (ulnar)
    4 and 5

165. Palmar Interossei for   C8–T1 (ulnar)
digits 2, 4, and 5

164. Dorsal Interossei for   C8–T1 (ulnar)
digits 2, 3, and 4

Finger Abduction

164. Dorsal Interossei:
    1st and 2nd, for   C8–T1 (ulnar)
    digits 2 and 3
    3rd and 4th, for digits
    3 and 4

154. Extensor digitorum   C7–C8 (radial)
(digits 2, 4, and 5)

Finger Adduction

165. Palmar Interossei:
    1st, 2nd, and 3rd, for C8–T1 (ulnar)
    digits 2, 4, and 5

155. Extensor indicis   C7–C8 (radial)
(for index finger)

Finger Motion: Little Finger

Flexion (Digit 5)

Carpometacarpal (CMC)

161. Opponens digiti minimi C8–T1 (ulnar)

Metacarpophalangeal (MP)

160. Flexor digiti minimi   C8–T1 (ulnar)
brevis

159. Abductor digiti minimi C8–T1 (ulnar)

163. 4th Lumbrical   C8–T1 (ulnar)

165. 3rd Palmar Interosseus C8–T1 (ulnar)

156. Flexor digitorum   C8–T1 (median)
superficialis for digit 5

157. Flexor digitorum   C8–T1 (ulnar)
profundus for digit 5

Proximal Interphalangeal (PIP)

156. Flexor digitorum   C8–T1 (median)
superficialis

157. Flexor digitorum   C8–T1 (ulnar)
profundus for digit 5

Distal Interphalangeal (DIP)

157. Flexor digitorum   C8–T1 (ulnar)
profundus for digit 5

Extension (Digit 5)

Metacarpophalangeal (MP)

154. Extensor digitorum   C7–C8 (radial)

158. Extensor digiti minimi C7–C8 (radial)

Proximal and Distal Interphalangeal (PIP and DIP)

154. Extensor digitorum   C7–C8 (radial)

158. Extensor digiti minimi C7–C8 (radial)

163. 4th Lumbrical   C8–T1 (ulnar)

165. 3rd palmar Interosseus C8–T1 (ulnar)

Abduction (Digit 5)

154. Extensor digitorum   C7–C8 (radial)
for 5th digit

159. Abductor digiti minimi C8–T1 (ulnar)

158. Extensor digiti minimi C7–C8 (radial)

161. Opponens digiti minimi C8–T1 (ulnar)

Adduction (Digit 5)

165. 3rd palmar Interosseus C8–T1 (ulnar)

Opposition (Digit 5)

159. Abductor digiti minimi C8–T1 (ulnar)

161. Opponens digiti minimi C8–T1 (ulnar)

160. Flexor digiti minimi   C8–T1 (ulnar)
brevis

163. 4th Lumbrical   C8–T1 (ulnar)

165. 3rd palmar Interosseus C8–T1 (ulnar)

LOWER EXTREMITY MOTIONS

Hip Motions

Hip Flexion

176. Iliacus   L2–L3 (femoral)

174. Psoas major   L2–L4 (often L1)

196. Rectus femoris   L2–L4 (femoral)

195. Sartorius   L2–L3 (femoral)

177. Pectineus	L2–L3 (femoral)	
179. Adductor longus	L2 or L3–L4 (obturator)	
180. Adductor brevis	L2–L4 (obturator)	
181. Adductor magnus (superior)	L2–L4 (obturator)	
185. Tensor fasciae latae	L4–S1 (superior gluteal)	
183. Gluteus medius (anterior)	L4–S1 (superior gluteal)	

Hip Extension

182. Gluteus maximus	L5–S2 (inferior gluteal)
192. Biceps femoris (long)	L5–S2 (sciatic [tibial])
193. Semitendinosus	L5–S2 (sciatic [tibial])
194. Semimembranosus	L5–S2 (sciatic [tibial])
181. Adductor magnus (inferior)	L2–L4 (sciatic [tibial])
183. Gluteus medius (posterior)	L4–S1 (superior gluteal)

Hip Abduction

183. Gluteus medius	L4–S1 (superior gluteal)
184. Gluteus minimus	L4–S1 (superior gluteal)
185. Tensor fasciae latae	L4–S1 (superior gluteal)
195. Sartorius	L2–L3 (femoral)
182. Gluteus maximus (upper)	L5–S2 (inferior gluteal)
186. Piriformis (hip flexed)	S1–S2 (nerve to Piriformis)
189. Gemellus superior (hip flexed)	L5–S1 (nerve to Obturator internus)
190. Gemellus inferior (hip flexed)	L5–S1 (nerve to Quadratus femoris)
187. Obturator internus (hip flexed)	L5–S1 (nerve to Obturator internus)

Hip Adduction

181. Adductor magnus	L2–L4 (sciatic [tibial] and obturator)

180. Adductor brevis	L2–L3 (obturator)
179. Adductor longus	L2 or L3–L4 (obturator)
177. Pectineus	L2–L3 (femoral)
178. Gracilis	L2–L3 (obturator)
188. Obturator externus	L3–L4 (obturator)
182. Gluteus maximus (lower)	L5–S2 (inferior gluteal)

Hip Internal Rotation (Medial rotation)

183. Gluteus medius (anterior)	L4–S1 (superior gluteal)
184. Gluteus minimus	L4–S1 (superior gluteal)
185. Tensor fasciae latae	L4–S1 (superior gluteal)
194. Semimembranosus	L5–S2 (sciatic [tibial])
193. Semitendinosus	L5–S2 (sciatic [tibial])
181. Adductor magnus[29]	L2–L4 (obturator, sciatic [tibial])
179. Adductor longus	L2 or L3–L4 (obturator)

Hip External Rotation (Lateral rotation)

182. Gluteus maximus	L5–S2 (inferior gluteal)
188. Obturator externus	L3–L4 (obturator)
191. Quadratus femoris	L5–S1 (nerve to Quadratus femoris)
189. Gemellus superior	L5–S1 (nerve to Obturator internus)
190. Gemellus inferior	L5–S1 (nerve to Quadratus femoris)
187. Obturator internus	L5–S1 (nerve to Obturator internus)
186. Piriformis	S1–S2 (nerve to Piriformis)
195. Sartorius	L2–L3 (femoral)
192. Biceps femoris (long)	L5–S2 (sciatic [tibial])
183. Gluteus medius (posterior)	L4–S1 (superior gluteal)
174. Psoas major	L2–L4
202. Popliteus (tibia fixed)	L4–S1 (tibial)

Knee Motions

Knee Flexion

194. Semimembranosus	L5–S2 (sciatic [tibial])
193. Semitendinosus	L5–S2 (sciatic [tibial])
192. Biceps femoris:	
Long	L5–S2 (sciatic [tibial])
Short	L5–S2 (sciatic, common peroneal)
178. Gracilis	L2–L3 (obturator)
195. Sartorius	L2–L3 (femoral)
202. Popliteus	L4–S1 (tibial)
185. Tensor fasciae latae (via iliotibial band) (after 30° knee flexion)	L4–S1 (superior gluteal)
207. Plantaris	S1–S2 (tibial)
205. Gastrocnemius	S1–S2 (tibial)

Knee Extension

196–200. Quadriceps femoris (all):	L2–L4 (femoral)
196. Rectus femoris	
197. Vastus lateralis	
198. Vastus intermedius	
199. Vastus medialis longus	
200. Vastus medialis oblique	
185. Tensor fasciae latae	L4–S1 (superior gluteal)

Knee Internal Rotation (Knee flexed)

194. Semimembranosus	L5–S2 (sciatic [tibial])
193. Semitendinosus	L5–S2 (sciatic [tibial])
195. Sartorius	L2–L3 (femoral)
178. Gracilis	L2–L3 (obturator)
202. Popliteus	L4–S1 (tibial)

Knee External Rotation (Knee flexed)

192. Biceps femoris:	
Long head	L5–S2 (sciatic [tibial])
Short head	L5–S2 (sciatic, common peroneal)
185. Tensor fasciae latae	L4–S1 (superior gluteal)

Ankle and Foot Motions

Ankle Plantar Flexion

205. Gastrocnemius	S1–S2 (tibial)
206. Soleus	S1–S2 (tibial)
204. Tibialis posterior	L4–L5 (tibial)
208. Peroneus longus	L5–S1 (superficial peroneal)
209. Peroneus brevis	L5–S1 (superficial peroneal)
207. Plantaris	S1–S2 (tibial)
222. Flexor hallucis longus	L5–S2 (tibial)
213. Flexor digitorum longus	L5–S2 (tibial)

Ankle Dorsiflexion

203. Tibialis anterior	L4–L5 (deep peroneal)
210. Peroneus tertius	L5–S1 (deep peroneal)
221. Extensor hallucis longus	L5 (deep peroneal) (L4–S1 also cited)
211. Extensor digitorum longus	L5–S1 (deep peroneal)

Foot Inversion

204. Tibialis posterior	L4–L5 (tibial)
203. Tibialis anterior	L4–L5 (deep peroneal)
221. Extensor hallucis longus	L5 (deep peroneal)
222. Flexor hallucis longus	L5–S2 (tibial)
213. Flexor digitorum longus	L5–S2 (tibial)
206. Soleus	S1–S2 (tibial)

Foot Eversion

208. Peroneus longus	L5–S1 (superficial peroneal)
209. Peroneus brevis	L5–S1 (superficial peroneal)

205. Gastrocnemius (medial head)   S1–S2 (tibial)

210. Peroneus tertius   L5–S1 (deep peroneal)

211. Extensor digitorum longus   L5–S1 (deep peroneal)

Motions of the Hallux

Great Toe Flexion

Proximal Joint (MP)

223. Flexor hallucis brevis   S1–S2 (medial plantar)

222. Flexor hallucis longus   L5–S2 (tibial)

224. Abductor hallucis   S1–S2 (medial plantar)

225. Adductor hallucis   S2–S3 (lateral plantar)

Distal Joint (IP)

222. Flexor hallucis longus   L5–S2 (tibial)

Great Toe Extension (Toe 1)

Proximal Joint (MP)

221. Extensor hallucis longus   L5 (deep peroneal) (L1–S4 also cited)

212. Extensor digitorum brevis   L5–S1 (deep peroneal)

Distal Joint (IP)

221. Extensor hallucis longus   L5 (deep peroneal)

Great Toe Abduction (Away from toe 2)

224. Abductor hallucis   S1–S2 (medial plantar)

Great Toe Adduction (Toward toe 2)

225. Adductor hallucis   S2–S3 (lateral plantar)

Motions of Toes 2, 3, and 4

Toe Flexion

MP Joints

218. Lumbricales:

1st, for digit 2   L5–S1 (medial plantar)

2nd, 3rd, and 4th, for digits 3, 4, and 5   S2–S3 (lateral plantar)

220. Plantar Interossei:
1st and 2nd, for digits 3 and 4   S2–S3 (lateral plantar, deep branch)

3rd, for digit 5   S2–S3 (lateral plantar, superficial branch)

219. Dorsal interossei, 1st to 4th, for digits 2 to 5   S2–S3 (lateral plantar)

214. Flexor digitorum brevis   S1–S2 (medial plantar)

213. Flexor digitorum longus   L5–S2 (tibial)

PIP Joints

214. Flexor digitorum brevis   S1–S2 (medial plantar)

213. Flexor digitorum longus   L5–S2 (tibial)

DIP Joints

213. Flexor digitorum longus   L5–S2 (tibial)

217. Quadratus plantae   S1–S3 (lateral plantar)

Toe Extension

Proximal Joints (MP)

211. Extensor digitorum longus   L5–S1 (deep peroneal)

212. Extensor digitorum brevis   L5–S1 (deep peroneal)

Middle and Distal Joints (PIP and DIP)

211. Extensor digitorum longus   L5–S1 (deep peroneal)

212. Extensor digitorum brevis   L5–S1 (deep peroneal)

218. Lumbricales:
1st for digit 2   L5–S1 (medial plantar)

2nd, 3rd, and 4th, for digits 3, 4, and 5   S2–S3 (lateral plantar)

220. Plantar Interossei for digits 3 to 5   S2–S3 (lateral plantar)

219. Dorsal Interossei for digits 2 to 5   S2–S3 (lateral plantar)

Toe Abduction *(Away from axial line through digit 2)*

219. Dorsal Interossei, 2nd, 3rd, and 4th, for digits 2, 3, and 4   S2–S3 (lateral plantar)

Toe Adduction *(Toward axial line through digit 2)*

220. Plantar interossei, 1st, 2nd, and 3rd, for digits 3, 4, and 5   S2–S3 (lateral plantar)

Motions of the Little Toe

Little Toe Flexion

MP Joint

216. Flexor digiti minimi brevis   S2–S3 (lateral plantar)

215. Abductor digiti minimi   S1–S3 (lateral plantar)

218. Lumbrical, 4th   S2–S3 (lateral plantar)

220. Interosseus, 3rd plantar   S2–S3 (lateral plantar)

214. Flexor digitorum brevis   S1–S2 (medial plantar)

213. Flexor digitorum longus   L5–S2 (tibial)

PIP Joint

214. Flexor digitorum brevis   S1–S2 (medial plantar)

213. Flexor digitorum longus   L5–S2 (tibial)

DIP Joint

213. Flexor digitorum longus   L5–S2 (tibial)

217. Quadratus plantae (Flexor digitorum accessorius)   S1–S3 (lateral plantar)

Little Toe Extension

Proximal Joint (MP)

211. Extensor digitorum longus   L5–S1 (deep peroneal)

Middle and Distal Joints (PIP and DIP)

211. Extensor digitorum longus   L5–S1 (deep peroneal)

218. Lumbrical, 4th   S2–S3 (lateral plantar)

220. Interosseus, 3rd plantar   S2–S3 (lateral plantar)

Little Toe Abduction *(Away from digit 4)*

215. Abductor digiti minimi   S1–S3 (lateral plantar)

Little Toe Adduction *(Toward digit 4)*

220. Interosseus, 3rd plantar   S2–S3 (lateral plantar)

PART 5. CRANIAL AND PERIPHERAL NERVES AND THE MUSCLES THEY INNERVATE

The sources used to report muscle innervations often cite very variable nerve supply to a given muscle in a human population. Such variability may occur because of individual differences in the distribution of peripheral nerves; or population differences; or the presence of injury (known or unknown) in the peripheral nerve pattern, among other things.

Among individuals, the patterns of nerve branching can vary considerably. An injury to a nerve may occur high or low along the pathway so that fibers not "caught" in the injury, or arising above it, may not show signs of dysfunction, leading to clinical ambiguity.

Objective data for a given muscle may not be available because the muscle is not available for thorough study; for example, the small and deep muscles of the hip, such as the Obturator externus and Gemellus superior. Thus, assignment of specific innervation levels often draws from conjecture as much as fact.

Readers should not be distraught at differences in segmental innervation sources from text to text, or author to author as these are most likely minor irritations and not noteworthy errors.

CRANIAL NERVES

Oculomotor (III)

Superior Division

- 3 Levator palpebrae superioris
- 6 Rectus superior

Inferior Division

- 7 Rectus inferior
- 8 Rectus medialis
- 11 Obliquus inferior

Trochlear (IV)

- 10 Obliquus superior

Trigeminal (V) *(largest of the cranial nerves)*

Mandibular Division

- 28 Masseter (masseteric branch)
- 29 Temporalis (deep temporal branch)
- 30 Lateral pterygoid (nerve to Lateral pterygoid)
- 31 Medial pterygoid (nerve to Medial pterygoid)
- 78 Digastric, anterior belly (inferior alveolar nerve)
- 75 Mylohyoid (inferior alveolar nerve, nerve to Mylohyoid)
- 46 Tensor veli palatini (nerve to Medial pterygoid)

Abducent (VI)

- 9 Rectus lateralis

Facial (VII) (see Fig. 9–10)

- 1 Occipitofrontalis (posterior auricular nerve)
  Frontalis (temporal branch)
  Occipitalis (posterior auricular nerve, occipital branch)
- 2 Temporoparietalis (temporal branch)
- 4 Orbicularis oculi (temporal and zygomatic branches)
- 5 Corrugator supercilii (temporal branch)
- 12 Procerus (buccal branch)
- 13 Nasalis (zygomatic branch)
- 14 Depressor septi (buccal branch)
- 15 Levator labii superioris (buccal branch)
- 16 Levator labii superioris alaeque nasi (buccal branch)
- 17 Levator anguli oris (buccal branch)
- 18 Zygomaticus major (buccal branch)
- 19 Zygomaticus minor (buccal branch)
- 20 Risorius (marginal mandibular branch)
- 21 Mentalis (marginal mandibular branch)
- 22 Transversus menti (marginal mandibular branch)
- 23 Depressor anguli oris (marginal mandibular branch)
- 24 Depressor labii inferioris (marginal mandibular branch)
- 25 Orbicularis oris (buccal and marginal mandibular branches)
- 26 Buccinator (buccal branch)
- 27 Auriculares posterior to posterior auricular nerve; Auriculares, anterior and superior (temporal branch)
- 78 Digastric, posterior belly (digastric branch)
- 76 Stylohyoid (stylohyoid branch)
- 88 Platysma (cervical branch)

Glossopharyngeal (IX)

44 Stylopharyngeus

Vagus (X)

36 Palatoglossus (via pharyngeal plexus)

41 Inferior pharyngeal constrictor (via pharyngeal plexus, including accessory [XI] nerve)

42 Middle pharyngeal constrictor (via pharyngeal plexus, including accessory [XI] nerve)

43 Superior pharyngeal constrictor (via pharyngeal plexus, including accessory [XI] nerve)

45 Salpingopharyngeus (via pharyngeal plexus, including accessory [XI] nerve)

49 Palatopharyngeus (via pharyngeal plexus)

46 Levator veli palatini (via pharyngeal plexus, including accessory [XI], vagus (X), and glossopharyngeal (IX) nerves)

48 Musculus uvulae (via pharyngeal plexus)

50 Cricothyroid (external laryngeal nerve)

51 Posterior cricoarytenoid (recurrent laryngeal nerve)

52 Lateral cricoarytenoid (recurrent laryngeal nerve)

53 Transverse arytenoid (recurrent laryngeal nerve)

54 Oblique arytenoid (recurrent laryngeal nerve)

55 Thyroarytenoid (recurrent laryngeal nerve)

Accessory (XI) (*with the vagus forms the pharyngeal plexus*)

48 Musculus uvulae (via pharyngeal plexus)

46 Levator veli palatini (via pharyngeal plexus)

43 Superior pharyngeal constrictor (via pharyngeal plexus)

42 Middle pharyngeal constrictor (pharyngeal plexus)

41 Inferior pharyngeal constrictor (via pharyngeal plexus)

45 Salpingopharyngeus (via pharyngeal plexus)

83 Sternocleidomastoid (spinal part and communication with C2–C3)

124 Trapezius (with fibers from C3–C4)

49 Palatopharyngeus (via pharyngeal plexus)

Hypoglossal (XII) (*motor nerve to the tongue*)

32 Genioglossus (muscular branch)

33 Hyoglossus (muscular branch)

34 Chondroglossus (muscular branch)

35 Styloglossus (muscular branch)

37 Superior longitudinal (muscular branch)

38 Inferior longitudinal (muscular branch)

39 Transverse lingual (muscular branch)

40 Vertical lingual (muscular branch)

77 Geniohyoid (nerve to Geniohyoid with fibers from 1st cervical nerve)

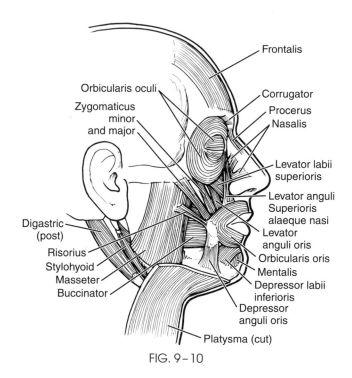

FIG. 9–10

Table 9-1 THE CRANIAL NERVES

Nerve	Origin	Branches (Motor)	Muscles Innervated
Olfactory (I) (all sensory)	Olfactory mucosa, high nasal cavity to olfactory bulb	Filamentous	No motor innervation
Optic (II) (central pathway connecting retina with brain)	Retina (ganglionic layer) and ends in optic chiasm	Peripheral nerves are in layers of retina (rod and cone receptors)	No motor innervation
Oculomotor (III)	Complex of nuclei in midbrain gray matter	*Superior division*	Levator palpebrae superioris Rectus superior
		Inferior division	Rectus inferior Inferior oblique Rectus medius
Trochlear (IV)	Nucleus is in cerebral aqueduct gray matter just above pons	Bilateral nerves	Superior oblique
Trigeminal (V) (largest cranial nerve, both motor and sensory)	Nuclei in lateral reticular formation of pons near floor of 4th ventricle	*Mandibular nerve*	Lower face and muscles of Mastication
		Anterior trunk Inferior alveolar nerve, mylohyoid branch	Digastric (anterior belly) Mylohyoid
		Nerve to Medial pterygoid Nerve to Lateral pterygoid Masseteric nerve Deep temporal nerve	Medial pterygoid Tensor veli palatini[13] Lateral pterygoid Masseter Temporalis
		Posterior trunk (Mainly sensory except for a few motor fibers to the) Mylohyoid	Mylohyoid
Abducent (VI)	Abducent nucleus (floor of 4th ventricle) dorsal to pons	Bilateral nerves	Rectus lateralis
Facial (VII) (predominantly motor) (sensory root called *nervus intermedius*) (Readers should know that there are untold variations in the pattern of branching of the facial (VII) nerve and the muscles innervated by each)	Motor nucleus lies in the reticular formation of the pons (lower border) Motor nucleus has 3 subnuclei: (1) Lateral (buccal) (2) Intermediate (orbital, temporal, and zygomatic facial branches) (3) Medial (auricular and cervical rami) Motor fibers also arise in superior salivatory nucleus (to muscles around eyes and forehead)	*Motor root* Posterior auricular nerve Occipital branch Digastric branch Stylohyoid branch Temporal branches Zygomatic branch	All muscles of facial expression Auriculares (posterior) Occipitofrontalis (occipital belly) Digastric (posterior belly) Stylohyoid Auriculares (Superior and anterior) Occipitofrontalis (frontal belly) Corrugator Orbicularis oculi, upper half Nasalis Orbicularis oculi, lower half

Table continued on following page

Table 9-1 THE CRANIAL NERVES *Continued*

Nerve	Origin	Branches (Motor)	Muscles Innervated

NOTE:
The buccal branches of nerves V and VII intermingle in the buccal area with their connective tissue sheaths fusing to form a buccal plexus. Rarely is it possible to trace individual motor branches from V or VII through the plexus to a specific muscle. Sensory fibers also are involved in the plexus.
		Buccal branch	Muscles of the nose and upper lip:
			  Procerus
			  Depressor septi
			  Levator labii superioris
			  Levator anguli oris
			Zygomatic major and minor
			Buccinator
			Orbicularis oris
			Levator labii superioris alaque nasi

		Marginal mandibular branch	Risorius Mentalis Depressor labii inferioris Orbicularis oris Depressor anguli oris
		Cervical branch	Platysma
Vestibular (XIII) (contains two fiber systems: vestibular and cochlear)	Central from groove between pons and medulla Vestibular ganglion in outer part of internal auditory meatus	No motor nerves	Maintains equilibrium and posture; orientation in space No skeletal muscle innervation
Glossopharyngeal (IX) (both motor and sensory)	Medulla (upper) nucleus ambiguous (rostral part)	Muscular branch	Stylopharyngeus Middle and inferior pharyngeal constrictors
Vagus (X) (both motor and sensory)	Medulla Vagal portion of nucleus ambiguous (to striated muscle)	Recurrent laryngeal Superior laryngeal External laryngeal Pharyngeal plexus (Joins with external pharyngeal n. and glossopharyngeal n. to form pharyngeal plexus with contributions from Hypoglossal n.)	Striated muscles of larynx Cricothyroid and Inferior constrictor Muscles of palate, pharynx No innervation to Stylopharyngeus or Tensor veli palatini
Accessory (XI) (The accessory part of this nerve is accessory to the vagus. The cranial part cannot be distinguished from the vagus.)	Caudal portion of the nucleus ambiguous in medulla Dorsal efferent nucleus Accessory nuclei in ventral horn from medulla to C6	Spinal (accessory) part (ramus externus) Blends especially with pharyngeal and superior laryngeal branches of the vagus. Unites with C2 and C3 and forms plexus with C3 and C4.	Pharyngeal muscles Intrinsic muscles of larynx (few slips) Arytenoids Sternocleidomastoid Trapezius

Hypoglossal (XII)
(all motor)
	Medulla
	Hypoglossal nuclei
	  Medial division
	  Lateral division
	Communicates with vagus and contributes to Pharyngeal plexus
		Descending branch
		  Upper root (C1–C3) of ansa cervicalis
		Muscular branch
		Nerve to thyrohyoid
		Nerve to geniohyoid (includes fibers from C1)
			Omohyoid
			Sternohyoid
			Sternothyroid
			Tongue muscles
			  Extrinsic and Intrinsic
			(no innervation to palatoglossus)
			Thyrohyoid
			Geniohyoid

PERIPHERAL NERVES

Nerves from Cervical and Brachial Plexuses (Upper Extremity Muscle Innervation)

 Cervical Plexus (Fig. 9–11)

1. Ventral primary divisions of first four cervical nerves (C1–C4).
2. C2, C3, and C4 divide into superior and inferior branches.
3. The cervical plexus communicates with three motor cranial nerves (vagus, hypoglossal, accessory).
4. Special nerves often leave both the cervical and brachial plexuses and supply motor innervation to individual muscles. These special nerves, when named, are usually named for the muscle they supply (e.g., nerve to Rectus capitis anterior). These nerves are listed under the appropriate spinal nerves (myotomes) in Part IV of this chapter.

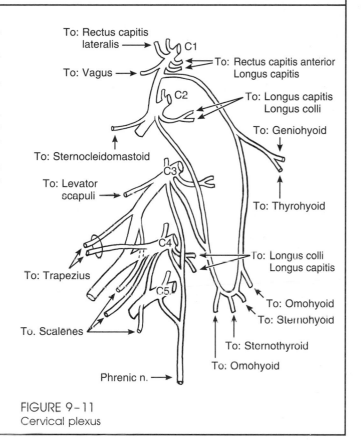

FIGURE 9–11
Cervical plexus

Brachial Plexus (Fig. 9–12)

1. Comprises the ventral primary divisions of the last four cervical (C5–C8) and the first thoracic (T1) nerves.
2. Supplies the nerves to the upper extremity.

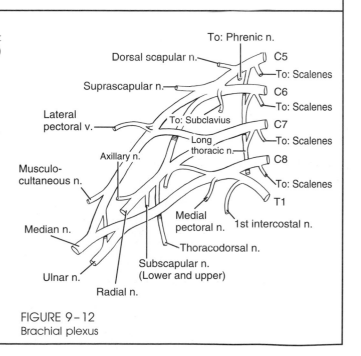

FIGURE 9–12
Brachial plexus

The Cervical Plexus (see Fig. 9–11)

Suboccipital Nerve (C1; first cervical dorsal ramus)

56 Rectus capitis posterior major

57 Rectus capitis posterior minor

58 Obliquus capitis superior

59 Obliquus capitis inferior

Greater Occipital Nerve (C1–C2, second cervical dorsal ramus)

Medial branch:

62 Semispinalis capitis

Lateral branch:

61 Splenius capitis

60 Longissimus capitis

62 Semispinalis capitis

Inferior Root of Ansa cervicalis C2–C3

84 Sternothyroid

86 Sternohyoid

87 Omohyoid (inferior belly)

Superior Root of Ansa cervicalis C1

85 Thyrohyoid

77 Geniohyoid

87 Omohyoid (superior belly)

Muscular Branches (deep branches, medial)

73 Rectus capitis lateralis C1–C2

72 Rectus capitis anterior C1–C2

74 Longus capitis C1–C3

79 Longus colli C2–C6

Muscular Branches (deep branches, lateral)

83 Sternocleidomastoid C2–C4

124 Trapezius C3–C4 (lower fibers)

127 Levator scapulae C3–C5

81 Scalenus medius C3–C8

Phrenic Nerve (C4; contributions from C3 and C5)

101 Diaphragm

The Brachial Plexus (see Fig. 9–12)

Cervical Spinal Roots

80 Scalenus anterior C4–C6 (ventral rami)

81 Scalenus medius C3–C8 (ventral rami)

82 Scalenus posterior C6–C8 (ventral rami)

Dorsal Scapular Nerve (C5, ventral ramus)

127 Levator scapulae

125 Rhomboid major

126 Rhomboid minor

Long Thoracic Nerve (C5–C7, ventral rami)

128 Serratus anterior

Suprascapular Nerve (C5–C6)

135 Supraspinatus

136 Infraspinatus

Nerve to Subclavius (C5–C6, ventral rami)

132 Subclavius

Lateral Pectoral Nerve (C5–C6, ventral rami)

131 Pectoralis major (clavicular portion)

129 Pectoralis minor

Medial Pectoral Nerve (C8–T1, ventral rami)

131 Pectoralis major (sternocostal portion)

129 Pectoralis minor

Subscapular Nerve (superior and inferior) (C5–C6, ventral rami)

34 Subscapularis	C5–C6 (superior and inferior)
138 Teres major	C5–C6 (inferior)

Thoracodorsal Nerve (C6–C8, ventral rami)

130 Latissimus dorsi

Musculocutaneous Nerve (C5–C7, ventral rami)

140 Biceps brachii (both heads)	C5–C6
141 Brachialis	C5–C6
139 Coracobrachialis	C5–C7

Axillary Nerve (C5–C6, ventral rami)

137 Teres minor (posterior branch)

133 Deltoid (anterior and posterior branches)

Median Nerve (C6–T1)

Supplies most of the flexor muscles of the forearm and the thenar muscles of the hand. The nerve has no branches above the elbow except on occasion when the nerve to the Pronator teres arises there. It arises from two roots:

Lateral (C5–C7, ventral rami)
Medial (C8–T1, ventral rami)

Muscular Branches in Forearm:

151	Flexor carpi radialis	C6–C7
146	Pronator teres	C6–C7
152	Palmaris longus	C7–C8
156	Flexor digitorum superficialis	C8–T1

Anterior Interosseus Nerve:

169	Flexor pollicis longus	C7–C8
157	Flexor digitorum profundus (lateral part)	C8–T1
147	Pronator quadratus	C7–C8

Muscular Branches in Hand (lateral terminal branch)

171	Abductor pollicis brevis	C8–T1
172	Opponens pollicis	C8–T1
170	Flexor pollicis brevis (superficial head)	C8–T1

Common Palmar Digital nerves (has four or five such)
1st and 2nd Common Palmar Digital Nerves

163	1st and 2nd Lumbricales	C8–T1

Radial Nerve (C5–C8)

This largest of the branches of the brachial plexus arises from the posterior cord, roots C5–T1. It supplies the extensor muscles of the arm and forearm. Its motor branches are the muscular and the posterior interosseous.

Muscular Branches

141	Brachialis	C7
142	Triceps brachii	C6–C8
144	Anconeus	C7–C8
143	Brachioradialis	C5–C6
148	Extensor carpi radialis longus	C6–C7

Posterior Interosseous Nerve

145	Supinator	C6–C7
149	Extensor carpi radialis brevis	C7–C8
158	Extensor digiti minimi	C7–C8
150	Extensor carpi ulnaris	C7–C8
154	Extensor digitorum	C7–C8
155	Extensor indicis	C7–C8
167	Extensor pollicis longus	C7–C8
168	Extensor pollicis brevis	C7–C8
166	Abductor pollicis longus	C7–C8

Ulnar Nerve (C8–T1)

Rises from the posterior cord to supply the muscles on the ulnar side of the forearm and hand. Its branches are the muscular, superficial terminal, and deep terminal

173	Adductor pollicis	C8–T1 (deep branch)
159	Abductor digiti minimi	C8–T1 (deep branch)
161	Opponens digiti minimi	C8–T1 (deep branch)
160	Flexor digiti minimi brevis	C8–T1 (deep branch)
157	Flexor digitorum profundus (medial part)	C8–T1 (muscular branch)
163	Lumbricales, 3rd and 4th	C8–T1 (deep branch)
153	Flexor carpi ulnaris	C7–T1 (muscular branch)
162	Palmaris brevis	C8–T1 (superficial branch)
164	Dorsal Interossei	C8–T1 (deep branch)
165	Palmar Interossei	C8–T1 (deep branch)
170	Flexor pollicis brevis (deep head)	C8–T1 (deep branch)
172	Opponens pollicis	C8–T1 (terminal branch)

Nerves of the Thoracic and Abdominal Regions

The muscles innervated by the thoracic and abdominal nerves are those that connect adjacent ribs (the intercostals); those that span a number of ribs between their attachments (the subcostals); and those that connect the ribs to the sternum (Transversus thoracis) and the ribs to the vertebrae (Levator costarum, Serratus posterior superior and posterior inferior).

Superior Thoracic Nerves (T1–T6, ventral rami)

Thoracic Intercostal Nerves

102	Intercostales interni	T1–T11
103	Intercostales externi	T1–T11
107	Levatores costarum	T1–T11 (dorsal rami)
108	Serratus posterior superior	T2–T5
106	Transversus thoracis	T2–T11

Lower Thoracic Nerves (T7–T12, ventral rami)

Thoracoabdominal Intercostal Nerves

102	Intercostales interni	T1–T11
103	Intercostales externi	T1–T11
104	Intercostales intimi	T1–T11
105	Subcostales	T7–T11

Spinal Nerves

110	Obliquus externus abdominis	T7–T12

111	Obliquus internus abdominis	T7–T12 (intercostal, ilioinguinal, and iliohypogastric nerves)
112	Transversus abdominis	T7–L1 (ilioinguinal, iliohypogastric)
113	Rectus abdominis	T7–T12
109	Serratus posterior inferior	T9–T12

Subcostal Nerve (T12)

114	Pyramidalis	T12
112	Transversus abdominis	T7–T12

Nerves from Lumbar and Sacral (Including Pudendal) Plexuses (Lower Extremity and Perineal Muscle Innervation)

Muscles Innervated Directly off Lumbar Plexus (Fig. 9–13)

100	Quadratus lumborum	T12–L3
174	Psoas major	L2–L4
175	Psoas minor	L1

Iliohypogastric (L1[T12])

112	Transversus abdominis	L1 (and T7–T12)
111	Obliquus internus abdominis	L1 (and T7–T12)

Ilioinguinal (L1)

112	Transversus abdominis	L1 (and T7–T12)
111	Obliquus internus abdominis	L1 (and T7–T12)

Genitofemoral (L1–L2)

117	Cremaster	L1–L2

Accessory Obturator (L3–L4) (When Present)

177	Pectineus	L3 (and femoral, L2–L3)

Obturator Nerve (L2–L4)

Anterior Branch

180	Adductor brevis	L2 or L3–L4
179	Adductor longus	L2–L4
178	Gracilis	L2–L3
177	Pectineus (often)	L2–L3

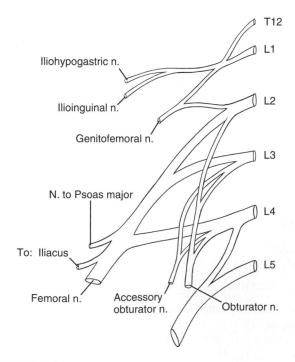

FIGURE 9–13
Lumbar plexus

Posterior Branch

181	Adductor magnus (superior and middle)	L2–L4
188	Obturator externus	L3–L4
180	Adductor brevis (unless supplied by anterior branch)	

Femoral Nerve (L2–L4)

176	Iliacus	L2–L3
177	Pectineus	L2–L3
195	Sartorius	L2–L3
196	Rectus femoris	L2–L4
198	Vastus intermedius	L2–L4
197	Vastus lateralis	L2–L4
199	Vastus medialis longus	L2–L4
200	Vastus medialis oblique	L2–L4
201	Articularis genus	L2–L4

Muscles Innervated via Sacral Plexus

Nerve to Quadratus femoris

191	Quadratus femoris	L5–S1
190	Gemellus inferior	L5–S1

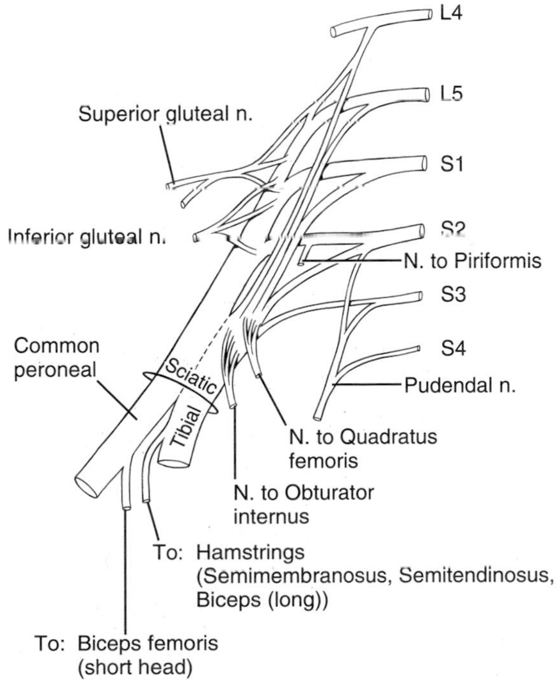

FIGURE 9–14
Sacral plexus

Nerve to Obturator internus

187	Obturator internus	L5–S1
189	Gemellus superior	L5–S1

Nerve to Piriformis

186	Piriformis	S1–S2

Superior Gluteal (L4–S1)

Superior Branch

184	Gluteus minimus	L4–S1

Inferior Branch

183	Gluteus medius	L4–S1
185	Tensor fasciae latae	L4–S1

Inferior Gluteal (L5–S2)

182	Gluteus maximus	L5–S2

Sciatic Nerve (L4–S3)

This is the largest nerve in the body, and it innervates the muscles of the posterior thigh and all of the muscles of the leg and foot. The sciatic trunk has a tibial component and a common peroneal component, which innervate five muscles before dividing to form the tibial and common peroneal nerves.

Common Peroneal Division (dorsal divisions L4–L5 and S1–S2)

192	Biceps femoris (short head)	L5–S2

Tibial Division (ventral divisions L4–L5 and S1–S3)

181	Adductor magnus (inferior)	L2–L4
192	Biceps femoris (long head)	L5–S2
194	Semimembranosus	L5–S2
193	Semitendinosus	L5–S2

Tibial Nerve (Medial Popliteal Nerve) (L4–S3)

This larger of the two main divisions of the sciatic nerve sends branches high in the leg to the posterior leg muscles (Triceps surae) and Popliteus. Lower branches supply motor innervation to the more distal posterior muscles. Its named branches are the lateral and medial plantar nerves.

High Branches

205	Gastrocnemius (both heads)	S1–S2
207	Plantaris	S1–S2
206	Soleus	S1–S2
202	Popliteus	L4–S1

Low Branches

206	Soleus	S1–S2
204	Tibialis posterior	L4–L5
213	Flexor digitorum longus	L5–S2
222	Flexor hallucis longus	L5–S2

Lateral Plantar Nerve (S2–S3)

| 217 | Quadratus plantae (Flexor digitorum accessorius) | S1–S3 |
| 215 | Abductor digiti minimi | S1–S3 |

Deep Branch

218	Lumbricales, 2nd, 3rd, and 4th	S2–S3
225	Adductor hallucis	S2–S3
219	Dorsal Interossei, 1st, 2nd, and 3rd	S2–S3
220	Plantar Interossei, 1st and 2nd	S2–S3

Superficial Branch

216	Flexor digiti minimi brevis	S2–S3
219	Dorsal interossei, 4th	S2–S3
220	Plantar interossei, 3rd	S2–S3

Medial Plantar Nerve (L5–S1)

218	Lumbrical, 1st	L5–S1
224	Abductor hallucis	S1–S2
223	Flexor hallucis brevis	S1–S2
214	Flexor digitorum brevis	S1–S2

Common Peroneal Nerve (L4–S2)

This smaller of the two divisions of the sciatic nerve divides into the deep and superficial peroneal nerves.

Deep Peroneal Nerve

203	Tibialis anterior	L4–L5
221	Extensor hallucis longus	L5
211	Extensor digitorum longus	L5–S1
212	Extensor digitorum brevis	L5–S1
210	Peroneus tertius	L5–S1
219	2nd Dorsal Interosseous	S2–S3

Superficial Peroneal Nerve

| 208 | Peroneus longus | L5–S1 |
| 209 | Peroneus brevis | L5–S1 |

Pudendal Plexus (Part of the Sacral Plexus)

Muscular Branches (S2–S4)

115	Levator ani	S2–S3
116	Coccygeus	S3–S4
123	Sphincter ani externus	S2–S3

Perineal Branch (S2–S4)

118	Transversus perinei superficialis	S2–S4
119	Transversus perinei profundus	S2–S4
120	Bulbocavernosus	S2–S4
121	Ischiocavernosus	S2–S4
122	Sphincter urethrae	S2–S4
123	Sphincter ani externus	S4

PART 6. MYOTOMES

THE MOTOR NERVE ROOTS AND THE MUSCLES THEY INNERVATE

In this portion of the Ready Reference chapter, the spinal roots for the axial and trunk skeletal muscles are outlined, along with the muscles innervated by each root. There are many variations of these innervation patterns, but this text presents a consensus derived from classic anatomy and neurology texts.

The muscles are presented here as originating from the dorsal or ventral primary rami. Each muscle is always preceded by its reference number for cross-reference. Named peripheral nerves for individual muscles are listed in parentheses (e.g., thoracodorsal) after the muscle. Specific muscle or part is in brackets.

The spinal nerves arise in the spinal cord and exit from it via the intervertebral foramina. There are 31 pairs: cervical (8), thoracic (12), lumbar (5), sacral (5), and coccygeal (1). These innervations are especially variable.

Each spinal nerve has two roots that unite to form the nerve: the *ventral root* (motor), which exits the cord from the ventral (anterior) horn, and the *dorsal root* (sensory), which enters the cord from the dorsal (posterior) horn. This text will address only the motor roots.

Each motor root divides into two parts:

1. *Primary ventral rami* (Fig. 9–15)
   The ventral rami supply the ventral and lateral trunk muscles and all limb muscles. The cervical, lumbar, and sacral ventral rami merge near their origin to form plexuses. The thoracic ventral rami remain individual and are distributed segmentally.
2. *Primary dorsal rami*
   The dorsal rami supply the muscles of the dorsal neck and trunk. The dorsal primary rami do not join any of the plexuses.

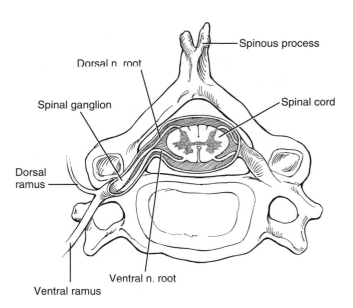

FIGURE 9–15
Rami of spinal nerves

The major plexuses formed by the cervical, lumbar, and sacral nerves are as follows:

Cervical plexus (ventral primary rami of C1–C4 and connecting cranial nerves)
Brachial plexus (ventral primary rami of C5–T1 and connections from C4 and T2)
Lumbosacral plexus (ventral primary rami of lumbar, sacral, pudendal, and coccygeal nerves)
Lumbar plexus (ventral primary rami of L1–L4 and communication from T12)
Sacral plexus (ventral primary rami of L4–L5 and S1–S3)
Pudendal plexus (ventral primary rami of S2–S4)
Coccygeal plexus (S4–S5)

THE CERVICAL ROOTS AND NERVES

C1

Ventral Primary Ramus

72 Rectus capitis anterior

73 Rectus capitis lateralis

74 Longus capitis

77 Geniohyoid

84 Sternothyroid

85 Thyrohyoid

86 Sternohyoid

87 Omohyoid

Dorsal Primary Ramus (of C1)

56 Rectus capitis posterior major

57 Rectus capitis posterior minor

58 Obliquus capitis superior

59 Obliquus capitis inferior

C2

Ventral Primary Ramus

72 Rectus capitis anterior

73 Rectus capitis lateralis

74 Longus capitis

79 Longus colli

83 Sternocleidomastoid

84 Sternothyroid

86 Sternohyoid

87 Omohyoid

Dorsal Primary Ramus[2,3]

60 Longissimus capitis

62 Semispinalis capitis

65 Semispinalis cervicis

94 Multifidi

C3

Ventral Primary Ramus

70 Intertransversarii cervicis

74 Longus capitis

79 Longus colli

84 Sternothyroid

86 Sternohyoid

87 Omohyoid

127 Levator scapulae (dorsal scapular)

81 Scalenus medius

83 Sternocleidomastoid

101 Diaphragm (C4)

124 Trapezius

Dorsal Primary Ramus (of C3)

60 Longissimus capitis

61 Splenius capitis

62 Semispinalis capitis

63 Spinalis capitis

64 Longissimus cervicis

65 Semispinalis cervicis

68 Spinalis cervicis

69 Interspinales cervicis

70 Intertransversarii cervicis [posterior]

71 Rotatores cervicis

94 Multifidi

C4

Ventral Primary Ramus

79 Longus colli

70 Intertransversarii cervicis [anterior]

127 Levator scapulae (dorsal scapular)

80 Scalenus anterior

81 Scalenus medius

101 Diaphragm (phrenic)

Dorsal Primary Ramus

61 Splenius capitis

62 Semispinalis capitis

63 Spinalis capitis

64 Longissimus cervicis

65 Semispinalis cervicis

66 Iliocostalis cervicis

67 Splenius cervicis

68 Spinalis cervicis

69 Interspinalis cervicis

70 Intertransversarii cervicis [posterior]

71 Rotatores cervicis

94 Multifidi

C5

Ventral Primary Ramus

79 Longus colli

70 Intertransversarii cervicis (anterior)

80 Scalenus anterior

81 Scalenus medius

132 Subclavius (n. to Subclavius)

101 Diaphragm

127 Levator scapulae (dorsal scapular)

125 Rhomboid major (dorsal scapular)

126 Rhomboid minor (dorsal scapular)

128 Serratus anterior (long thoracic)

129 Pectoralis minor (medial and lateral pectoral)

131 Pectoralis major [clavicular head] (lateral pectoral)

135 Supraspinatus (suprascapular)

136 Infraspinatus (suprascapular)

134 Subscapularis (subscapular, upper and lower)

138 Teres major (subscapular, lower)

133 Deltoid (axillary)

137 Teres minor (axillary)

139 Coracobrachialis (musculocutaneous)

140 Biceps brachii (musculocutaneous)

141 Brachialis (musculocutaneous)

143 Brachioradialis (radial)

Dorsal Primary Ramus (of C5)

60 Longissimus capitis

61 Splenius capitis

62 Semispinalis capitis

63 Spinalis capitis

64 Longissimus cervicis

65 Semispinalis cervicis

66 Iliocostalis cervicis

67 Splenius cervicis

68 Spinalis cervicis

69 Interspinalis cervicis

70 Intertransversarii cervicis [posterior]

72 Rotatores cervicis

94 Multifidi

C6

Ventral Primary Ramus

79 Longus colli

70 Intertransversarii cervicis [anterior]

80 Scalenus anterior

81 Scalenus medius

82 Scalenus posterior

130 Latissimus dorsi (thoracodorsal)

132 Subclavius (n. to Subclavius)

128 Serratus anterior (long thoracic)

131 Pectoralis major [clavicular head] (lateral pectoral) [Sternocostal head] (medial and lateral pectorals)

129 Pectoralis minor (medial and lateral pectorals)

136 Infraspinatus (suprascapular)

135 Supraspinatus (suprascapular)

134 Subscapularis (subscapular, upper and lower)

138 Teres major (subscapular, lower)

133 Deltoid (axillary)

137 Teres minor (axillary)

139 Coracobrachialis (musculocutaneous)

140 Biceps brachii (musculocutaneous)

141 Brachialis (musculocutaneous)

142 Triceps brachii (radial)

143 Brachioradialis (radial)

144 Anconeus (radial)

145 Supinator (radial)

148 Extensor carpi radialis longus (radial)

146 Pronator teres (median)

151 Flexor carpi radialis (median)

Dorsal Primary Ramus (of C6)

60 Longissimus capitis

61 Splenius capitis

62 Semispinalis capitis

63 Spinalis capitis

64 Longissimus cervicis

65 Semispinalis cervicis

66 Iliocostalis cervicis

67 Splenius cervicis

68 Spinalis cervicis

69 Interspinales cervicis

70 Intertransversarii cervicis [posterior]

71 Rotatores cervicis

93 Multifidi

C7

Ventral Primary Ramus

70 Intertransversarii cervicis [anterior]

81 Scalenus medius

82 Scalenus posterior

128 Serratus anterior (long thoracic)

130 Latissimus dorsi (thoracodorsal)

131 Pectoralis major, sternocostal head (medial and lateral pectorals)

129 Pectoralis minor (medial and lateral pectorals)

139 Coracobrachialis (musculocutaneous)

141 Brachialis (radial)

142 Triceps brachii (radial)

144 Anconeus (radial)

145 Supinator (radial)

148 Extensor carpi radialis longus (radial)

149 Extensor carpi radialis brevis (radial)

150 Extensor carpi ulnaris (radial)

154 Extensor digitorum (radial)

155 Extensor indicis (radial)

158 Extensor digiti minimi (radial)

166 Abductor pollicis longus (radial)

167 Extensor pollicis longus (radial)

168 Extensor pollicis brevis (radial)

146 Pronator teres (median)

147 Pronator quadratus (median)

151 Flexor carpi radialis (median)

152 Palmaris longus (median)

153 Flexor carpi ulnaris (median)

169 Flexor pollicis longus (median)

Dorsal Primary Ramus (of C7)

60 Longissimus capitis

62 Semispinalis capitis

63 Spinalis capitis

64 Longissimus cervicis

65 Semispinalis cervicis

66 Iliocostalis cervicis

67 Splenius cervicis

68 Spinalis cervicis

69 Interspinales cervicis

70 Intertransversarii cervicis [posterior]

71 Rotatores cervicis

94 Multifidi

C8

Ventral Primary Ramus

70 Intertransversarii cervicis [anterior]

81 Scalenus medius

82 Scalenus posterior

130 Latissimus dorsi (thoracodorsal)

131 Pectoralis major, sternocostal (lateral and medial pectorals)

129 Pectoralis minor (medial and lateral pectorals)

142 Triceps brachii (radial)

144 Anconeus (radial)

149 Extensor carpi radialis brevis (radial)

150 Extensor carpi ulnaris (radial)

154 Extensor digitorum (radial)

155 Extensor indicis (radial)

158 Extensor digiti minimi (radial)

166 Abductor pollicis longus (radial)

167 Extensor pollicis longus (radial)

168 Extensor pollicis brevis (radial)

147 Pronator quadratus (median) (C8)

152 Palmaris longus (median)

156 Flexor digitorum superficialis (median)

157 Flexor digitorum profundus, digits 2 and 3 (median)

163 Lumbricales, 1st and 2nd (median)

169 Flexor pollicis longus (median)

170 Flexor pollicis brevis, superficial head (median)

171 Abductor pollicis brevis (median)

172 Opponens pollicis (median, ulnar)

170 Flexor pollicis brevis, deep head (ulnar)

173 Adductor pollicis (ulnar)

153 Flexor carpi ulnaris (ulnar)

157 Flexor digitorum profundus, digits 4 and 5 (ulnar)

163 Lumbricales, 3rd and 4th (ulnar)

164 Interossei, dorsal (ulnar)

165 Interossei, palmar (ulnar)

159 Abductor digiti minimi (ulnar)

161 Opponens digiti minimi (ulnar)

160 Flexor digiti minimi brevis (ulnar)

162 Palmaris brevis (ulnar)

Dorsal Primary Ramus (of C8)

60 Longissimus capitis

62 Semispinalis capitis

63 Spinalis capitis

64 Longissimus cervicis

65 Semispinalis cervicis

66 Iliocostalis cervicis (variable)

67 Splenius cervicis

68 Spinalis cervicis (variable)

69 Interspinales cervicis

70 Intertransversarii cervicis [posterior]

71 Rotatores cervicis

94 Multifidi

THE THORACIC ROOTS AND NERVES

There are 12 pairs of thoracic nerves arising from the ventral primary rami: T1 to T11 are called the *intercostals* and T12 is called the *subcostal nerve*. These nerves are not part of a plexus. T1 and T2 innervate the upper extremity as well as the thorax; T3–T6 innervate only the thoracic muscles; the lower thoracic nerves innervate the thoracic and abdominal muscles.

T1

Ventral Primary Ramus

107 Levatores costarum

102 Intercostales externi

103 Intercostales interni

104 Intercostales intimi

131 Pectoralis major [sternocostal head] (medial and lateral pectoral)

129 Pectoralis minor (medial and lateral pectorals)

147 Pronator quadratus (median)

156 Flexor digitorum superficialis (median)

157 Flexor digitorum profundus, digits 2 and 3 (median)

163 Lumbricales, 1st and 2nd (median)

170 Flexor pollicis brevis [superficial head] (median)

171 Abductor pollicis brevis (median)

172 Opponens pollicis (median and ulnar)

153 Flexor carpi ulnaris (ulnar)

157 Flexor digitorum profundus, digits 4 and 5 (ulnar)

159 Abductor digiti minimi (ulnar)

160 Flexor digiti minimi brevis (ulnar)

161 Opponens digiti minimi (ulnar)

162 Palmaris brevis (ulnar)

163 Lumbricales, 3rd and 4th (ulnar)

164 Interossei, dorsal (ulnar)

165 Interossei, palmar (ulnar)

170 Flexor pollicis brevis [deep head] (ulnar)

173 Adductor pollicis (ulnar)

Dorsal Primary Ramus (of T1)

62 Semispinalis capitis

65 Semispinalis cervicis

93 Semispinalis thoracis

64 Longissimus cervicis

91 Longissimus thoracis

63 Spinalis capitis (highly variable)

92 Spinalis thoracis

89 Iliocostalis thoracis

66 Iliocostalis cervicis (variable)

94 Multifidi

99 Intertransversarii thoracis

95 Rotatores thoracis

97 Interspinales thoracis

T2

Ventral Primary Ramus

107 Levatores costarum

102 Intercostales externi

103 Intercostales interni

104 Intercostales intimi

108 Serratus posterior superior

106 Transversus thoracis

Dorsal Primary Ramus (of T2)

65 Semispinales cervicis (variable)

93 Semispinalis thoracis

64 Longissimus cervicis

91 Longissimus thoracis

92 Spinalis thoracis

66 Iliocostalis cervicis (variable)

89 Iliocostalis thoracis

94 Multifidi

95 Rotatores thoracis

97 Interspinales thoracis

99 Intertransversarii thoracis

T3

Ventral Primary Ramus

107 Levatores costarum

102 Intercostales externi

103 Intercostales interni

104 Intercostales intimi

108 Serratus posterior superior

106 Transversus thoracis

Dorsal Primary Ramus

93 Semispinalis thoracis

64 Longissimus cervicis (variable)

65 Semispinalis cervicis

91 Longissimus thoracis

92 Spinalis thoracis

66 Iliocostalis cervicis

89 Iliocostalis thoracis

94 Multifidi

95 Rotatores thoracis

97 Interspinales thoracis

99 Intertransversarii thoracis

T4, T5, T6

Ventral Primary Ramus

107 Levatores costarum

102 Intercostales externi

103 Intercostales interni

104 Intercostales intimi

106 Transversus thoracis

108 Serratus posterior superior (to T5)

Dorsal Primary Ramus

65 Semispinalis cervicis

89 Iliocostalis thoracis

93 Semispinalis thoracis

91 Longissimus thoracis

92 Spinalis thoracis

94 Multifidi

95 Rotatores thoracis

99 Intertransversarii thoracis

T7

Ventral Primary Ramus

107 Levatores costarum

103 Intercostales interni

102 Intercostales externi

104 Intercostales intimi

105 Subcostales

106 Transversus thoracis

110 Obliquus externus abdominis

111 Obliquus internus abdominis

112 Transversus abdominis

113 Rectus abdominis

Dorsal Primary Ramus

93 Semispinalis thoracis

91 Longissimus thoracis

92 Spinalis thoracis

89 Iliocostalis thoracis

94 Multifidi

95 Rotatores thoracis

99 Intertransversarii thoracis

T8

Ventral Primary Ramus

107 Levatores costarum

103 Intercostales interni

102 Intercostales externi

104 Intercostales intimi

105 Subcostales

106 Transversus thoracis

110 Obliquus externus abdominis

111 Obliquus internus abdominis

112 Transversus abdominis

113 Rectus abdominis

Dorsal Primary Ramus

93 Semispinalis thoracis

91 Longissimus thoracis

92 Spinalis thoracis

89 Iliocostalis thoracis

94 Multifidi

95 Rotatores thoracis

99 Intertransversarii thoracis

T9, T10, T11

Ventral Primary Ramus

107 Levatores costarum

103 Intercostales interni

102 Intercostales externi

104 Intercostales intimi

105 Subcostales

106 Transversus thoracis

109 Serratus posterior inferior

110 Obliquus externus abdominis

111 Obliquus internus abdominis

112 Transversus abdominis

113 Rectus abdominis

Dorsal Primary Ramus

93 Semispinalis thoracis

91 Longissimus thoracis

92 Spinalis thoracis

89 Iliocostalis thoracis

94 Multifidi

95 Rotatores thoracis

97 Interspinales thoracis

99 Intertransversarii thoracis

T12

Ventral Primary Ramus

100 Quadratus lumborum

112 Transversus abdominis

109 Serratus posterior inferior

110 Obliquus externus abdominis

111 Obliquus internus abdominis

113 Rectus abdominis

114 Pyramidalis

Dorsal Primary Ramus

93 Semispinalis thoracis

91 Longissimus thoracis

92 Spinalis thoracis

89 Iliocostalis thoracis

94 Multifidi

95 Rotatores thoracis

97 Interspinales thoracis

99 Intertransversarii thoracis

THE LUMBAR ROOTS AND NERVES

The lumbar plexus is formed by the first four lumbar nerves and a communicating branch from T12. The fourth lumbar nerve gives its largest part to the lumbar plexus and a smaller part to the sacral plexus. The fifth lumbar nerve and the small segment of the fourth lumbar nerve form the lumbosacral trunk, which is part of the sacral plexus.

L1

Ventral Primary Ramus

100 Quadratus lumborum

175 Psoas minor

112 Transversus abdominis

111 Obliquus internus abdominis

117 Cremaster (genitofemoral)

Dorsal Primary Ramus

90 Iliocostalis lumborum

91 Longissimus thoracis

96 Rotatores lumborum

94 Multifidi

98 Interspinales lumborum

99 Intertransversarii lumborum

L2

Ventral Primary Ramus

100 Quadratus lumborum

174 Psoas major

176 Iliacus

117 Cremaster (genitofemoral)

177 Pectineus (femoral)

178 Gracilis (obturator)

179 Adductor longus (obturator)

180 Adductor brevis (obturator)

181 Adductor magnus
Superior and middle fibers (obturator)
Inferior fibers (sciatic, tibial)

195 Sartorius (femoral)

196–200 Quadriceps femoris (femoral)

    196 Rectus femoris

    197 Vastus intermedius

    198 Vastus lateralis

    199 Vastus medialis longus

    200 Vastus medialis obliquus

201 Articularis genus (femoral)

Dorsal Primary Ramus

90 Iliocostalis lumborum (variable)

96 Rotatores lumborum

94 Multifidi

98 Interspinales lumborum

99 Intertransversarii lumborum

L3

Ventral Primary Ramus

100 Quadratus lumborum

174 Psoas major

176 Iliacus (femoral)

177 Pectineus (femoral)

178 Gracilis (obturator)

179 Adductor longus (obturator)

180 Adductor brevis (obturator)

181 Adductor magnus, superior and medial fibers (obturator)
Inferior fibers (sciatic, tibial)

188 Obturator externus (obturator)

195 Sartorius (femoral)

196–200 Quadriceps femoris (femoral)

    196 Rectus femoris

    197 Vastus intermedius

    198 Vastus lateralis

    199 Vastus medialis longus

    200 Vastus medialis obliquus

201 Articularis genus (femoral)

Dorsal Primary Ramus

90 Iliocostalis lumborum

96 Rotatores lumborum

94 Multifidi

98 Interspinales lumborum

99 Intertransversarii lumborum

L4

Ventral Primary Ramus

175 Psoas major

179 Adductor longus (obturator)

181 Adductor magnus
Superior and middle fibers (obturator)
Lower fibers (sciatic, tibial)

183 Gluteus medius (superior gluteal)

184 Gluteus minimus (superior gluteal)

185 Tensor fasciae latae (superior gluteal)

188 Obturator externus (obturator)

195–200 Quadriceps femoris (femoral)

    196 Rectus femoris

    197 Vastus lateralis

    198 Vastus intermedius

    199 Vastus medialis longus

    200 Vastus medialis obliquus

201 Articularis genus (femoral)

202 Popliteus (tibial)

203 Tibialis anterior (deep peroneal)

204 Tibialis posterior (tibial)

Dorsal Primary Ramus

90 Iliocostalis lumborum

96 Rotatores lumborum

94 Multifidi

98 Interspinales lumborum

99 Intertransversarii lumborum

L5

Ventral Primary Ramus

182 Gluteus maximus (inferior gluteal)

183 Gluteus medius (superior gluteal)

184 Gluteus minimus (superior gluteal)

185 Tensor fasciae latae (superior gluteal)

187 Obturator internus (n. to Obturator internus)

189 Gemellus superior (n. to Obturator internus)

190 Gemellus inferior (n. to Quadratus femoris)

191 Quadratus femoris (n. to Quadratus femoris)

192 Biceps femoris, short head (sciatic, common peroneal)
long head (sciatic, tibial)

194 Semimembranosus (sciatic, tibial)

193 Semitendinosus (sciatic, tibial)

202 Popliteus (tibial)

204 Tibialis posterior (tibial)

213 Flexor digitorum longus (tibial)

222 Flexor hallucis longus (tibial)

203 Tibialis anterior (deep peroneal)

210 Peroneus tertius (deep peroneal)

211 Extensor digitorum longus (deep peroneal)

212 Extensor digitorum brevis (deep peroneal)

221 Extensor hallucis longus (deep peroneal)

208 Peroneus longus (superficial peroneal)

209 Peroneus brevis (superficial peroneal)

218 Lumbricales, 1st [foot] (medial plantar)

Dorsal Primary Ramus

90 Iliocostalis lumborum

96 Rotatores lumborum

94 Multifidi

99 Intertransversarii lumborum

THE LUMBOSACRAL ROOTS AND NERVES

The intermingling of the ventral primary rami of the lumbar, sacral, and coccygeal nerves is known as the lumbosacral plexus. There is uncertainty about any motor innervation from the dorsal primary rami below S3. The nerves branching off this plexus supply the lower extremity in part and also the perineum and coccygeal areas via the pudendal and coccygeal plexuses.

S1

Ventral Primary Ramus

182 Gluteus maximus (inferior gluteal)

183 Gluteus medius (superior gluteal)

184 Gluteus minimus (superior gluteal)

185 Tensor fasciae latae (superior gluteal)

186 Piriformis (n. to Piriformis)

187 Obturator internus (nerve to Obturator internus)

189 Gemellus superior (nerve to Obturator internus)

190 Gemellus inferior (nerve to Quadratus femoris)

191 Quadratus femoris (nerve to Quadratus femoris)

192 Biceps femoris
Short head (sciatic, common peroneal n.)
Long head (sciatic, tibial n.)

194 Semimembranosus (sciatic, tibial division)

193 Semitendinosus (sciatic, tibial division)

205 Gastrocnemius (tibial)

207 Plantaris (tibial)

202 Popliteus (tibial)

204 Tibialis posterior (tibial)

206 Soleus (tibial)

213 Flexor digitorum longus (tibial)

222 Flexor hallucis longus (tibial)

223 Flexor hallucis brevis (tibial)

203 Tibialis anterior (deep peroneal [often])

210 Peroneus tertius (deep peroneal)

211 Extensor digitorum longus (deep peroneal)

212 Extensor digitorum brevis (deep peroneal)

208 Peroneus longus (superficial peroneal)

209 Peroneus brevis (superficial peroneal)

215 Abductor digiti minimi (lateral plantar)

217 Quadratus plantae [Flex. Dig. accessorius] (lateral plantar)

214 Flexor digitorum brevis (medial plantar)

224 Abductor hallucis (medial plantar)

218 Lumbricales, 1st [foot] (medial plantar)

Dorsal Primary Rami

94 Multifidi

99 Intertransversarii lumborum

S2

Ventral Primary Ramus

182 Gluteus maximus (inferior gluteal)

186 Piriformis (Nerve to Piriformis)

192 Biceps femoris
Short head (sciatic, common peroneal n.)
Long head (sciatic, tibial n.)

194 Semimembranosus (sciatic, tibial division)

193 Semitendinosus (sciatic, tibial division)

205 Gastrocnemius (tibial)

206 Soleus (tibial)

207 Plantaris (tibial)

213 Flexor digitorum longus (tibial)

222 Flexor hallucis longus (tibial)

214 Flexor digitorum brevis (medial plantar)

224 Abductor hallucis (medial plantar)

217 Quadratus plantae [Flex. dig. accessorius] (lateral plantar)

215 Abductor digiti minimi (lateral plantar)

216 Flexor digiti minimi brevis [foot] (lateral plantar)

225 Adductor hallucis (lateral plantar)

218 Lumbricales 2nd, 3rd, and 4th [foot] (lateral plantar)

219 Interossei, dorsal (lateral plantar)

220 Interossei, plantar (lateral plantar)

115 Levator ani (pudendal)

118 Transversus perinei superficialis (pudendal)

119 Transversus perinei profundus (pudendal)

120 Bulbocavernosus (pudendal)

121 Ischiocavernosus (pudendal)

122 Sphincter urethrae (pudendal)

123 Sphincter ani externus (pudendal)

Dorsal Primary Rami

94 Multifidi

S3

Ventral Primary Ramus

217 Quadratus plantae [Flex. Dig. accessorius] (lateral plantar)

215 Abductor digiti minimi (lateral plantar)

216 Flexor digiti minimi brevis [foot] (lateral plantar)

225 Adductor hallucis (lateral plantar)

218 Lumbricales 2nd, 3rd, and 4th [foot] (lateral plantar)

219 Interossei, dorsal (lateral plantar)

220 Interossei, plantar (lateral plantar)

115 Levator ani (pudendal)

116 Coccygeus (pudendal)

118 Transversus perinei superficialis (pudendal)

119 Transversus perinei profundus (pudendal)

120 Bulbocavernosus (pudendal)

121 Ischiocavernosus (pudendal)

122 Sphincter urethrae (pudendal)

123 Sphincter ani externus (pudendal)

S4 and S5

Ventral Primary Ramus

116 Coccygeus (to S4, pudendal)

123 Sphincter ani externus (to S4, perineal)

118 Transversus perinei superficialis (to S4, pudendal)

119 Transversus perinei profundus (to S4, pudendal)

120 Bulbocavernosus (to S4, pudendal)

121 Ischiocavernosus (to S4, pudendal)

122 Sphincter urethrae (to S4, pudendal)

123 Sphincter ani externus (to S4, perineal)

References

1. Clemente CD. *Gray's Anatomy,* 30th (American) ed. Philadelphia: Lea & Febiger, 1985.
2. Williams PL. *Gray's Anatomy,* 38th (British) ed. London: Churchill-Livingstone, 1995.
3. Figge FHJ. *Sobotta's Atlas of Human Anatomy,* Vol. 1. *Atlas of Bones, Joints and Muscles,* 8th English ed. New York: Hafner, 1968.
4. Clemente CD. *Anatomy: A Regional Atlas of the Human Body.* Baltimore: Urban & Schwarzenberg, 1998.
5. Netter FH, Colacino S. *Atlas of Human Anatomy.* Summit, NJ: Ciba Geigy, 1974.
6. Jenkins DB. *Hollingshead's Functional Anatomy of the Limbs and Back.* Philadelphia: WB Saunders, 1998.
7. Grant JCB. *An Atlas of Anatomy,* 10th ed. Baltimore: Lippincott Williams & Wilkins, 1999.
8. Moore KL. *Clinically Oriented Anatomy,* 3rd ed. Baltimore: Williams & Wilkins, 1992.
9. Haerer AF. *DeJong's The Neurological Examination,* 5th ed. Philadelphia: JB Lippincott, 1992.
10. DuBrul EL. *Sicher and DuBrul's Oral Anatomy,* 8th ed. St Louis, Ishiyaku EuroAmerica, 1990.
11. Nairn RI. The circumoral musculature: Structure and function. Br Dent J 138:49–56, 1975.
12. Lightoller GH. Facial muscles: The modiolus and muscles surrounding the rima oris with remarks about the panniculus adiposus. J Anat 60:1–85, 1925.
13. Keller JT, Saunders MC, Van Loveren H, Shipley MT. Neuroanatomical considerations of palatal muscles: tensor and levator palatini. Cleft palate J 21:70–75, 1984.
14. Perry J, Nickel VL. Total cervical-spine fusion for neck paralysis. J Bone Joint Surg [Am] 41:37–60, 1959.
15. Moyers RE. Electromyographic analysis of certain muscles involved in temporomandibular movement. Am J Orthodont 36:481–515, 1950.
16. deSousa OM. Estudoelectromiografico do m. platysma. Folia Clin Biol 33:42–52, 1964.
17. Jones DS, Beargie RJ, Pauly JE. An electromyographic study of some muscles of costal respiration in man. Anat Rec 117:17–24, 1953.
18. Soo KC, Guiloff RF, Pauly JE. Innervation of the Trapezius muscle: A study in patients undergoing neck dissections. Head Neck 12:488–495, 1990.
19. Basmajian JV. *Muscles Alive,* 2nd ed. Baltimore: Williams & Wilkins, 1967.
20. Sodeberg GL. *Kinesiology: Application to Pathologic Motion.* Baltimore: Williams & Wilkins, 1997.
21. Doody SG, Freedman L, Waterland JC. Shoulder movements during abduction in the scapular plane. Arch Phys Med Rehabil 10:595–604, 1970.
22. Perry J. Muscle control of the shoulder. In Rowe CR (ed). *The Shoulder.* New York: Churchill-Livingstone, 1988, pp. 17–34.
23. Ip M, Chang KS. A study of the radial supply of the human Brachialis muscle. Anat Rec 162:363–371, 1968.
24. Basmajian JV, DeLuca CJ. *Muscles Alive,* 5th ed. Baltimore: Williams & Wilkins, 1985.
25. Basmajian JV, Travill AA. Electromyography of the pronator muscles of the forearm. Anat Rec 139:45–49, 1961.
26. Flatt AE. *Kinesiology of the Hand.* Am Acad Orthop Surg Instructional Course Lectures XVIII. St. Louis: CV Mosby, 1961.
27. Muller T. Variations in the Abductor pollicis longus and Extensor pollicis brevis in the South African Bantu. South Afr J Lab Clin Med 5:56–62, 1959.
28. Martin BF. The annular ligament of the superior radio-ulnar joint. J Anat 92:473–482, 1958.
29. Day MH, Napier JR. The two heads of the Flexor pollicus brevis. J Anat 95:123–130, 1961.
30. Harness D, Sekales E, Chaco J. The double motor innervation of the Opponens pollicis: An electromyographic study. J Anat 117:329–331, 1974.
31. Forrest WJ. Motor innervation of human thenar and hypothenar muscles in 25 hands: A study combining EMG and percutaneous nerve stimulation. Canad J Surg 10:196–199, 1967.
32. McKibben B. Action of the iliopsoas muscle in the newborn. J Bone Joint Surg [Br] 50:161–165, 1968.
33. DeSousa OM, Vitti M. Estudio electeromiografica de los musculos adductores largo y mayor. Arch Mex Anat 7:52–53, 1966.
34. Janda V, Stara V. The role of thigh adductors in movement patterns of the hip and knee joint. Courier 15:1–3, 1965.
35. Kaplan EB. The iliotibial tract. Clinical and morphological significance. J Bone Joint Surg [Am] 40:817–831, 1958.
36. Pare EB, Stern JT, Schwartz JM. Functional differentiation within the Tensor fasciae latae. J Bone Joint Surg [Am] 63:1457–1471, 1981.
37. Sneath R. Insertion of the Biceps femoris. J Anat 89:550–553, 1955.
38. Lieb FJ, Perry J. Quadriceps function: An anatomical and mechanical study using amputated limbs. J Bone Joint Surg [Am] 50:1535–1548, 1968.
39. Lieb FJ, Perry J. Quadriceps function: An electromyographic study under isometric conditions. J Bone Joint Surg [Am] 53:749–758, 1971.
40. Last RJ. The Popliteus muscle and the lateral meniscus. J Bone Joint Surg [Br] 32:93–99, 1950.
41. Cummins EJ, Anson BJ, Carr BW, Wright RR. Structure of the calcaneal tendon (of Achilles) in relation to orthopedic surgery; with additional observations of the Plantaris muscle. Surg Gynecol Obstet 83:107–116, 1946.
42. Lewis OJ. The comparative morphology of m. flexor accessorius and the associated flexor tendons. J Anat 96:321–333, 1962.

Index

Note: Page numbers followed by the letter b refer to boxed material; those followed by f refer to figures, and those followed by t refer to tables.